Over recent years, general or office practice has come to be recognised as the most suitable place for the majority of minor surgical procedures. Vija Sodera, both a general practitioner and hospital casualty surgeon, has the ideal background to communicate effectively the relevant skills necessary to develop this set-up in your own practice. A gifted teacher and accomplished artist, Vija Sodera combines these talents to take the reader through all the procedures applicable to UK practice and more – a comprehensive approach which will appeal to doctors worldwide.

Detailed step by step descriptions of over 160 techniques and procedures are clearly presented along with their medico-legal aspects. Among the many aspects covered in detail are:

Operating room fixtures and fittings

Operating equipment choice

Patient and doctor preparation including Hepatitis B and HIV precautions

Local anaesthetics

Steroid injections

Operative techniques including cryotherapy, the use of electrocautery and diathermy

Operative complications

Clinical and histological appearances of common skin lesions

Minor surgical procedures

Minor casualty problems

Beautifully and extensively illustrated throughout, this work includes clear anatomical drawings and photographs. As the most comprehensive text of its kind, it is sure to become and remain a standard on the subject for many years to come.

Minor surgery in practice

Minor surgery in practice

VIJA K. SODERA MB ChB FRCS(Ed)
White Lodge Surgical Clinic, Aldwick, Bognor Regis
Casualty Surgeon, Bognor Regis War Memorial Hospital, Bognor Regis

All illustrations and clinical photographs by

Vija K. Sodera

Photographs of instruments and injection techniques by

Roy Gardner

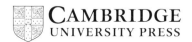
CAMBRIDGE
UNIVERSITY PRESS

Published by the Press Syndicate of the University of Cambridge
The Pitt Building, Trumpington Street, Cambridge CB2 1RP
40 West 20th Street, New York, NY 10011-4211, USA
10 Stamford Road, Oakleigh, Melbourne 3166, Australia

© Cambridge University Press 1994

First published 1994

Printed in Great Britain at
the University Press, Cambridge

A catalogue record for this book is available from the British Library

Library of Congress cataloguing in publication data

Sodera, Vija K.
Minor surgery in practice / Vija K. Sodera : all illustrations by
Vija K. Sodera.
p.   cm.
Includes bibliographical references.
ISBN 0-521-44466-7 (hc)
1. Surgery, Minor.   2. Ambulatory surgery.   I. Title.
[DNLM: 1. Surgery, Minor – methods.   2. Ambulatory Surgery –
– methods.   3. Ambulatory Care Facilities – organization &
administration.   WO 192 S679m   1994]
RD111.S66   1994
617′.024 – dc20   93-31378 CIP

ISBN 0 521 44466 7 hardback

This book is dedicated to my darling wife Margaret
and to my dear daughters Melanie and Lisa.

Contents

Foreword

For the hospital consultant, minor surgery in general practice can result in a welcome reduction in the workload. For the patient, minor surgery provides a valuable service that should result in improved health care. For the general practitioner, minor surgery offers an extra dimension of interest and allows the frustrated surgeon to keep a hand in.

Vija Sodera has taken a very special interest in the minor surgery field. He is a highly competent general surgeon who finds the art of minor surgery both challenging and satisfying. This excellent book, superbly illustrated by the author, is the culmination of many years' work, during which time Vija Sodera has striven to promote quality minor surgery. Clearly, he has succeeded in his aim.

This book provides a comprehensive and safe working platform from which general practitioners can develop their minor operative services. There is no substitute for experience, and all general practitioners should know their limits and keep well within them. However, with the help of the excellent text and illustrations, already competent general practitioners should be able to strengthen their working knowledge and move forward to more complex procedures. For surgical beginners, there is much basic help to entice them into the field of minor surgery.

Without doubt, this book will become a standard text for all those working in the field of minor surgery, an area of general practice which should continue to flourish, providing general practitioners with additional clinical satisfaction and the patient with a valuable and much needed service.

Dr Andrew Naylor MB BS
General Practitioner
Pagham, West Sussex

Preface

Everyone is now agreed that the proper place for the majority of minor surgical procedures is in the general practice setting and not in hospital. The aim of this book is to take the reader through all the procedures applicable to general practice in the United Kingdom and more. Thus, there are included many procedures that some doctors will not feel confident to handle and there are other procedures that interested and *experienced* doctors might like to add to their repertoires.

Minor surgical procedures should not be performed without the doctor having a prior understanding of the possible outcomes (both good and bad), and their immediate management. Therefore, throughout this book, particular emphasis is given to detailing practical problems, pitfalls, and complications that may be encountered, along with their solutions. In addition a specific chapter is included on wound healing and complications.

In the chapter on minor skin surgery, specific details and photographs are provided of common and important skin lesions. Although it is not suggested that general practitioners should undertake surgery of squamous cell carcinoma or malignant melanoma, the clinical photographs and histological sections will help to ensure their familiarity with the appearances of these clinical conditions and thus to avoid inappropriate surgery on suspicious lesions.

Throughout this book, I would emphasise that doctors should only perform procedures that they are capable of handling *easily*. In *general practice* the old surgical adage *'if in doubt, cut it out'* is quite inappropriate. It should be replaced by simply: *'if in doubt . . . don't'*.

V.K.S. 1994

Acknowledgements

I would like to express my grateful thanks to: my wife, Margaret, for her painstaking help with the manuscript, and also her endless patience and support; also my daughters Melanie and Lisa for being so tolerant when I have had one eye and one cerebral hemisphere on my computer while they tried to talk with their dad.

Special thanks must be given to my good friend Mr Michael Saleh for his support, encouragement and helpful comments. In writing this book I have used many ideas (particularly on local anaesthetics and surgical technique) for which he should take the credit, and which have been previously published in our *Illustrated Handbook of Minor Surgery and Operative Technique* (Heinemann 1987).

I am indebted to Mr Harry Sunderland, Mr Wyn Morris-Jones and the late Professor Frank O'Gorman for teaching me so much in my early days in surgery; all the doctors at Grove House Surgery in Nyetimber for their helpful comments, Professor M. N. Naylor for his helpful comments and detailed examination of the manuscript; Dr Lynda Tempest, Dr Paul Archer and Dr Caroline Archer for checking the manuscript and adding their helpful comments; Mr John Hoggan for his advice on dental problems; Mr Philip Perkins for his helpful contribution; Dr Tariq Sadiq for his assistance; Dr Sylvia Ellis for her comments on IUCDs; Dr Geoff Smith for so generously giving his time to offer his advice and comments on histopathology and also for providing the histological sections; Mr Mick Eaton for producing the actual photomicrographs; Dr Sarah Thomas for her kind help in providing the colour photographs of skin lesions; Mr Roy Gardner for his great help in producing the photographs of surgical instruments, equipment and injection techniques; Mr Peter Rowles and Melanie Sodera for their photographic help; Mr Stephen Trowbridge for his help with some of the operative photographs; Mrs Anne Wood for her help and support with the computer; Mr Mike Bosely for his help with the printing; all the manufacturers and suppliers who have kindly provided photographs; all the nursing staff in the Casualty Department at Bognor Regis War Memorial Hospital who have always been so helpful and supportive; Dr Richard Barling, Medical Editor at Cambridge University Press, for all his help and encouragement; Dr Jocelyn Foster and Stephanie Thelwell at CUP for all their hard work throughout the production of this book; Dr Penny McLaughlan for her painstaking editing of the manuscript; and finally, all the patients who have kindly allowed me to photograph their problems.

I am indebted to all the above, but nevertheless, the responsibility for any errors or omissions must remain mine.

SECTION I

1

Introduction

Minor surgery can be both a challenging and a satisfying aspect of general medical practice and the patient also has the benefit of being seen in familiar surroundings with familiar staff. In addition, performing minor operations in the doctor's surgery rather than in hospital can result in significant cost savings. It is also reassuring to know that when comparing hospital and general practice settings, and given similar types of minor surgical operations, it is found that there are no significant differences in the healing times or rate of complications such as wound infection or wound breakdown [1].

What can be done

Although a wide range of procedures can be performed in the general practice setting, the most important thing to know is one's capability and to stay within it. The inexperienced doctor should *never* undertake surgery in malignant tumours, where there is doubt about the diagnosis, where wound closure may be difficult, and on patients or sites of the body where a poor scar is likely to result. It is important to bear in mind that surgery should be performed only if it is indicated. That may sound obvious but many lesions *do not* need to be excised and often patients come only for a diagnosis. Inappropriate surgery can be avoided by adherence to a simple basic rule: *'if unsure, just refer'*.

There are two fundamental groups of techniques and procedures that are appropriate for general practice. The first group is shown in Table 1.1 and includes the types of conditions that almost any doctor should be able to handle *easily* and without requiring the use of any special expertise or equipment. Nevertheless, most doctors will confine their minor surgery to straightforward procedures such as simple injection techniques (Fig. 1.1), excisions of simple skin lesions (Fig. 1.2), cysts and the treatment of ingrowing toenails (Fig. 1.3). And rightly so, since more involved surgery should only be undertaken by properly trained, experienced and interested practitioners. Thus, it may be appropriate for one partner (who has a sound basic surgical training) of a group practice to provide minor surgical services for the patients of other partners, who themselves might have other special interests and skills.

As their interest and experience grows, doctors might add further techniques and procedures to their repertoire. The second group comprises advanced techniques and procedures which should only be undertaken by doctors with experience and a special interest in surgery (Fig. 1.4). These techniques and

Fig. 1.1. Injection for tennis elbow is a simple technique.

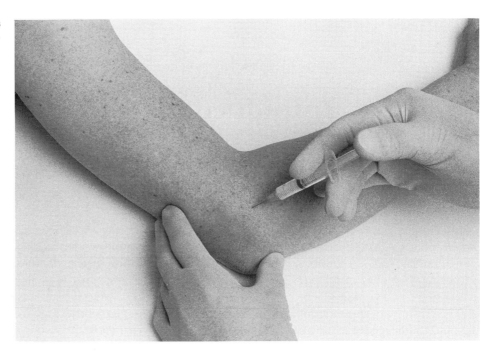

Fig. 1.2. This naevus can be easily removed by shave excision or elliptical skin excision. All excised lesions should be sent for histological examination.

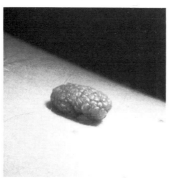

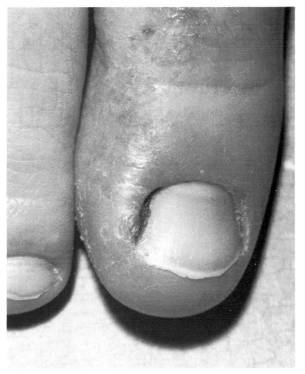

Fig. 1.3. Ingrowing toenails can be easily and quickly treated in the surgery.

procedures are exemplified in Table 1.2. For example, only very small basal cell carcinomas that are in sites with plenty of spare skin should be excised in the doctor's surgery. Larger basal cell carcinomas, squamous cell carcinomas and suspicious pigmented lesions, should always be referred to a dermatologist or surgeon.

Table 1.1. *Simple minor surgery*

Examples of techniques and procedures that almost any doctor should be able to handle easily and without requiring the use of any special expertise or equipment.

Aspiration of hydrocoele/breast cyst/ganglion
Steroid injections of soft tissues
Cryotherapy of *benign* skin lesions
Excision biopsy of *benign* skin lesions
Excision of sebaceous cyst and lipoma
Segmental phenolisation of nail bed
Suture of simple lacerations
Drainage of superficial abscesses
Nasal cautery for epistaxis

Table 1.2. *Advanced minor surgery*

These are examples of some additional types of procedure that can be handled given adequate time, facilities and skill.
These procedures should not be undertaken without appropriate surgical experience.

Steroid injection of joints
Excision of lesions on face, eyelids, or neck
Excision of basal cell carcinoma
Excision of meibomian cyst
Marsupialisation of Bartholin's cyst
Vasectomy
Varicose vein ligation

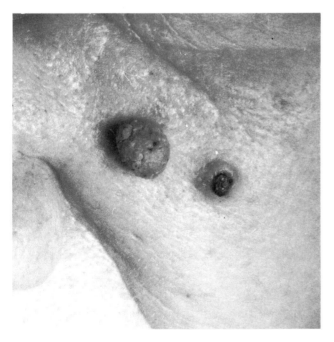

Fig. 1.4. Although clinically they looked quite different, both of these lesions on the cheek turned out to be basal cell carcinomas.

Some procedures, such as vasectomy, may look simple when demonstrated but can be extremely difficult to perform when the operator has no experience and training. These should not be attempted by the inexperienced doctor.

Safety is of paramount importance and therefore no procedure should be undertaken unless there are adequate facilities and equipment available, and the possible immediate complications can be dealt with. Although it is advisable always to have a nurse in attendance, most of the routine procedures can be done without an assistant.

Rules for safe surgery

1. Obtain consent and ensure patient is fully informed before operating.
2. Stay within your capabilities.
3. Do not operate where the diagnosis or treatment options are unclear.
4. Obtain histological diagnosis before obliterative techniques (i.e. cryotherapy, electrocautery, diathermy) are used.
5. Do not operate on malignant tumours.
6. Take a representative sample (or samples) for histological examination if there are numerous similar lesions.
7. Identify all subcutaneous structures and do not make any cut except under direct vision.
8. Send all excised lesions for histological examination.
9. Ensure all histology reports are checked and acted upon.
10. If unsure, just refer.

Practical training and experience are essential and it is important to attend instruction and refresher courses where appropriate. Hospital colleagues will generally be only too happy to offer guidance and the opportunity for practitioners to look in on particular procedures. There should certainly be no embarrassment in asking for help and advice. With regard to steroid injections, the inexperienced doctor should start with simple soft tissue injections and obtain advice from specialist colleagues.

Although dependent on the workload, it is generally advisable to arrange a specific morning or afternoon session for a list of four or five cases. However, a number of simple conditions can be dealt with just as easily when the cases present in the ordinary surgery, provided the drugs and equipment are readily available. This applies particularly to steroid injections and cryotherapy applications.

Minor surgery requiring the use of general anaesthetics necessitates far more time, experience, equipment and facilities than is usually available in general practice. This is the domain of the specialist or the experienced doctor and such procedures are outside the scope of this book.

Medico-legal aspects

It is true that there is no such thing as minor surgery, only minor surgeons. No less care should be taken when planning and performing minor surgery than any other surgery. However, no matter how simple an operation or procedure may be, or how well it is carried out, there will always be the possibility of something going wrong. For example, a simple surgical wound may unexpectedly break down or a blister may become infected after cryotherapy. Thus, although the aim is always to minimise the risk of complications, problems are not completely avoidable. It is therefore, essential to ensure that medical protection insurance is up to date and covers general practice operative surgery.

In general practice medico-legal problem areas are likely to be related to the excision of an unexpected skin malignancy, scars, damage to peripheral nerves and tendons, and with more involved procedures such as vasectomy.

Apart from the hazards of operative surgery, equal care should be taken to use the correct doses and concentrations of different preparations. For example, the injection of haemorrhoids with 80% phenol (instead of 5%) can cause severe necrosis and ulceration [2].

Surgical expertise

It is imperative that no procedure should be undertaken unless the surgeon is fully conversant with the operation, and with the management of any possible immediate complications. When there is a claim of negligence applied to the performance of an operation, the courts will apply the following generally established rule: 'A practitioner will not be guilty of negligence if he or she acted in accordance with a practice accepted as proper by a reasonable body of medical people' [3].

Consent

The more fully informed the patient is before any procedure, the less likely it will be that the practitioner will be held responsible for any problem or failure of the operation. Prior to giving written consent, the patient should be given enough information to make an informed decision to agree to the proposed procedure. The nature of the procedure, possible outcomes and any likely complications should be explained in appropriate detail. Particularly when skin lesions are being removed for cosmetic purposes, the patient should be informed of scar maturation and fading times, expected final appearance and risk of keloid, etc.

Written consent is not necessary for very minor procedures such as cryotherapy or steroid injections but written consent should be obtained for biopsies and for more involved procedures. It is necessary to obtain written consent for vasectomy prior to the operation (although written consent from both partners is not legally necessary, some lawyers would advise that it should be obtained from both partners).

Informed verbal consent should be noted in the patient's file [4]. In addition to specifying the name of the procedure, it is advisable to insert on any consent form a clause which states that the patient has been fully informed of any likely effects, complications or risks of the operation.

Consent

1. Consent is only valid if patient has been fully informed.
2. Oral consent is adequate for most minor procedures but this should be recorded in the patient's file.
3. Written consent should be obtained for involved procedures.
4. Consent should be obtained by the practitioner and should not be delegated.

Sample consent form

Mr V. K. Sodera MB ChB FRCSEd
WHITE LODGE CLINIC
OPERATION CONSENT FORM

I,

of:

consent to the operation of:

....

the nature and purpose of which has been fully explained to me by Mr Sodera. I also understand the risks and possible complications that can occur.

Signature: .... Date: ....
(Patient/Parent/Guardian)

Skin lesions

Although the vast majority of lesions excised as an outpatient procedure are benign, [5,6,7], excised lesions should always be sent for histological examination. Obtaining an histological diagnosis is also extremely helpful for on-going self-education. Not uncommonly, in a patient with multiple benign lesions such as skin tags or seborrhoeic warts, it is not practical for every lesion to be placed into a separate container, numbered and located. In such circumstances it is reasonable to select and send only a representative sample for histological examination. However, it cannot be overemphasised that extreme diligence must always be exercised and practice should always err on the side of caution. For example, basal cell carcinoma is often difficult to distinguish from innocent skin blemishes in its early stages and there has been at least one report of the removal of a *pale* pedunculated skin lesion in a *teenager* in which the specimen was not sent for histological examination and the patient developed a virulent malignant melanoma 18 months later [4].

The management of inadequately excised skin lesions is fully discussed in chapter 15.

Scars following surgery

Patients should be warned that scars are inevitable after any surgery. Remember that minor surgery can have major cosmetic consequences (Fig. 1.5). In particular, warning should be given that scars following excision of benign naevi may stretch in areas where there is unavoidable movement or tension (see chapter 9) (Fig. 1.6).

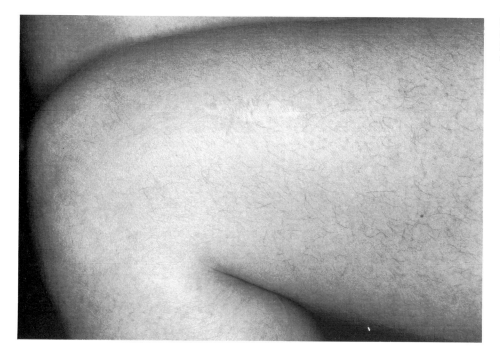

Fig. 1.5. This stretched scar followed removal of a simple dermatofibroma. Note that it is not in line with the natural skin creases.

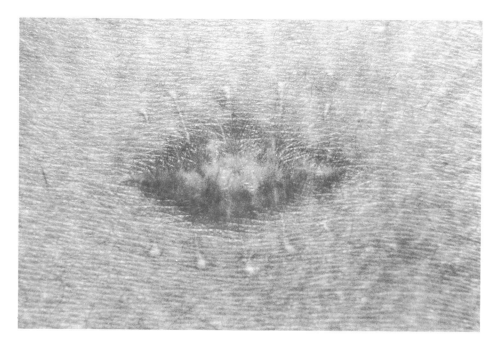

Fig. 1.6. This scar followed removal of a benign pigmented naevus on the back. The patient was not known to be susceptible to hypertrophic scarring.

Peripheral nerve injury

Damage to nerves is a not uncommon cause of litigation as subcutaneous lesions excised under local anaesthesia can be close to nerves, or in the case of neurofibromata, actually arising from nerves. It is essential to bear in mind the anatomy of peripheral nerves when performing minor surgery (Fig. 1.7). Many nerve injuries follow operations such as biopsy of lymph nodes in the posterior triangle of the neck where the spinal accessory nerve is vulnerable [8]. Vulnerable nerves and structures are discussed more fully in chapter 8.

Fig. 1.7. Beware of lesions near nerves. This lesion could be a simple inclusion dermoid or a neuroma arising from the digital nerve and should be referred to a specialist.

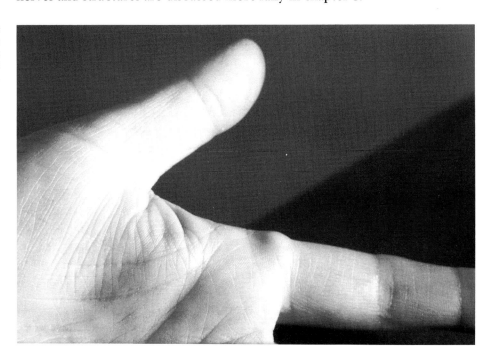

Vasectomy

Vasectomy is designed to result in permanent sterility. However, any vasectomy adequately performed with due care by experienced surgeons will have a risk of failure. Thus, when counselling patients it is important not to express or imply a *guarantee* of sterility. In addition, it must be made clear that there is always a small risk of natural reversal [9]. Finally, any alternatives to vasectomy must also be discussed with the patient.

Minor casualties

Doctors dealing with minor casualties need to be alert to the possibility of tendon injuries as these can often follow simple lacerations (see chapter 11). Extreme diligence must be maintained when one is dealing with infected or contaminated minor wounds because serious problems such as gas gangrene [10] can occur if a thorough wound toilet is not carried out. Such cases should be referred to an accident and emergency department.

Safety in the surgery

It is important to ensure that all electrical and sterilising equipment is safe and properly maintained. In particular, caustic and dangerous chemicals and drugs should be kept well out of the way where children cannot have access. All chemicals and medicines should be clearly labelled and the labels should be read before use. Particular care should be taken when chemicals are supplied in identical bottles: it has been known for 80% phenol, rather than adhesive remover, to be accidentally rubbed onto the skin after removal of a dressing (Fig. 1.8).

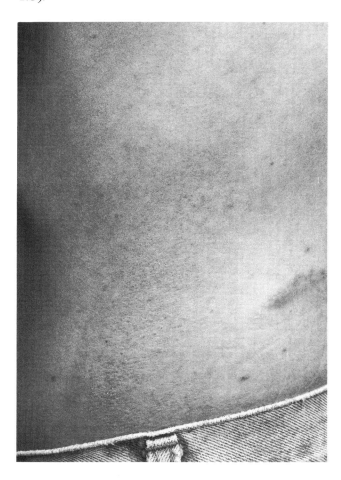

Fig. 1.8. This patient had phenol accidentally applied to the skin instead of adhesive remover. The photograph shows the appearance 9 months after the incident.

References

1. Cost effectiveness of minor surgery in general practice: a prospective comparison with hospital practice. O'Cathain, A., Brazier, J. E., Milner, P. C. & Fall, M. *British Journal of General Practice* (1992), **42**, 13–17.

2. Errors in prescribing and giving drugs – wrong dilution. Ferner, R. E. *Journal of the Medical Defence Union* (1992), no. 3, 62.

3. Liability for failed sterilisation. Childs, M. *Journal of the Medical Defence Union* (1992), no. 3, 64.

4. Litigation and plastic surgery. Hiles, R. *Journal of the Medical Defence Union* (1992), no. 4, 79–81.

5. Do all minor excised lesions require histological examination? Discussion paper. Paraskevopoulos, J. A., Hosking, S. W. & Johnson, A. G. *Journal of the Royal Society of Medicine* (1988), **81**, 583–584.
6. Carcinomatous change in cysts of the skin. McDonald, L. W. *Archives of Dermatology* (1963), **87**, 208–211.
7. Subcutaneous liposarcoma. Weitzner, S. *International Journal of Dermatology* (1973), **12**, 283–284.
8. Day surgery. Birch, R. *Journal of the Medical Defence Union* (1992), no. 3, 71.
9. Department of Health sued after husband's vasectomy. Dyer, C. *British Medical Journal* (1992), **305**, 912.
10. Gas gangrene following puncture wound in foot. Case history: 'GP admits notes were not contemporaneous'. *Journal of the Medical Defence Union* (1992), no. 4, 87–88.

2

Operating room and equipment

Operating room

Fixtures and fittings

Most minor procedures can be performed in a clean uncluttered room (Fig. 2.1). A wash basin should be fitted with elbow taps. There must be easily cleaned surfaces on which to put necessary items and a trolley for surgical instruments. A pedal bin is needed for clinical waste and disposables. A 'sharps' bin should be placed in such a position that needles and syringes can be discarded immediately and near to their point of use. Tall sharps bins are preferable to the shorter types because they allow needles to fall safely away from the opening. Necessary drugs should be kept in a lockable cupboard, which should be unlocked during an operating session to allow for immediate access. Spare unsterilised instruments should preferably be protected and kept in a closed cupboard or drawer.

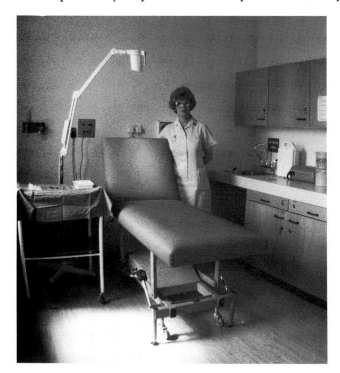

Fig. 2.1. Most minor procedures can be performed in a clean uncluttered room.

There must be good temperature control and ventilation as there will undoubtedly be times when a patient will feel faint and other times when the surgeon will feel uncomfortable because of an operative difficulty in a patient who is awake and able to appreciate the situation.

An intercom can be extremely useful and a radio tuned to a music station with the volume set low is relaxing for both the surgeon and the patient.

Lighting

Good lighting is essential. For safety reasons, British Standards prohibit the use of mains voltage-adjustable lamps in clinical situations, hence lamps should be purpose-made to 12 or 24 volts and use an integral mains transformer. A free-standing mobile lamp is both economical to purchase and versatile in use (Fig. 2.2). Wall- or ceiling-mounted operating lights are useful but unnecessary for minor surgery and are considerably more expensive. A ring light with a magnifying lens is essential for adequate inspection and treatment of conditions such as corneal and subtarsal foreign bodies (Fig. 2.3).

Fig. 2.2. Daray standard mobile light.

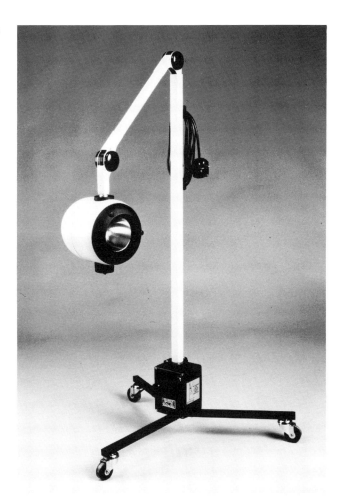

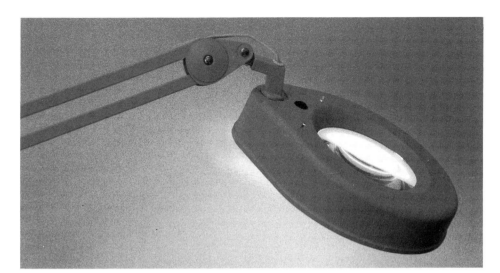

Fig. 2.3. Ring light with magnifying lens.

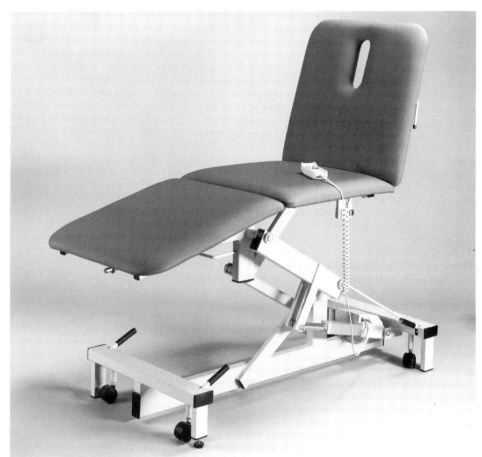

Fig. 2.4. The Plinth Co. height adjustable couch.

Operating table

Operating theatre tables are unnecessary and far too expensive. As an alternative, there are a number of height-adjustable couches available which cost considerably less (Fig. 2.4). However, a simple standard couch is quite adequate for most minor procedures. The only practical drawback is the lack of height adjustment. This can cause problems of backache if the surgeon stands and the patient is supine or prone for all procedures. However, operating on the head and neck with the head end of the couch tilted up allows for a good working height. For operations on the body and limbs the use of a typist's chair with gas-height adjustment and castors can make life more comfortable for the surgeon.

Resuscitation equipment

It is essential to have basic resuscitation equipment including airways, masks and self-inflating bag (e.g. an Ambubag) at hand, although they will be only very rarely required (Fig. 2.5). An intravenous line and saline, and drugs such as adrenaline, salbutamol, aminophylline, chlorpheniramine and hydrocortisone should be available to treat any collapse or reaction to injected drugs (see chapter 6).

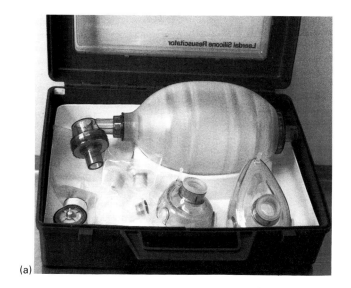

(a)

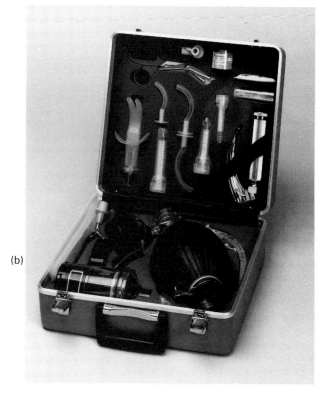

(b)

Fig. 2.5. (a) and (b) Portable cases containing resuscitation equipment.

Surgical instruments

The majority of minor surgical procedures can be performed with a basic pack consisting of only a few types of instrument (Fig. 2.6). It is quite unnecessary to purchase a large variety of instruments. Although top-quality instruments are not necessary for most minor surgery, the purchase of cheap and inferior-functioning instruments is false economy and should be avoided.

Basic minor surgery pack

Instrument	Size	Number
Needle holder	5 in.	1
Scalpel handle	no. 3	1
Dissecting forceps		
Fine non-toothed forceps	5 in.	1
Fine toothed forceps	5 in.	1
Medium non-toothed forceps	5 in.	1
Medium toothed forceps	5 in.	1
Scissors		
Dissecting, curved	$4\frac{1}{2}$ in.	1
Straight, stitch	5 in.	1
Artery clips, curved	5 in.	2

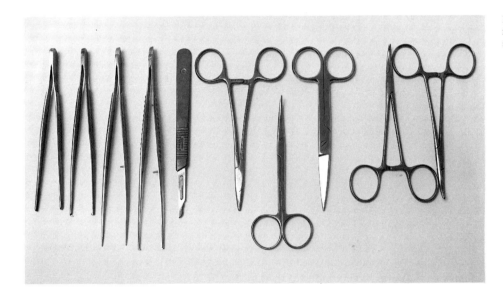

Fig. 2.6. This basic pack is suitable for both minor surgery and the suture of simple lacerations.

Purchasing surgical instruments

1. Get good quality instruments.
2. Get instruments with boxed hinges. Avoid instruments with screw hinges.
3. Get *curved* artery clips. Avoid straight or bulky artery clips.
4. Avoid crude dissecting scissors and forceps.

Needle holder A good quality box needle holder such as a 5 in. Halsey will comfortably handle 3/0 down to 5/0 sutures. Only very occasionally is a larger needle holder necessary (Fig. 2.7). Needle holders with tungsten carbide-lined jaws do reduce wear but they are significantly more expensive than those with

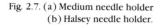

Fig. 2.7. (a) Medium needle holder
(b) Halsey needle holder.

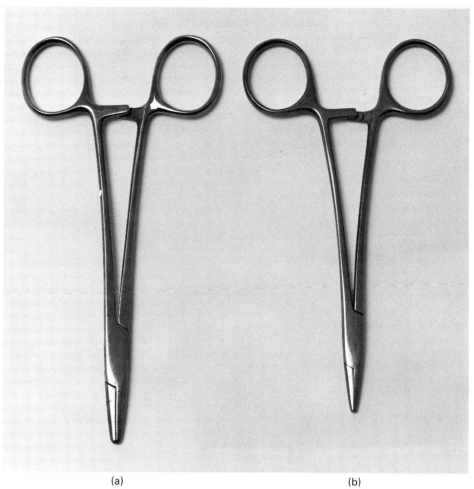

(a)   (b)

plain stainless steel jaws, which are quite adequate for minor surgery. However, it is important to purchase instruments that have good-fitting teeth and jaws. Some cheap instruments have crude teeth that do not grip fine needles properly and others have sharp ridges that have been known to cut through sutures when instrument ties are attempted. Purchasing such instruments is false economy.

There are some alternatives to the standard type of needle holder, although the choice is entirely one of personal preference. (Fig. 2.8). The Gillies needle holder has inbuilt scissors in its blades but has no rachet mechanism and is preferred by some surgeons as its use avoids the necessity to palm instruments. The McPhail needle holder sits comfortably in the palm and has a rachet that is disengaged with the little finger.

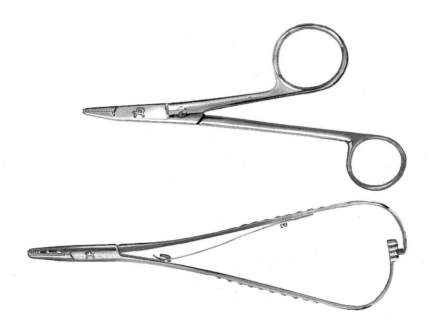

Fig. 2.8. (a) Gillies needle holder (b) McPhail needle holder.

(a)
Gillies
needle holder

(b)
McPhail
needle holder

Scalpel handle A no. 3 handle is all that is needed (Fig. 2.9). This can take no. 10, 11 and 15 blades (Fig. 2.10). The no. 10 blade has a large curved cutting edge and is suitable for larger incisions. The pointed no. 11 blade can be used for stab incisions, e.g. when lancing abscesses. The no. 15 blade has a small curved cutting edge that is ideal for the majority of minor surgical cases. To minimise risk of accidental injury, scalpel blades should be held in an artery clip or needle holder while being attached to and removed from a scalpel handle.

Disposable scalpels are available in packs of 10. They are convenient but in the long run are more expensive than using steel handles and disposable blades.

Fig. 2.9. (BELOW, LEFT) Disposable scalpel and steel scalpel handle.

Fig. 2.10. (BELOW) Scalpel blades nos. 11,10,15.

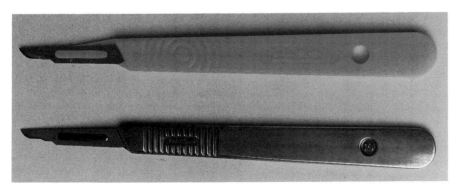

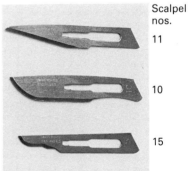

Scalpel
nos.

11

10

15

Dissecting forceps Medium 5 in. non-toothed forceps can be used to hold cotton-wool balls for skin preparation and can be used for crude or gauze dissection (Fig. 2.11). Fine 5 in. toothed and fine non-toothed forceps can be used for the majority of minor procedures (Fig. 2.12). Medium 5 in. toothed forceps are sometimes required when suturing larger incisions or wounds. Small (4 in.) forceps are used for very fine work (Fig. 2.13).

Fig. 2.11. Medium non-toothed forceps (5 in.) and medium toothed forceps (5 in.).

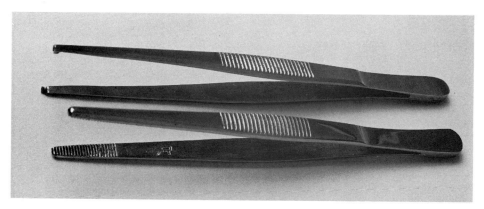

Fig. 2.12. Fine non-toothed forceps (5 in.) and fine toothed forceps (5 in.).

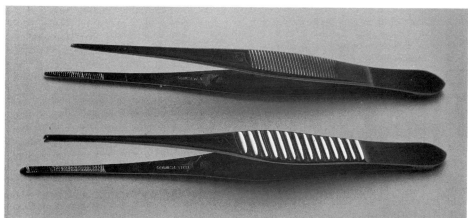

Fig. 2.13. Small non-toothed forceps (4 in.) and small toothed forceps (4 in.).

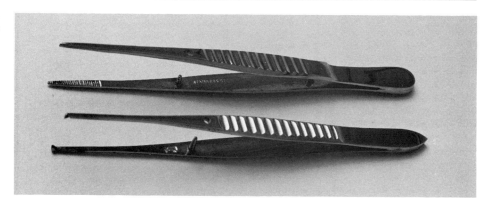

Scissors Curved dissecting scissors such as the strabismus scissors ($4\frac{1}{2}$ in.) are ideal for dissecting in small and medium sized wounds (Fig. 2.14). Straight stitch scissors (5 in.) are suitable for most non-dissecting purposes and are adequate for cutting most nails. Small, fine-pointed scissors are useful for delicate surgery.

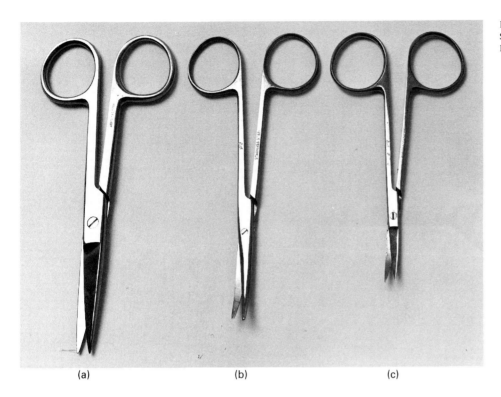

(a)   (b)   (c)

Fig. 2.14. (a) Stitch scissors (b) Strabismus dissecting scissors (c) Fine pointed curved scissors.

Artery clips Artery clips (or forceps) can be used for many different purposes. A number of small curved artery clips are available but there are no practical differences between them. The 5 in. Halsted mosquito is ideal for most minor surgical applications (Fig. 2.15). Instruments with more bulky tips such as the Spencer Wells have little application and are not recommended.

There is no practical use for straight artery clips in minor surgery because curved clips are essential for haemostasis, can be used for blunt dissection, are more versatile than straight clips, and will not be damaged when used in non-dissecting roles from removing all but thickened toenails, to securing a rubber

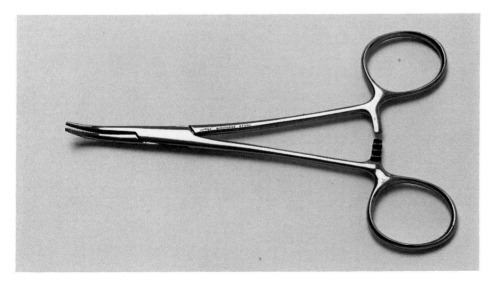

Fig. 2.15. Halsted mosquito artery clip.

band tourniquet. It is advisable only to use instruments with *boxed* hinges as these have a superior function and are less liable to entangle sutures (Fig. 2.16).

Nail clippers and bone nibblers Nail clippers ($5\frac{1}{2}$ in.) and bone nibblers (6 in.) are useful for cutting and reducing thick nails and onychogryphosis (Fig. 2.17).

Fig. 2.16. Artery clips with boxed and non-boxed hinges.

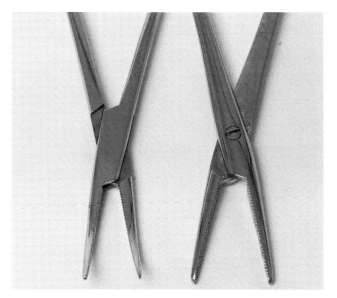

Fig. 2.17. (a) Nail clippers (b) Paton bone nibblers.

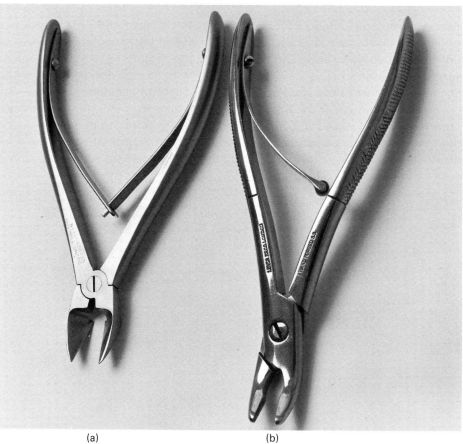

(a)   (b)

Allis forceps These are well suited for isolating and delivering the vas during vasectomy (Fig. 2.18).

Curette A sharp, general-purpose, double-ended curette is useful for scraping surface skin lesions and abscess cavities (Fig. 2.19).

Eyelid clamp (Chalazion ring clamp) These are essential for dealing with meibomian cysts (Fig. 2.20).

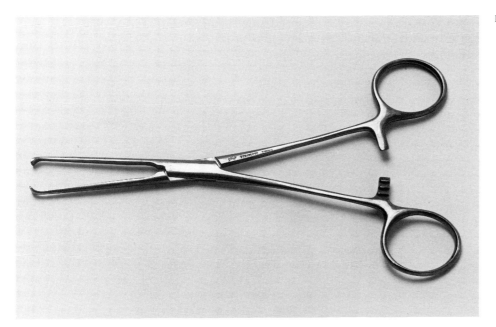

Fig. 2.18. Allis forceps.

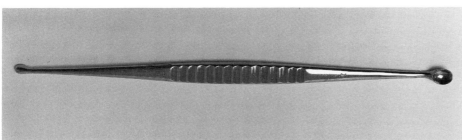

Fig. 2.19. Volkman's double-ended curette.

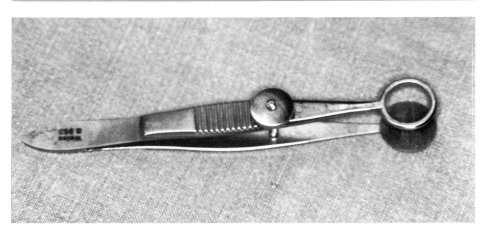

Fig. 2.20. Chalazion ring clamp.

Sinus forceps These are useful for emptying and packing haematoma and abscess cavities (Fig. 2.21a).

Splinter forceps These forceps are able to grasp effectively with their tips and are very useful for removing splinters (Fig. 2.21b).

Probes Disposable steel probes (5 in.) are available for exploring sinuses and abscesses (Fig. 2.21c).

Retractors If an assistant is required, small hand retractors are useful, and a small self-retaining retractor such as a West $5\frac{1}{2}$ in. is occasionally required when deeper structures need to be exposed (Fig. 2.22).

Fig. 2.21. (a) Sinus forceps (b) Splinter forceps (c) Disposable probe.

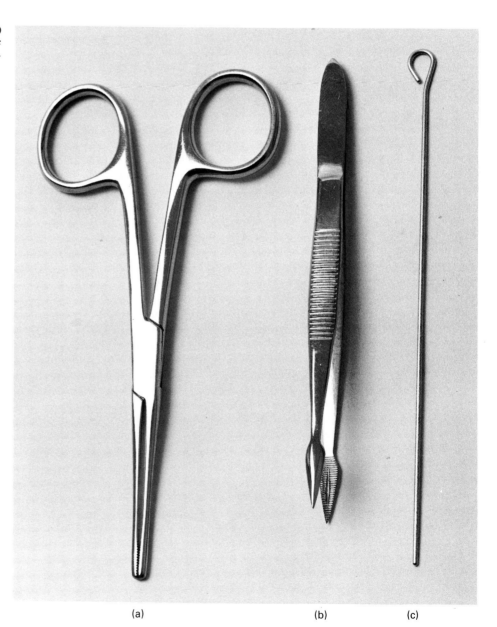

(a)   (b)   (c)

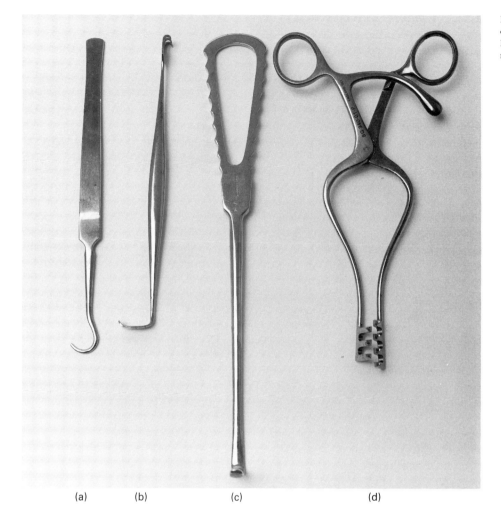

Fig. 2.22. (a) Single hook (b) Kilner double-ended retractors (c) Small Langenbeck (d) West self-retaining retractor.

(a)   (b)   (c)   (d)

Sutures

Although there is a large selection of sutures to choose from, only a few types are necessary for the majority of minor surgical procedures (Fig. 2.23). For example, 5/0 and 3/0 nylon sutures are ideal for skin closure of small and larger wounds, respectively, and 3/0 plain catgut is perfectly sufficient for subcutaneous suturing of most small wounds.

Although silk is the easiest material to tie, most doctors find that monofilament nylon is a superior material for a number of reasons (see chapter 10). Some of the newer sutures, such as Novafil (polybutester), have even better handling characteristics than does nylon. The synthetic absorbable sutures such as Dexon, Dexon II (polyglycolic) and Vicryl (polyglactin) are superior to catgut in strength and handling and are preferred when wound support is required for longer periods of time. A selection of appropriate sutures is listed in Table 2.1.

Table 2.1. *Suture materials*

Suture	Size	Needle	
	USP (Metric)	Ethicon	Davis & Geck
Non-absorbable sutures			
Monofilament sutures		Code No.	Code No.
Nylon	5/0 (1)	15 mm W526	16 mm 4401-23
Nylon	3/0 (2)	26 mm W320	24 mm 4403-43
Polybutester	5/0 (1)		19 mm 4402-23
Polybutester	3/0 (2)		24 mm 4418-43
Braided sutures			
Nylon	2/0 (3)	30 mm W5333	25 mm 6325-46
Silk	5/0 (1)	13 mm W468	16 mm 1078-21
Silk	3/0 (2)	35 mm W666	24 mm 1076-51
Absorbable sutures			
Catgut plain	3/0 (2)	22 mm W510	24 mm　268-41
Catgut chromic	2/0 (3)	30 mm W441	30 mm　430-51
Polyglycolic	3/0 (2)	—	25 mm 6325-86
Polyglactin	3/0 (1.5)	20 mm W9786 (undyed) —	

Fig. 2.23. Needles and sutures (needle size in parentheses).

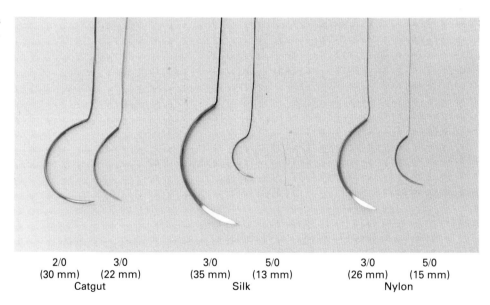

Electrocautery

Electrocautery is used primarily in the treatment of superficial skin lesions. The mains-operated desk-top units are both sturdy and inexpensive (Figs. 2.24, 2.25). Battery-operated portable hand-held units are also available and can be used with rechargeable batteries (Fig. 2.26). Trickle chargers can ensure that the cautery unit is always ready for use.

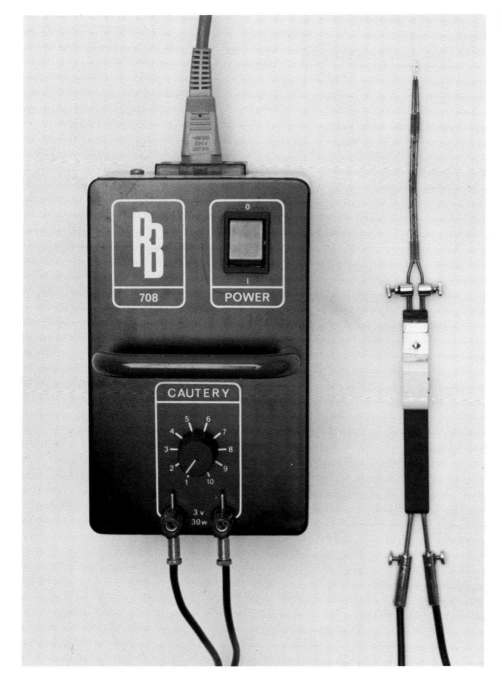

Fig. 2.24. Standard cautery
equipment.

The standard wire loop is a general-purpose cautery tip. The flat tip can be used
for amputation of a pedunculated papilloma and, along with the ball-ended tip, for
cautery of the raw bed after curettage. The cold point cautery tip is useful for
dealing with small lesions such as the central vessel in a spider naevus.

After each case the cautery should be left red hot for a short time to burn off any
tissue debris. Thus, the tips are self-sterilising.

Fig. 2.25. Cautery tips.

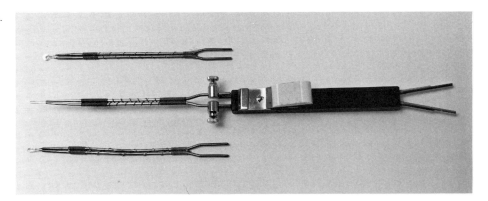

Fig. 2.26. (a) and (b) Portable
cautery equipment.

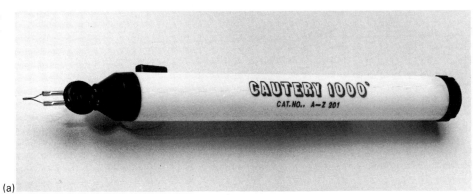

(a)

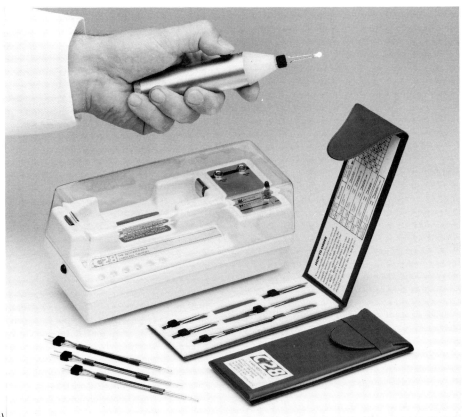

(b)

Diathermy

Usually when the word 'diathermy' is mentioned thoughts turn to the large units found in hospital operating theatres. However, small diathermy units are very easy to use in minor surgery and are recommended in preference to electrocautery units, since diathermy can fulfil all the functions of an electrocautery and is far more controllable and versatile. A small diathermy unit such as the Birtcher hyfrecator (Fig. 2.27) allows both bipolar use (where current only flows between the tips of the special bipolar forceps) and unipolar use (where current flows through the patient) (Fig. 2.28a).

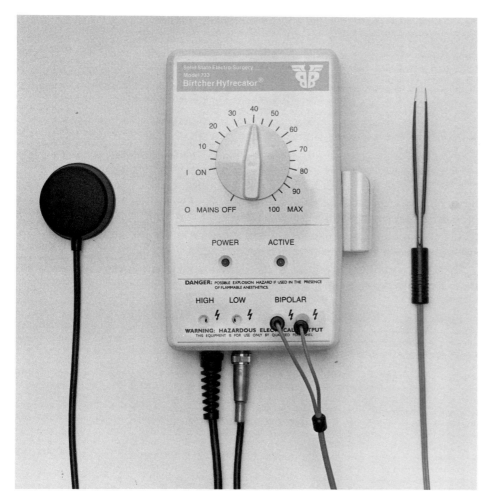

Fig. 2.27. Birtcher hyfrecator in bipolar mode.

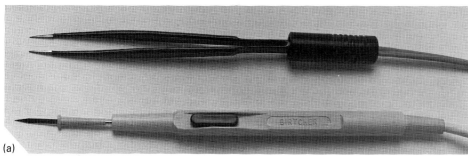

(a)

Fig. 2.28a. Bipolar forceps and unipolar handle.

Bipolar forceps have to be sterilised in an autoclave. In addition to their use in treating skin lesions, bipolar forceps are safer to use than electrocautery in confined situations such as during control of epistaxis and can be conveniently used to obtain haemostasis within a wound.

Cryotherapy equipment

Liquid nitrogen is colourless, odourless, non-inflammable and inert to most chemicals. It can be readily obtained and delivered on a regular basis and is conveniently stored in 30–50 l stainless steel Dewar flasks (Fig. 2.28b) and poured into the cryospray or cryoprobe canisters when required for treatment sessions. Depending on the workload, 50 l may last several months before a refill is required.

Liquid nitrogen should only be transported in purpose-made vehicles or in open-backed vehicles. It *should not* be transported inside the passenger compartment of a car because of the serious risk to the driver of any fumes causing hypoxia or obstruction of vision.

Because of the risk of cold injury from splashes, it is advisable to wear protective gloves and goggles when pouring liquid nitrogen from the storage container into the cryospray or cryoprobe canisters [1] (Fig. 2.29). Note that rapid unscrewing of a container of liquid nitrogen can result in the explosive release of the liquid nitrogen, especially when the container has been overfilled or shaken. Thus, the pressure should first be relieved using the release valve. It should be remembered that transient exposure to very cold fumes can produce discomfort in breathing and can provoke an asthmatic attack in susceptible individuals.

There are a number of methods of using liquid nitrogen. For a treatment session it can be poured into a small Dewar flask and used with a cotton bud (Fig. 2.30).

Fig. 2.28b. (BELOW, LEFT) Stainless steel Dewar flasks.

Fig. 2.29. (BELOW, CENTRE AND RIGHT) (a) and (b) Protective goggles and gloves should be used when pouring liquid nitrogen to avoid splashes.

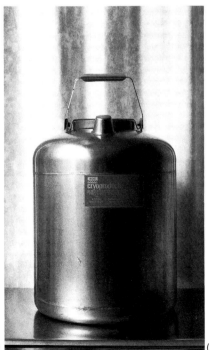
(b)

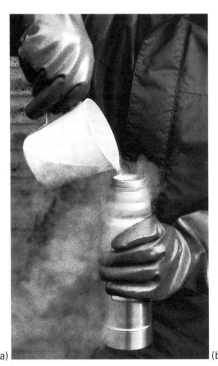
(a)

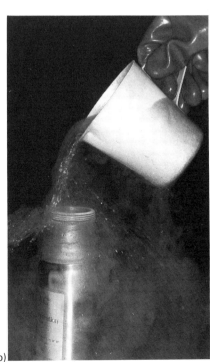
(b)

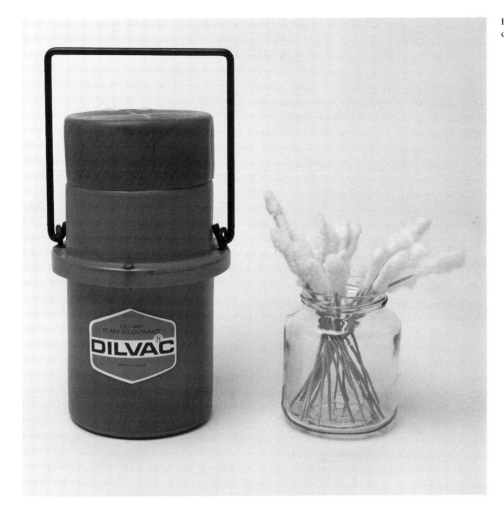

Fig. 2.30. Liquid nitrogen flask and cotton buds.

However, for the routine treatment of skin lesions and verrucae, the cryospray is certainly the quickest and a most efficient method of using liquid nitrogen (Fig. 2.31). The cryospray apparatus comprises a hand-held container with a trigger and valve system that allows the liquid nitrogen to escape as a spray through a fine nozzle.

Cryoprobe units allow the liquid nitrogen to pass within the probe head itself and out through a waste tube, cooling the probe head as it does so (Fig. 2.32).

An alternative to liquid nitrogen is the use of disposable aerosol coolant sprays such as the Histofreezer (Fig. 2.33).

Disposables

Syringes

For injecting sclerosant into varicose veins and for injecting steroids into finger and hand joints 1 ml (diabetic), syringes are used. For most steroid injections 2 ml syringes are useful. For injecting local anaesthetic 5 ml and 10 ml syringes are useful. In addition, 10 ml syringes are also used for aspiration of a ganglion

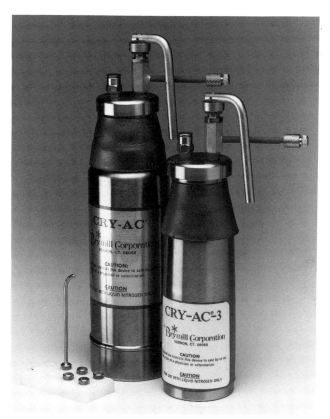

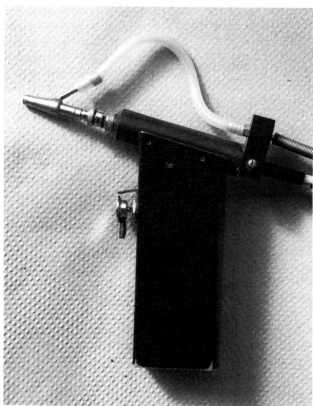

Fig. 2.31. (ABOVE) CRY-AC
equipment.

Fig. 2.32. (ABOVE, RIGHT)
Cryoprobe hand unit.

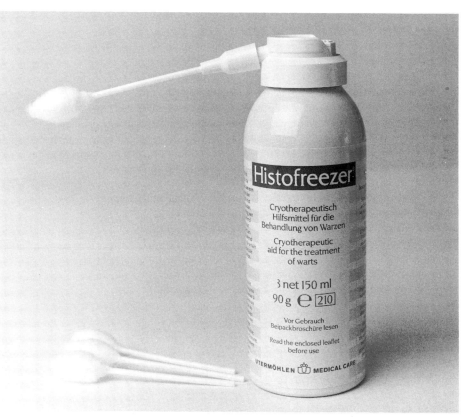

Fig. 2.33. Histofreezer.

(adequate suction is often not possible with smaller syringes) and 20 ml syringes are used for aspirating large joints and hydrocoeles. Some doctors use dental syringes (which use local anaesthetic cartridges) in preference to disposable syringes.

Needles

Orange 23G 25 mm needles are used for local anaesthetic injections. The general purpose green 21G needles are used for drawing up of local anaesthetics and steroids and also for aspirating large joints. Cream 19G needles are used for aspirating large volumes e.g. from hydrocoeles. Blue 21G needles are unnecessary.

Intravenous cannulae are useful for aspirating and injecting hydrocoeles and ganglions.

Dressing packs

Many commercial dressing packs are available (Fig. 2.34). They all commonly include a paper towel that can be used as a drape, a plastic tray in which skin

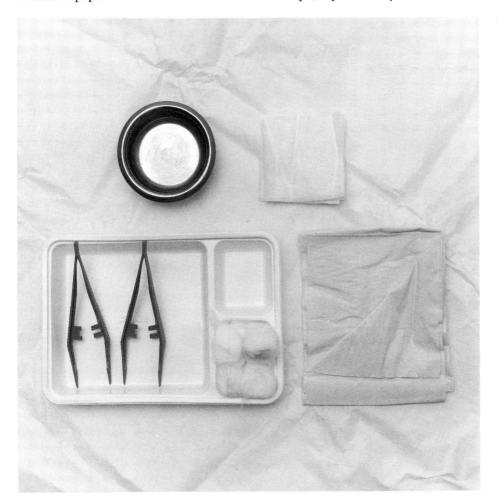

Fig. 2.34. Dressing pack.

preparation can be poured, disposable plastic forceps and cotton wool balls with which the skin preparation can be applied, and some gauze swabs. Most of the items are available individually wrapped.

Reference

1. *Care with Cryogenics. The Safe Use of Low Temperature Liquified Gases.* (Information brochure.) British Oxygen Company, The Priestley Centre, 10 Priestley Road, Surrey Research Park, Guildford, Surrey GU2 5XY.

3

Sterilisation

Heat sterilisation of instruments

Ideally, most surgical instruments should be sterilised with steam, under pressure in an autoclave. Bacteria and spores will be destroyed by heating to 121°C for 15 min. When dry heat is used this process requires heating to 160°C for 60 min. Boiling should not be used as it is a means of disinfection only (i.e. it will not kill spores) [1,2].[1]

It is essential to remove any adherent blood and tissues with a hard brush and the instruments should be rinsed in running water prior to sterilisation [3]. Gloves should be worn throughout the pre-sterilisation cleaning process.

Sterilisation times		
	Temperature (°C)	Time (min)
Autoclave	121	15
	126	10
	134	3
Dry heat	160	60
	170	40
	180	20

These times refer to holding times, *which commence only when the instruments to be sterilised have reached the required temperature* [2].

When assessing sterilisation times, it is important to allow for the heating up and cooling down times, which together can be considerable and may affect the way an operating session is organised.

Hot air sterilisers

Hot air sterilisers (Fig. 3.1) have the disadvantage that they are much more time-consuming in use and cannot be used for delicate instruments such as bipolar

---

[1] Disinfection refers to the inactivation of vegetative bacteria, viruses and fungi, but not bacterial spores. Sterilisation refers to the complete destruction of all organisms and spores.

Fig. 3.1. Hot air steriliser.

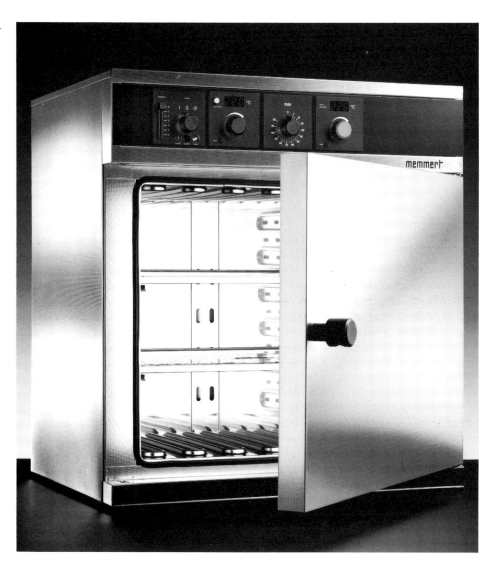

forceps because of their insulating coating. Another disadvantage is that instruments sterilised with hot air cannot be stored in a sterile state after removal from the unit. However, hot air sterilisation remains an effective method and may be adequate for some doctors. It is important that all aspects of the heat chamber achieve sterilisation temperatures and only units which are fan-assisted are to be recommended.

Sterilisation essentials

1. Use an autoclave or Central Sterile Supply Department.
2. Ensure regular servicing.
3. Ensure adequate insurance.
4. Maintain log of sterilisation cycles.

Autoclaves

Autoclaves take far less time than hot air sterilisers to complete a sterilisation cycle (Figs. 3.2, 3.3). At 121 °C the sterilisation time is 15 min but to this has to be added the loading and cooling times. Thus, after the time for the sterilisation temperature to be reached has been taken into account, it takes at least 20 min before instruments can be used. As with all sterilisers, it is important that instruments are loaded properly so that all the surfaces are exposed to the steam. Some autoclaves feature rack systems to keep all the instruments separated.

After completion of the autoclave cycle the instruments should be left to cool down and then used immediately. If they are not to be used immediately after sterilisation, autoclaved instruments should be put on a trolley laid with sterile paper and covered with a sterile cloth or sterile paper. They must then be used within a 3 hour period.

Fig. 3.2. Prestige autoclave.

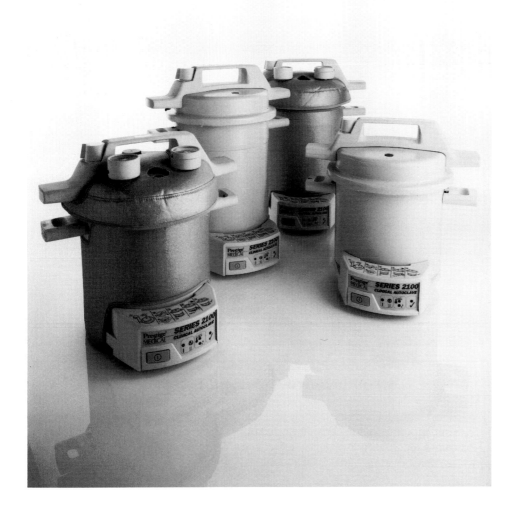

Fig. 3.3. SES 2000 autoclave.

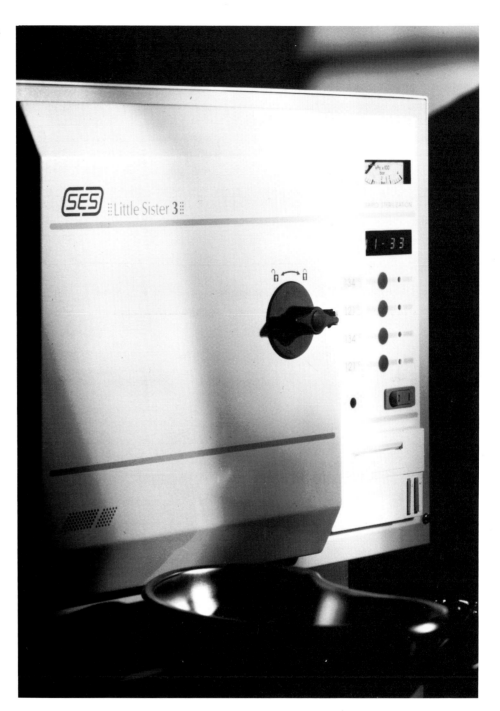

Recommended features for autoclaves

1. Preset automatic cycle.
2. Unit should provide separate indication of both temperature and pressure.
3. Unit should have a thermocouple entry point for control and monitoring during servicing.

At the present time, it is advised by the Department of Health that, since adequate penetration of steam cannot be guaranteed, wrapped instruments should only be passed through autoclaves featuring a prevacuum cycle. Such prevacuum cycles are not found in any of the small autoclaves commonly available.

It is recommended that only distilled or deionised water should be used because tap water will leave residual salts in the autoclave.

Being pressure systems, autoclaves in the United Kingdom are required by law to be inspected at least four times a year [4] and a written protocol is required detailing how and when pressure tests are to be carried out [5]. Since accidents can always happen, it is essential to take out third party insurance cover [6] against injuries due to accidental explosion.

All sterilisers should have thorough tests at installation, along with regular thermometric testing (using a thermocouple) and annual servicing and testing. The sterilisation cycle number should be recorded in the patient's notes.

Instrument packs

Since sterilisation cycles, even with an autoclave, can take at least 20 min, this can cause significant delays during an operating session. If it can be arranged, it can be a more convenient and economical option to get basic packs of instruments regularly sterilised, packed and delivered by a local hospital Central Sterilisation and Supply Department (CSSD). This would require the purchase of a number of sets of the basic instruments and a steriliser could be used simply to sterilise instruments on an *ad hoc* basis, for example instruments that have been dropped, or those that are infrequently used.

Chemical disinfection of instruments

Chemical disinfection is an uncertain process and should only be used for low-risk instruments used for low-risk procedures. For example: a proctoscope, or a vaginal speculum when used for colposcopy are low-risk instruments; a vaginal speculum used for insertion of an intra-uterine contraceptive device is a high risk instrument.

Hypochlorites have good microbiocidal properties. Sodium hypochlorite (bleach) can be used as a ready liquid or sodium dichloroisocyanurate (NaDCC) can be made up from tablets when required. It is usually easier to use tablets as they are stable and the resultant strength of solution is reliable. Although glutaraldehyde is no longer recommended (because of its irritant vapour) consideration should be given to the use of nitrile rubber gloves because ordinary household gloves may be permeable to such chemicals.

Care must be taken because hypochlorite, iodine and phenol may corrode instruments and surfaces, and may be inactivated by organic matter and detergents.

Immersion for 10 min in 70% (v/v) isopropyl alcohol can be used to disinfect items such as thermometers. Note that alcohol preparations are inflammable.

References

1. Adequacy of general practitioner's premises for minor surgery. Humphreys, H. & Dearden, D. A. *British Medical Journal* (1991), **302**, 1468.

2. *A Code of Practice for Sterilisation of Instruments and Control of Cross Infection.*(Information booklet.) British Medical Association: London (1989).

3. Adequacy of general practitioner's premises for minor surgery. Hoffman, P. N., Taylor, L. J. & Cookson, B. D. *British Medical Journal* (1991), **302**, 1468–1469.

4. *Health Technical Memorandum* (HTM10) (United Kingdom) (1980). Department of Health, Medical Devices Directorate, 14 Russell Square, London WC1B 4EP.

5. Performance test certificate (BS 3970 Part 4) (United Kingdom) (1990). *Specification for Transportable Steam Sterilisers for Unwrapped Instruments and Utensils.* British Standards Institute publication.

6. Department of Health Safety Action Bulletin No. 82, SAB(92)27, (United Kingdom) (1990). *Transportable Steam Sterilisers: Maintenance, Inspection and Insurance.* Department of Health, Medical Devices Directorate, 14 Russell Square, London WC1B 4EP.

4

Preoperative preparation and postoperative care

Patient preparation

History and examination

As with any surgery, there should be an appropriate review of the patient's history prior to any procedure. Any allergy to local anaesthetics, antibiotics or dressings should be established and made clear at the head of the clinical notes.

Special care should be taken to assess patients with diabetes and those with peripheral vascular disease prior to distal limb surgery. Patients with a history of rheumatic fever, or who have a prosthetic heart valve, joint prosthesis or cardiac pacemaker should be given an antibiotic cover 1 hour prior to the operation. It has been recommended that a single oral dose of flucloxacillin should be used in patients with abnormal native valves, and this should be supplemented with intramuscular or intravenous gentamicin in patients with prosthetic valves. Patients allergic to penicillin may be given a single 500 mg dose of vancomycin [1].

Because of the necessity for leg bandaging, it is advisable for women to stop taking oral contraceptives 4–6 weeks prior to having varicose vein injections or multiple ties. However, it is important to ensure an alternative form of contraception during the time when the patient is not taking the oral contraceptive. However, cessation of oral contraceptives is not necessary for other forms of minor surgery [2,3,4].

Informed consent should be obtained (see chapter 1). Most patients will need reassurance that the operation will be free from pain after the initial anaesthetic injection. However, it should be mentioned that the local anaesthetic will only numb the operative site and that the surrounding skin will retain normal sensation.

It is important to re-examine and mark the site of any subcutaneous lesion prior to the injection of local anaesthetic, as the volume of the injected fluid can make the lesion difficult to define.

Premedication

Premedication is usually unnecessary for most minor procedures in adults, but may be used in children, anxious adults and for more complicated or lengthy surgical procedures. Keeping a relaxed, reassuring and jovial atmosphere is more important than a sedative.

A simple regime in adults is to use Temazepam 10–30 mg 1 hour before surgery. In children, diazepam 2.5–5 mg or trimeprazine 3–4 mg/kg may be used 1–2 h before surgery [5]. Note that trimeprazine is liable to cause postoperative restlessness when pain is present.

Patient information leaflet

It can be most helpful for patients to have some simple leaflets to read while waiting for their operation appointment. An example leaflet is shown opposite.

Surgeon preparation

Clothing

No hat or mask or special clothing is necessary for the majority of minor procedures. For simple skin surgery ordinary clothing may be protected by a disposable plastic apron. When operating on a list of patients it may be appropriate but not essential to wear dedicated loose trousers and top. It is advisable to wear dedicated clothing for more involved operations such as vasectomy or varicose vein ligation.

Scrubbing up

There is no need to scrub up for most minor surgical procedures. The hands can be simply washed using either 4% (w/v) chlorhexidine (Hibiscrub) detergent solution or 7.5% (w/v) povidone iodine (Betadine) detergent solution, dried with clean paper towels and gloves worn. Some doctors prefer to use only soap and water. However, a formal scrub should be undertaken prior to more involved or lengthy procedures.

Gloves

Gloves should be worn for all surgical procedures and whenever there is any risk of coming into contact with blood or body fluids. Standard surgeon's gloves (which are more durable and have tight cuffs to fit around gowns) are an unnecessary expense. Less expensive sterile 'procedure' gloves such as Premier are ideal (Fig. 4.1).

Latex rubber may induce a skin sensitivity reaction in some wearers but hypoallergenic gloves (such as Biogel) are widely available. It should be noted that there are reports of an increasing number of patients (particularly in the

Patient information leaflet
Minor surgery

On arrival

It is quite understandable that you will feel a little anxious so if you have any questions when you arrive for your operation, please feel free to ask any of the nurses or the doctor. Before proceeding, the doctor will explain the nature and purpose of the operation and you will then be asked to sign a consent form.

The operation

You will be awake and alert during the operation and you will be free to chat with your doctor and nurse at all times. You will feel some slight initial discomfort with the local anaesthetic but, once the injection is over, the procedure should be completely pain-free.

At the end of your operation, any incision may be closed with very fine nylon stitches or with surgical tape, depending on the procedure. Often (particularly around the face and scalp), no dressing is necessary.

After the operation

After your surgery you will be able to relax and have some refreshment, following which you should feel ready to go home.

Driving will not normally present any problems after minor surgery. However, with more involved operations and when sedation has been given, you will be advised to be driven home. If there is any reason why you should not return to work the same day, you will be advised accordingly.

Aftercare

In most cases, there will only be some soreness felt around the operation site and pain-killers will not normally be required. However, your doctor will prescribe them for you if necessary. Surgical wounds on the face, head and neck can be left exposed immediately. Most other sites on the body can be exposed for light washing after 48 hours even when sutures are present because by then the wounds and suture holes are sealed. At other times wounds can be covered for work, and to avoid soiling of clothing. Stitches are normally removed after 4 to 14 days, depending on the nature and site of the operation. You can be reassured that the removal of stitches is a simple and quick procedure and causes very little (if any) discomfort.

Could there be any complications?

Complications are rare.

Occasionally some unavoidable bruising may occur around the operation site. Normally this fades gradually over a period of 1 to 3 weeks after the operation.

Rarely, an infection may develop in a part of the wound and this may give rise to some unexpected discomfort and swelling. If so, the surgery should be contacted for advice. Treatment is usually a simple matter.

Although problems are uncommon, we would like you to feel free to contact the surgery if you have any worrying symptoms.

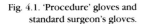
Fig. 4.1. 'Procedure' gloves and
standard surgeon's gloves.

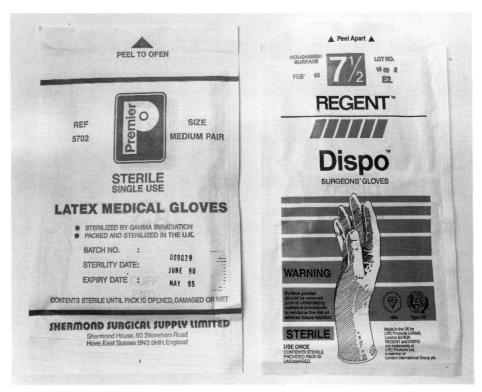

United States) who are allergic to latex and a number of cases of anaphylaxis have
been reported following pelvic examinations, and barium enemas using latex
catheters [6].

Protective glasses

Fine blood spots can be commonly found on surgeon's protective glasses even
after simple skin surgery and the use of diathermy. Consideration should therefore be given to the routine wearing of protective glasses for all routine minor
surgery [7].

Preoperative preparation

Skin shaving

The skin should be shaved with a disposable razor when the hair is long enough to
interfere with the operation or the application of a dressing. A useful technique for
removing hair cuttings is to apply a length of adhesive tape to the area. The hairs
simply stick to the tape and can be easily lifted away. Often on the scalp and chest
it may be possible simply to secure the hair flat and out of the way with adhesive
tapes. It is best to get the patient to shave the scrotal (but not the pubic) hair 48 h
before vasectomy. This allows any scratches to become sealed to avoid any
stinging sensation when spirit-based antiseptics are used.

Skin preparation

Infection and resistant organisms should not be a problem in the general practice setting and, for most minor skin biopsies and excisions, it is quite acceptable simply to cleanse the skin with 0.5% (w/v) aqueous chlorhexidine[1]. However, for other than simple skin surgery, spirit-based 10% povidone iodine or 4% chlorhexidine are the preferred antiseptic solutions and can be applied to the skin using the non-toothed disposable forceps that come with many dressing packs. When contaminated lesions such as keratoacanthoma or ulcerated basal cell carcinoma are excised, it is advisable to leave a cotton wool ball soaked in antiseptic solution directly on the lesion for several minutes prior to the surgery. This will help to minimise postoperative inflammation or wound infection.

Draping

Special towels are unnecessary for most minor cases. The sterile paper towels that come in most dressing packs are quite adequate and a central window can be cut to suit the size of the lesion. A medium-sized disposable paper towel with a central window ('circ' or circumcision towel) can be used for larger cases.

Postoperative care

Follow-up

Patients should be informed and instructed regarding any dressing changes they may have to do, and invited to seek advice if any problems arise after the operation. It is helpful for the surgeon to review selected cases some months after surgery to assess the appearance of the scar, benefit of treatment, etc., particularly in the early stages while he or she is building up experience.

Washing

Surgical wounds on the face, head and neck can generally be left exposed immediately, although they may require a light gauze dressing for a few hours to absorb any slight ooze. Most other sites on the body can be exposed for light washing after 24–48 h even when sutures are present because by then the wounds and suture holes are sealed. At other times wounds can be covered for work, and to avoid soiling of clothing and bedding.

Pain relief

The majority of minor procedures do not require post-operative analgesics. However, for those that do, Co-proxamol (paracetamol and dextropro-

---

[1] It is common practice to cleanse the skin with 0.5% aqueous chlorhexidine for simple skin surgery. In the author's experience this technique is perfectly safe and does not result in wound infection.

poxyphene) is usually adequate for pain relief. Patients with operations on the hands and feet will often benefit considerably from simple elevation of the limb. Vasectomy patients complain of heaviness and aching in the scrotum in addition to the soreness around the vas but, even so, Co-proxamol or a codeine preparation such as Codafen (codeine and ibuprofen) are quite adequate. It is unusual to require analgesia after the first 24 h.

Operating room log

A book should be kept in the operating room to record details of the date, patient's name, type of operation, pathology specimen and surgeon's name. A note should also be kept of stock numbers of all solutions used for injection (including local anaesthetics and steroid injectants).

Operation notes

Operation notes should be kept simple and succinct and include details of the clinical diagnosis, the procedure, any particular features or complications and the suture materials used. The proposed time for dressing changes and suture removal should be noted, along with any special postoperative instructions. A prominent note should be made of any material sent for histology.

Pathology specimens and results

All tissue specimens can be preserved in formalin (Fig. 4.2). The container must be clearly marked with the patient's name, the type of lesion, the site and side of

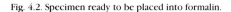

Fig. 4.2. Specimen ready to be placed into formalin.

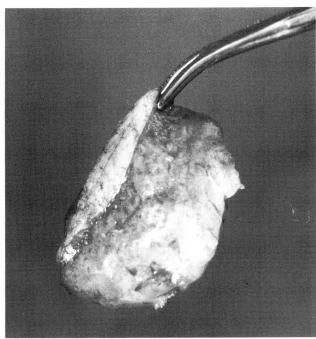

the body it came from and the date. The pathology form should give as much clinical detail as possible for the pathologist. The clinical appearance should be noted and a diagnosis should always be attempted, although this is not always possible. If the lesion is pigmented, a note should be made of any associated symptoms and signs such as itching, bleeding, irregularity or enlargement.

A separate record should be kept of all specimens that are sent for histological examination. This record should be checked regularly in order to confirm that reports have been received, to identify any pending pathology reports and to document that the patient has been informed of the result and any necessary action.

Audit and case analysis

Although not essential, it can be very helpful to document information such as clinical diagnosis, treatment, histological diagnosis and outcome for different types of case. If clearly documented, such information can be very informative and instructive with regard to both clinical and financial audit and may even be used as a basis for an article. Different practices will have different interests and it is, therefore, worth while spending a little time in defining exactly which parameters are to be recorded.

Example of case analysis for audit

Steroid injections

Date	Name	Age	M/F	Clinical diagnosis	Number of injections	Other treatment	Outcome	Other comments

Skin lesions

Date	Name	Age	M/F	Clinical diagnosis	Histological diagnosis	Wound appearance, infection	Other comments

Cryotherapy of warts

Date	Name	Age	M/F	Clinical extent	Number of treatments	Time needed for cure	Other comments

References

1. Endocarditis following skin procedures. Spelman, D. W., Weinmann, A. & Spicer, W. J. *Journal of Infection* (1993) **26**, 185–189.
2. Should the pill be stopped preoperatively? Sue-Ling, H. & Hughes, L. E. *British Medical Journal* (1988), **296**, 447–448.
3. Should the pill be stopped preoperatively? Guillebaud, J. *British Medical Journal* (1988), **296**, 786–787.
4. Should the pill be stopped preoperatively? Robinson, G., Cohen, H., Mackie, I. J. & Machin, S. J. *British Medical Journal* (1988), **296**, 787.
5. *British National Formulary 1993*. British Medical Association and Royal Pharmaceutical Society of Great Britain: London.
6. *General Practitioner* 7 August 1992 (Report).
7. Avoiding exposure to HIV and hepatitis: protective glasses and minor surgery. Hurren, J. S. *British Medical Journal* (1993), **306**, 335–336.

5

Precautions against hepatitis B and HIV infection

Hepatitis/AIDS precautions

The risk of infection to staff involved in general practice minor surgery should be extremely small provided a few simple precautions are taken and are universally applied *in all cases*.

Surveillance studies provide good evidence that human immunodeficiency virus (HIV) is not easily transmitted in the clinical health care setting. In the United States Communicable Disease Center Surveillance project the risk of acquiring HIV infection as a result of a single 'sharps' injury involving blood from a known HIV-infected patient was found to be less than 0.5%. This compares with a risk of hepatitis B transmission under parallel circumstances of the order of 20%. The majority of accidents arise from cuts and needlestick injuries. However, by August 1992 no HIV seroconversion after an injury from a suture needle or other solid needle used in the operating theatre had been reported [1].

Vaccination

It is important that all staff involved in surgery should receive active immunisation with hepatitis B vaccine. The risk of hepatitis B virus transmission to a health care worker who has been fully immunised and who has shown an immune response after vaccination is virtually zero [2]. If the subsequent antibody level is greater than 100 IU a booster dose should be given every 3–5 years. Non-converters should be vaccinated again and if they still fail to convert they should be tested for hepatitis B e antigen to identify infectious carriers. Staff who are e antigen positive or HIV positive should not participate in invasive procedures and should receive appropriate counselling [3].

Wounds and abrasions in staff

Any skin cuts, abrasions or open eczematous skin should be covered with a waterproof dressing and gloves should be worn whenever there is any risk of coming into contact with blood or other body fluids (Fig. 5.1).

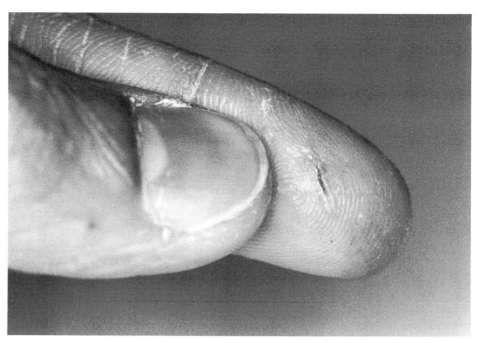

Fig. 5.1. All skin cuts should be covered with a waterproof dressing.

Essential routine precautions for staff to minimise risk of exposure to hepatitis B and HIV

Staff
Ensure vaccination against hepatitis B.
Cover all cuts, abrasions and eczematous areas.
Maintain high level of theatre discipline.

Sharps
Do not resheath needles.
Do not guide needles by hand.
Do not pass sharps hand to hand.
Dispose of sharps immediately at point of use.

Tissues and fluids
Clear and disinfect spillages promptly.
Ensure safe disposal of clinical waste.

Sharps

Sharps bins should be placed so that needles and blades can be disposed of immediately at their point of use. Needles should only be resheathed after use if required again (for example, with local anaesthetics) and only by scooping the sheath from a surface, one-handed. Otherwise the needle should be discarded unsheathed. Sharps boxes should not be over-filled and care should be taken to look before dropping needles and syringes into sharps boxes so as to avoid any used needles that may be inadvertently pointing upwards (Fig. 5.2).

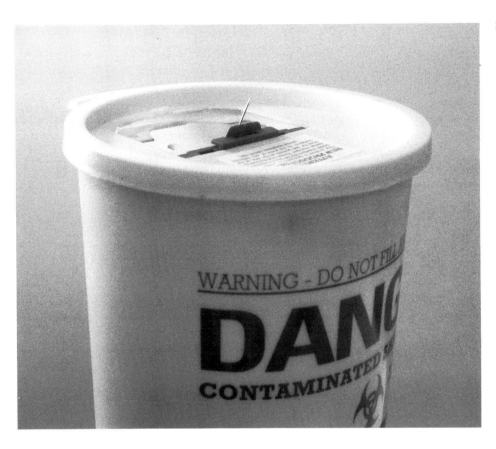

Fig. 5.2. Do not overfill sharps boxes.

The majority of glove perforations affect the index finger and thumb of the non-dominant hand, hence great care should be taken when handling suture needles [4].

Spilt blood and tissue fluids

Infectious cell-free HIV has been recovered from dried material after up to 3 days at room temperature, and after 15 days in an aqueous environment [5]. Spilt blood and other body fluids should be mopped up with disposable towels and the surface cleaned with 10% hypochlorite (bleach) or dichloroisocyanurate (Presept). It is recommended that the solution should be left on the surface for 3 min after which the surface should be rinsed and dried [6]. Inactivation of HIV by 70% ethanol is slow and its use is not recommended [7,8,9].

Cleaning of work surfaces

Gloves should be worn during all cleaning procedures. All work surfaces and trolleys should be routinely washed down with ordinary detergent and wiped with 70% isopropyl alcohol or 1000 ppm hypochlorite.

Operating on known hepatitis B and HIV carriers

It is preferable to refer known hepatitis B and HIV carriers to a local hospital for minor surgery where necessary equipment and facilities are already available and where clinical waste can be more easily disposed of.

However, should the situation arise where invasive procedures have to be performed in general practice a number of basic measures need to be taken for protection. All staff should wear protective clothing (goggles, plastic aprons, gloves and overshoes). Disposable items and equipment should be used if possible and sent for incineration immediately after use.

All pathological specimens must be double wrapped in polythene bags and clearly labelled as being hepatitis B or HIV positive.

It is advisable to send all reusable instruments to a local CSSD for sterilisation.

Accidental contact with hepatitis B or HIV

There is no risk to an individual by spillage of HIV blood onto intact skin. However, there is a risk from contact with mucous membranes and the eyes. Since the efficacy of current treatment for HIV is unclear, expert counselling and advice should be sought for treatment of contact with HIV blood or tissue [9,10].

Immediate action should be taken to reduce contamination to a minimum. Bleeding should be encouraged from the inoculation site. The skin should be thoroughly washed with soap and water. The eyes should be bathed with saline. Any contamination with hepatitis B virus may require treatment with hepatitis B specific immunoglobulin if the individual is sero-negative.

Immediate treatment of accidental staff contact with hepatitis B or HIV blood or tissues

1. Encourage bleeding from inoculation site.
2. Wash site with soap and water.
3. Bathe eyes with saline.
4. Consider hepatitis B specific immunoglobulin.
5. Obtain expert counselling.

References

1. Risks to surgeons and patients from HIV and hepatitis: guidelines on precautions and management of exposure to blood and body fluids. Joint Working Party of Hospital Infection Society and the Surgical Infection Study Group. *British Medical Journal* (1992), **305**, 1337–1343.
2. HIV, hepatitis B virus and other blood borne pathogens in health care setting: review of risk factors and guidelines for prevention. Hu, D. J., Kane, M. A. & Heymann, D. L. *Bulletin of the World Health Organization* (1991), **69**, 623–630.
3. Risks to surgeons and patients from HIV and hepatitis. Boxall, E. H. *British Medical Journal* (1993), **306**, 652–653.

4. Perforation of gloves in an accident and emergency department. Richmond, P. W., McCabe, M., Davies, J. P. & Thomas, D. M. *British Medical Journal* (1992), **304**, 879–880.

5. Stability and inactivation of HTLV-III/LAV under clinical and laboratory conditions. Resnick, L., Veren, K., Salahuddin, S. W., Tondreau, S. & Markham, P. D. *Journal of the American Medical Association* (1986), **255**, 1887–1891.

6. *A Code of Practice for Sterilisation of Instruments and Control of Cross Infection*. (Information booklet.) British Medical Association 1989.

7. Chemical inactivation of HIV on surfaces. Hanson, P. J. V., Gor, D., Jeffries, D. J. & Collins, J. V. *British Medical Journal* (1989), **298**, 862–864.

8. Inactivation of HIV on surfaces by alcohol. Burren, J. V., Cooke, E. A., Mortimer, P. P. & Simpson, R. A. *British Medical Journal* (1989), **299**, 459.

9. *Guidance for Clinical Health Care Workers: Protection against Infection with HIV and Hepatitis Viruses*. (1990). HMSO: London.

10. Further information can be obtained from the Department of Health booklet *AIDS–HIV Infected Health Care Workers* (1991). Department of Health: London.

SECTION II

6

Local anaesthetics

A large variety of procedures can be easily and safely performed using simple local anaesthetic techniques. Patients should be reassured that local anaesthesia only causes some slight initial discomfort, followed by complete numbness to pain in the area concerned. However, normal sensation will be retained in all areas other than the operative site. Anxious patients generally respond well to reassurance and rarely require premedication (see chapter 4).

After the injection of local anaesthetic the small diameter pain fibres are blocked before the larger fibres carrying touch sensation, which in turn are blocked before the largest motor fibres. The effect of the agent injected depends largely on the rate of blood perfusion in the tissue. For example, in the face, perfusion is rapid and reabsorption of the agent is fast unless a vasoconstrictor drug is added. After simple skin infiltration, anaesthesia begins to occur almost immediately. A digital nerve block may take up to 5 min to be complete, depending on the presence or absence of acute inflammation. Blocks of larger nerves take correspondingly more time.

Anecdotal evidence suggests that using lignocaine warmed to 37 °C results in less pain on injection than does lignocaine at room temperature. It is suggested that this may be due to the warm solution causing less nociceptor stimulation, which may also achieve a faster onset of neural blockade [1]. However, there are many variables involved with the discomfort felt with local anaesthetics, for example the pH of injected fluid, density of the tissue in the injection area, the rate of injection and the presence of inflammation near the injection site. A useful method of reducing the pain of injection is to use a counter-irritant such as pinching the nearby skin before and during the injection [2]. For practical purposes, when a fast-acting local anaesthetic such as lignocaine is used, probably the most important single factor in minimising the pain of injection is that of operator technique.

Drugs

Lignocaine

Lignocaine is inexpensive, very safe and is more stable than most other local anaesthetics (Fig. 6.1a). It readily diffuses through the tissues and its onset of action is rapid. The duration of action will depend on the site of administration

Table 6.1. *Maximum doses advised for plain (no adrenaline) lignocaine (dose in adults)*

Concentration % (mg/ml)	Maximum volume (ml)
0.5 (5)	40
1 (10)	20
2 (20)	10
4 (40)	5

Note: Although these doses are commonly exceeded by experienced anaesthetists, these figures allow a working safety margin.

Fig. 6.1a. Lignocaine vials and hyaluronidase.

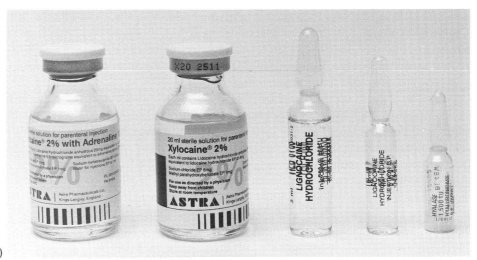

(a)

and local vascularity, and varies between 20 and 90 min. Plain lignocaine has a slight vasodilator effect, although in most circumstances this is of no significance. The use of adrenaline will reduce bleeding, and increase both the duration of action and also the maximum safe dosage by reducing the absorption rate. Although larger amounts can be used, it is suggested that the maximum volumes of drug used should not exceed the volumes listed in Table 6.1 [*3*]. Commonly a 0.5% or 1% solution should be used for skin infiltration. The 2% solution is usually unnecessary for routine minor surgery although it can be used to good effect, for example in order to reduce the volume of fluid injected when a digital nerve block is performed. In children, or cases of old age, debility, hepatic disease, renal impairment, epilepsy or heart block, lower doses must be used.

Lignocaine can be obtained in either ampoules or multidose vials, with or without adrenaline.

Prilocaine and bupivicaine

Although prilocaine is the safest drug for intravenous regional anaesthesia because of its slow reabsorption by the circulation, it has a slower onset of action than lignocaine and confers no benefit in general practice minor surgery. Bupivicaine has a much longer duration of action (4–6 h) compared with lignocaine (0.5–1.5 h) but it has a much slower onset of action than does lignocaine.

Adrenaline (epinephrine)

The addition of adrenaline can virtually eliminate bleeding in most cases and can be safely used for most sites except digits, the tip of the nose, the ear lobes and the shaft of the penis, or where there is circulatory impairment. Adrenaline is particularly useful in highly vascular areas such as the scalp and face. It is usually combined with lignocaine in a strength of 1:200000 (5 µg/ml). This solution is effective in producing a dry operative field in non-inflamed skin provided that the operator waits at least 5–10 min before making the skin incision (Fig. 6.1b). Note that when simple infiltration local anaesthesia is used adrenaline acts mainly on the small intradermal vessels. Bleeding can still be expected to appear from larger and deeper vessels, which will have to be either avoided or tied.

The use of 1:200000 adrenaline limits the safe volume of solution to 80 ml because of the risk of adrenaline toxicity.

Complications with adrenaline There is a risk of profound ischaemia if lignocaine with adrenaline is accidentally injected into, for example, a finger or toe. However, Astra Pharmaceuticals have had few reported cases of accidental injections and in these, no problems have resulted [4]. In addition, it is apparent that, among podiatrists in the United States at least, for many years there has been a widespread practice of injecting lignocaine with adrenaline into toes, seemingly without a high rate of complications [5].[1]

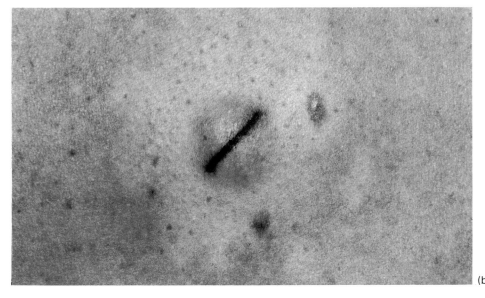

Fig. 6.1b. Effect of local anaesthetic with adrenaline infiltrated around a sebaceous cyst.

(b)

[1] In a questionnaire survey of 839 practitioners and over 2100000 injections of adrenaline-containing local anaesthetic, Roth found a low rate of complications [5]. Nevertheless, the overall incidence of loss of part or all of the involved toe or more radical amputation was one case per 132000 injections. However, no comparison was made with complication rates when plain anaesthetic solutions were used. Since bloodless toe surgery can be performed safely using plain lignocaine and a carefully applied tourniquet, adrenaline should not be used, however small the risk may be.

There is no specific treatment for accidental injection into a digit. Although warming the patient's hand might increase the blood supply to the digit, whether this has any significant benefit is unknown. Thus, prevention of accidents is better than attempted cure. Lignocaine with adrenaline is dispensed in bottles that have red lettering and to minimise risk of any error it should be kept separate from the plain solution. One method of reducing the risk of error is to keep lignocaine and adrenaline in a red tray and to replace the bottle in the tray immediately after drawing up.

Adrenaline should not be used in the following situations

Digits.
Tip of the nose.
Ear lobes.
Shaft of the penis.
Where there is circulatory impairment.

Hyaluronidase

This enzyme inactivates hyaluronic acid and aids diffusion of local anaesthetics. It is particularly useful where the skin is tightly bound down to the subcutaneous tissues (for example, the nose, palm, sole and scar tissue). The usual dose is 1500 IU. Adrenaline should be used with the anaesthetic drug, since the increased rate of diffusion will result in a shorter duration of action.

The local anaesthetic, adrenaline and hyaluronidase can be drawn up in the same syringe.

Systemic toxic reactions

Systemic toxic reactions may occur with any local anaesthetic agent. However, hypersensitivity reactions occur mainly with the ester-type local anaesthetics, such as amethocaine, benzocaine, cocaine and procaine. Reactions are less frequent with the amide types, such as lignocaine, bupivicaine, and prilocaine [6].

However, hypersensitivity may be due to preservatives and not due to the local anaesthetic drug itself (note that all plain local anaesthetics supplied in ampoules by Astra Pharmaceuticals are free of preservatives).

If, for example, a patient has a known hypersensitivity to lignocaine (an amide) it is likely that hypersensitivity will be found to both bupivicaine and prilocaine.[1] Although it may be possible in such a case to use instead an ester-type local anaesthetic such as procaine, any patient with a past history of some sort of reaction to a previous local anaesthetic injection should have their minor operation in hospital with full resuscitation facilities at hand.

Allergy and anaphylaxis are in fact very rare and the vast majority of reactions

---

[1] A protocol for testing for hypersensitivity to local anaesthetics (which should be done in hospital) may be obtained from Astra Pharmaceuticals, Home Park, Kings Langley, Hertfordshire WD4 8DH, United Kingdom.

are due to the use of large volumes of drug or injection directly into the circulation. Cardiac toxicity produces hypotension, bradycardia and heart block. Cerebral toxicity produces an excitable state followed by coma, convulsions and respiratory arrest. Before the start of any procedure where large total doses of agents may be used, an intravenous cannula should be inserted and resuscitation equipment should be readily available. However, any such procedure should not be performed in the general practice setting.

Anaphylaxis should be treated by giving adrenaline i.m., along with an anti-histamine such as chlorpheniramine i.v. and hydrocortisone i.v. Laryngeal oedema, brochospasm and hypotension should be treated with 0.5–1 mg (0.5–1 ml of 1 : 1000) adrenaline repeated every 10 min according to blood pressure and pulse measurements [6].

In view of the rapid and unpredictable onset of anaphylaxis treatment is not easily studied by controlled trials. Some would consider the standard dose of adrenaline too high and advocate a smaller dose of 0.3–0.5 mg [7].

In addition to the adrenaline an antihistamine such as chlorpheniramine 10–20 mg (diluted in 5–10 ml of blood or saline) should be given by slow intra-venous injection, along with intravenous fluids if hypotension persists. Intra-venous aminophylline 250 mg or nebulised salbutamol should be given for persistent brochospasm, along with intravenous hydrocortisone 100–300 mg (Fig. 6.2).

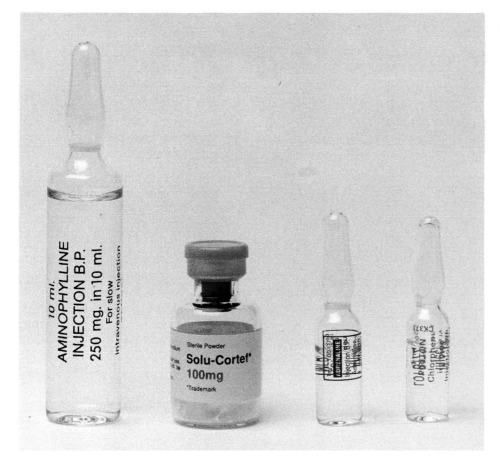

Fig. 6.2. Aminophylline, hydrocortisone, adrenaline, and chlorpheniramine.

Treatment of allergy and anaphylaxis

Adrenaline i.m. 0.5–1 ml of 1:1000, repeated after 10 min if necessary.
Hydrocortisone i.v. 100–300 mg.
Chlorpheniramine i.v. 10–20 mg.
Saline i.v. to maintain blood pressure.
Aminophylline i.v. 250 mg.
Or
Salbutamol in nebuliser for persistent bronchospasm.

Entonox (nitrous oxide)

Although it is not a local anaesthetic, Entonox is included here because it is useful in selected cases (Fig. 6.3). Entonox is a mixture of 50% nitrous oxide and 50% oxygen and stored in cylinders that are blue with a segmented white neck. Entonox can be of particular value in the treatment of painful lesions such as abscesses, multiple verrucae and wounds in small children. It causes a light

Fig. 6.3. Entonox delivery system.

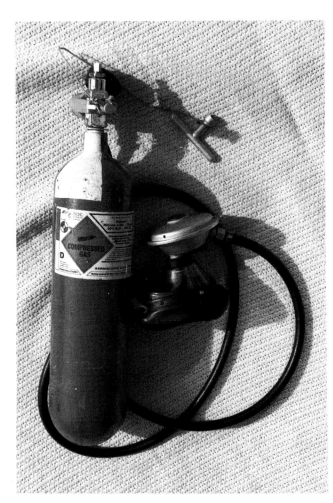

analgesia without loss of consciousness, although it can cause light-headedness. The delivery system has a demand valve, thus it is self-administered and regulated. Recovery following Entonox anaesthesia is usually rapid.

Local anaesthetic techniques

Topical anaesthesia (**Fig. 6.4**)

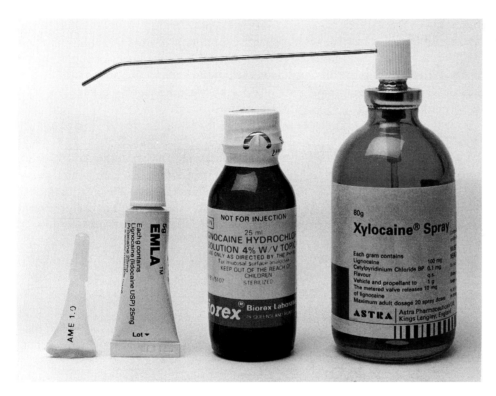

Fig. 6.4. Topical anaesthesia preparations: Amethocaine minims, EMLA cream, lignocaine hydrochloride, lignocaine spray.

Skin Lignocaine and prilocaine are mixed together as EMLA cream 5 % (w/v) in a water miscible base. It can be used in children prior to injection or venepuncture. A thick layer of the cream is applied under an occlusive dressing. Although the data sheet recommends a waiting time of at least 60 min, it is often possible to find useful surface anaesthesia within 20–30 min. The application is usually associated with a transient redness and oedema. Note that since EMLA cream provides only very superficial anaesthesia, it cannot be relied upon in the treatment of skin lesions with cryotherapy or cautery.

The traditional use of ethyl chloride spray prior to incision of abscesses is both very crude and unpredictable in its effect. In such cases, dome infiltration or wide infiltration of lignocaine is preferable.

Cornea and conjunctiva Amethocaine 0.5 % drops are used to anaesthetise the cornea and conjunctiva. Unfortunately, amethocaine causes intense pain on instillation, but fortunately anaesthesia commences rapidly after only a few minutes. Its duration of action may last up to 30–60 min. The anaesthetised eye should be protected with a patch until normal sensation is restored.

Nose A ribbon impregnated with 2 % lignocaine and adrenaline may be inserted into the nose to anaesthetise the nasal mucosa prior to cautery for epistaxis.

The traditional paste containing cocaine with its inherent vasoconstrictive effect has probably no additional benefit over the use of lignocaine in conjunction with adrenaline.

Mouth and throat Topical 4 % lignocaine or an aerosol spray of 10 % lignocaine may be used to anaesthetise areas in the mouth and throat. It has an extremely bitter taste. The patient should be warned against eating or drinking until the effect of the anaesthetic has worn off, as the numbness of the throat may interfere with swallowing. In addition, the patient should be warned to take care to avoid inadvertent biting of the anaesthetised area of buccal mucosa or tongue.

Local infiltration anaesthesia

Local infiltration requires no knowledge of anatomy. The anaesthetic is injected into the subcutaneous fat and blocks small cutaneous nerves and their nerve endings (Fig. 6.5). For the vast majority of injections, a 25 mm 25G needle is ideal. The shorter 12 mm 25G needles are too short and should be avoided. However, a finer 28G needle on a 1 ml syringe is kinder for delicate areas such as the nose or eyelids.

Fig. 6.5. The plane of injection.

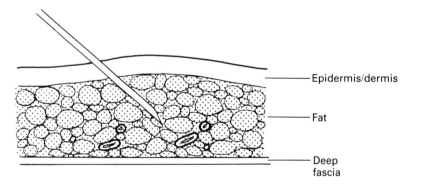

Epidermis/dermis

Fat

Deep fascia

In the scalp, it is easy to inadvertently inject the anaesthetic below the epicranial aponeurosis. This is likely to result in an incomplete block and can be recognised by the lack of resistance to the injection (Fig. 6.6).

It is always wise to re-examine any skin and subcutaneous lesions, and mark out the proposed skin incision prior to the injection, as the volume of injected fluid can easily obscure subcutaneous lesions and associated skin creases. The patient having been forewarned, the needle is inserted through the skin so as to lie in the subcutaneous fat underneath the dermis. The needle is then directed horizontally and small amounts injected as the needle is advanced. There should be no resistance to the injection. It is not necessary to pull back on the plunger of the syringe prior to injection, provided the needle is kept moving. Even if a small vessel is punctured, the amount of anaesthetic entering the circulation will be

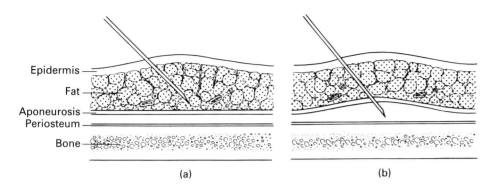

Fig. 6.6. Scalp infiltration, (a) correct (b) incorrect.

Epidermis

Fat

Aponeurosis

Periosteum

Bone

(a)   (b)

small and insignificant. Before the needle reaches the end of its travel it should be either withdrawn and redirected under the skin or inserted further along at a site already anaesthetised. Wherever possible, the needle should be inserted through an anaesthetised area (Fig. 6.7).

During operations below the deep fascia, further deep infiltrations will be necessary.

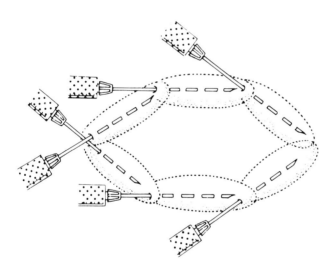

Fig. 6.7. Whenever possible, the needle should be inserted through anaestheised skin.

Local anaesthetic infiltration of lacerations When lacerations are anaesthetised, the injection is made directly into the subdermal plane from inside the wound. If the wound is contaminated or the skin is mobile, the percutaneous route is used, although this is more painful. Note that the injection of local anaesthetic should not be made into a wound until any nearby nerve and tendon function has been assessed.

With lacerations in children it can be helpful first to drip some local anaesthetic directly onto a gauze placed inside the wound and leave it for some 5–10 min. This will anaesthetise the internal surfaces of the wound and make subsequent injection into the wound more tolerable. It has been reported that often the topical instillation of local anaesthetic may result in anaesthesia of the skin extending into and away from the wound edges, such that skin suture is possible without the necessity for local anaesthetic injection [8]. However, the effect is quite variable and cannot be relied upon. Each case must be checked for numbness to pin-prick before skin suture is begun.

Dome infiltration anaesthesia This is extremely useful for draining abscesses and haematomata when the overlying skin is thin and not indurated (Fig. 6.8). The needle is injected horizontally directly into the dome of the abscess or haematoma. Only a small quantity of local anaesthetic (perhaps 0.25–0.5 ml) is necessary and this only causes a transient sharp pain. Almost immediately the dome can be punctured with a no. 11 blade, releasing the pus or blood.

Fig. 6.8. Dome infiltration anaesthesia.

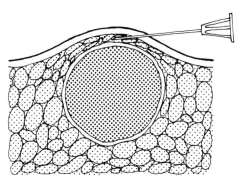

Local anaesthetic infiltration of the palm and the sole of the foot Injecting directly into the thick palmar or plantar skin is extremely painful and should always be avoided if possible. When injecting for example, a trigger finger, the palmar skin can be anaesthetised with an injection of local anaesthetic through the soft dorsal skin of the web space (see chapter 7) (Figs. 6.9, 6.10).

Fig. 6.9. Injection through the soft dorsal skin to anaesthetise the palmar skin prior to injection into trigger finger.

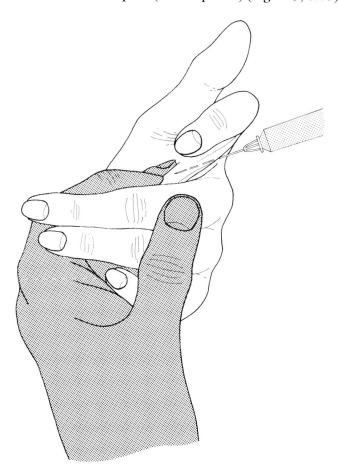

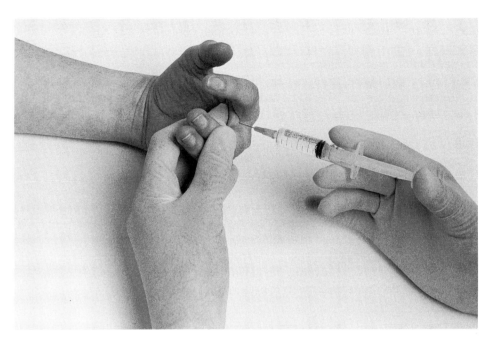

Fig. 6.10. Injection through the soft dorsal skin to anaesthetise the palmar skin prior to injection into trigger finger.

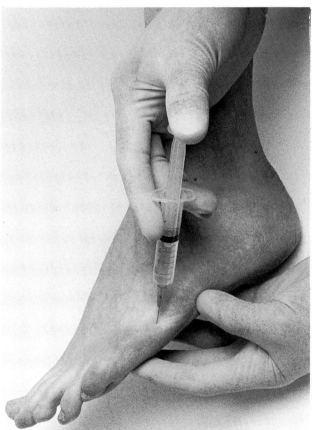

Fig. 6.11. Local anaesthetic injection through the side of the foot.

In the treatment of large solitary verrucae or other lesions on the sole of the foot, it is often possible to insert the needle through the softer skin on either the medial or lateral side of the foot and direct it towards the lesion (Fig. 6.11).

Local anaesthesia around the eye The cornea is supplied by the opthalmic nerve via the ciliary nerves. The whole ocular conjunctiva is supplied by the ophthalmic nerve and the sensation to the upper and lower eyelids is supplied by the ophthalmic and maxillary nerves, respectively. Thus, during an operation on the eyelids, the eyelid itself can be infiltrated with lignocaine but the ocular conjunctiva and cornea have to be anaesthetised separately with topical amethocaine (see above).

Peripheral nerve blocks

Digital nerve block The technique is similar for the fingers and toes. A 25G needle and 3 ml of 1 % *plain* lignocaine is used. Adrenaline must not be used. The approach at the transverse palmar crease that blocks the common digital nerves is not recommended as the palmar skin is thick and this makes the injection very painful (Fig. 6.12).

Instead, an approach blocking the separate digital nerves through the softer dorsal skin of the interdigital web is preferred (Figs. 6.13, 6.14).

Fig. 6.12. Digital nerve block, palmar approach.

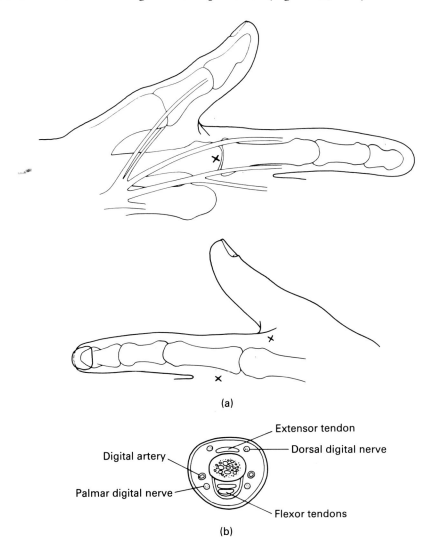

(a)

Fig. 6.13. Digital nerve block, dorsal approach.

Extensor tendon

Digital artery

Dorsal digital nerve

Palmar digital nerve

Flexor tendons

(b)

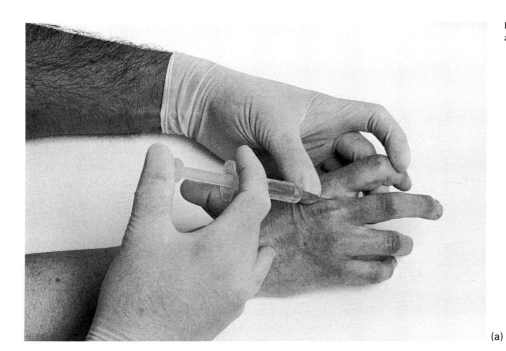

Fig. 6.14. Digital nerve block, dorsal approach: (a) finger and (b) toe.

(a)

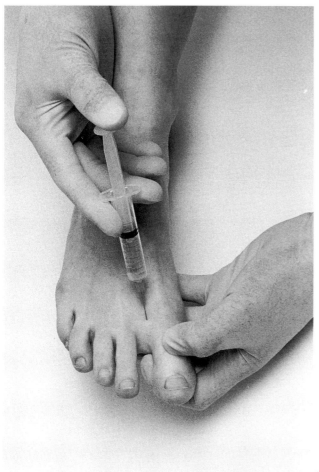

(b)

However, a more proximal block *is* indicated in the presence of severe infection, where the rise in tissue tension caused by the injection may compromise the arterial supply and venous drainage of the digit.

The needle is inserted through the interdigital web skin and 0.5 ml is injected under the point of the needle entry site to block the smaller dorsal digital nerve. The needle is then advanced until the resistance of the palmar skin is felt and 1 ml of solution injected as the needle is slightly withdrawn. The procedure is repeated on the other side of the digit.

It is often not necessary to block the dorsal nerves in the fingers and lesser toes as their areas of innervation seldom extend much beyond the proximal interphalangeal joint. However, in the thumb and great toe, the dorsal nerves must be blocked as they may supply a variable area up to and including the nail bed (Fig. 6.15).

Median nerve block The median nerve lies in the mid-line at the wrist, immediately below the palmaris longus tendon. The block is performed with the arm abducted, elbow extended and the forearm supinated. The palmaris longus tendon on the anterior surface of the wrist is identified by active wrist flexion against resistance. The needle is inserted at the ulnar border of the tendon, 2 cm proximal to the distal wrist crease (Figs. 6.16, 6.17, 6.18). If the tendon is absent,

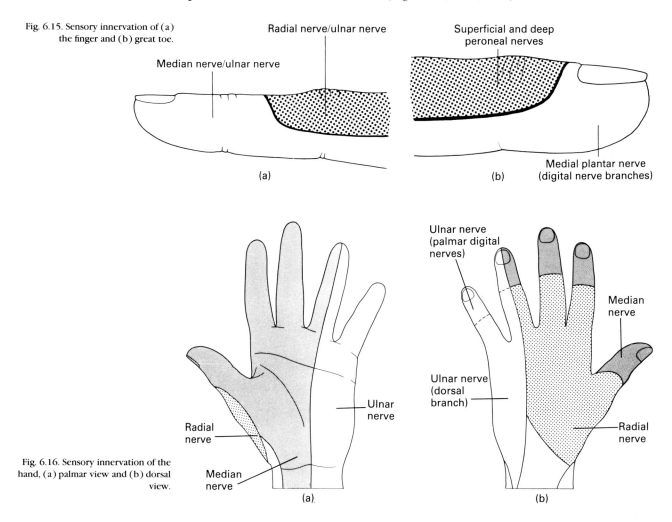

Fig. 6.15. Sensory innervation of (a) the finger and (b) great toe.

Fig. 6.16. Sensory innervation of the hand, (a) palmar view and (b) dorsal view.

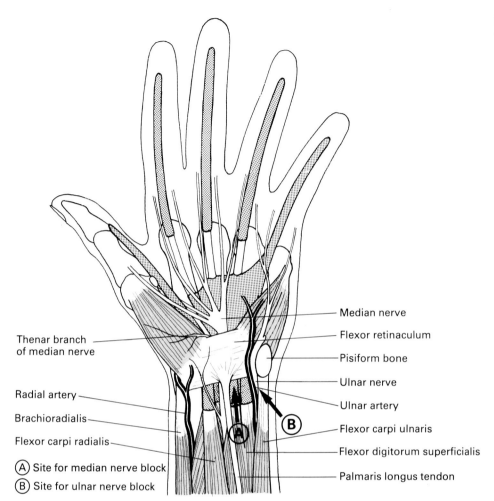

Fig. 6.17. Anaesthetic block of Ⓐ median nerve and Ⓑ ulnar nerve.

Thenar branch of median nerve

Radial artery

Brachioradialis

Flexor carpi radialis

Ⓐ Site for median nerve block

Ⓑ Site for ulnar nerve block

Median nerve

Flexor retinaculum

Pisiform bone

Ulnar nerve

Ulnar artery

Flexor carpi ulnaris

Flexor digitorum superficialis

Palmaris longus tendon

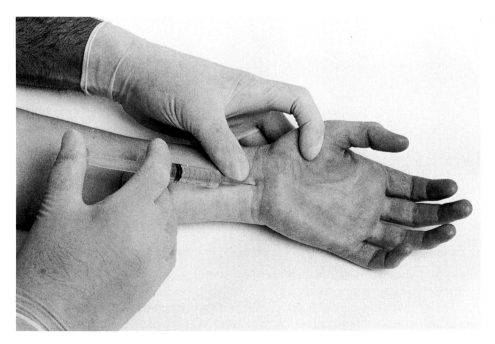

Fig. 6.18. Median nerve block.

the needle is inserted 0.5 cm medial to mid-line. This approach (to the side of the nerve) minimises the risk of intraneural injection. If paraesthesia occur and persist, the needle should be slightly withdrawn and adjusted to avoid an intraneural injection, and then 3–5 ml of 1% lignocaine solution (with adrenaline) is injected.

Ulnar nerve block The palmar cutaneous branch and the dorsal branch arise proximal to the wrist and must be blocked separately. The arm should be abducted, the elbow extended and the forearm supinated. The needle is inserted to the radial side of the flexor carpi ulnaris tendon and 3 cm proximal to the distal wrist crease (Figs. 6.17, 6.19). If paraesthesia occur and persist, the needle should be withdrawn slightly and adjusted to avoid an intraneural injection, and then 3–5 ml of 1% lignocaine solution (with adrenaline) is injected.

Anaesthesia of the palmar cutaneous and dorsal branches is achieved with a field block extending dorsally from the radial border of the flexor carpi ulnaris to the tip of the ulnar styloid.

Fig. 6.19. Ulnar nerve block.

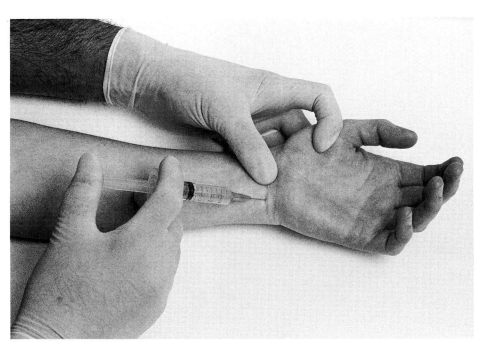

Posterior tibial nerve block This block is useful when dealing with lesions and lacerations on the plantar aspect of the foot. The needle is placed just anterior to the Achilles tendon at the level of the medial malleolus and 3–5 ml of 1% lignocaine solution (with adrenaline) is injected (Figs. 6.20, 6.21, 6.22).

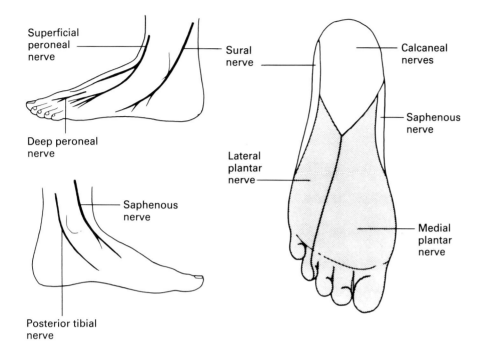

Fig. 6.20. Sensory innervation of the foot.

Calcaneal nerve block This block is useful in the treatment of lesions on the heel using liquid nitrogen, electrocautery, or during injection of steroids into anxious patients. The calcaneal nerves supply the bulk of the skin of the heel and can be blocked by a band of local anaesthetic injected horizontally into the skin below the level of the medial malleolus (Fig. 6.23).

Tourniquets

The use of exsanguination and a tourniquet is helpful for most operations on the digits as even a small amount of persistent bleeding can seriously obscure the operative field.

The tourniquet is applied prior to any skin preparation. Because of the small diameter of the fingers and toes it is not normally possible to exsanguinate the digit by merely squeezing the digit in the operator's hand. A simple and convenient method is repeatedly to fold a large tissue into a thick strip and wrap it around the digit (Fig. 6.24). This creates bulk that can then be squeezed effectively by the operator's hand thus exsanguinating the digit. Tension is then applied to a non-sterile elastic band placed around the base of the digit and the elastic band secured with an artery clip (Fig. 6.25).

The tourniquet should not be too tight or too loose. If the tourniquet is applied too tightly there is a risk of damage to the underlying digital nerves or vessels. If the tourniquet is applied too loosely (shown by a dusky blue tinge) the resulting congestion will lead to continued oozing from any cut tissues. Although there are no specific guidelines to define the maximal digital tourniquet time, most procedures take less than 30 min and this length of time is quite safe.

Fig. 6.21. Posterior tibial nerve block.

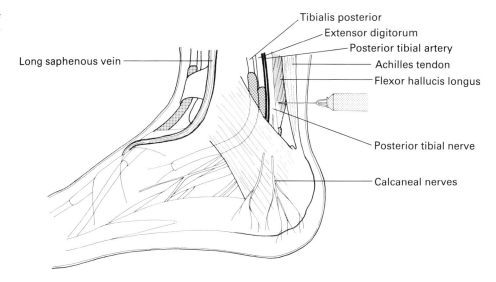

Tibialis posterior
Extensor digitorum
Posterior tibial artery
Achilles tendon
Flexor hallucis longus

Long saphenous vein

Posterior tibial nerve

Calcaneal nerves

Fig. 6.22. Posterior tibial nerve block.

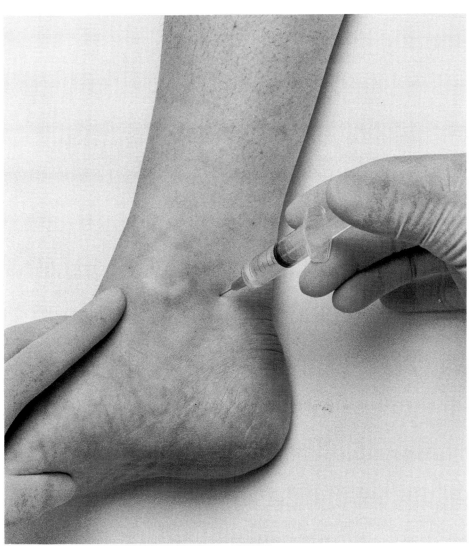

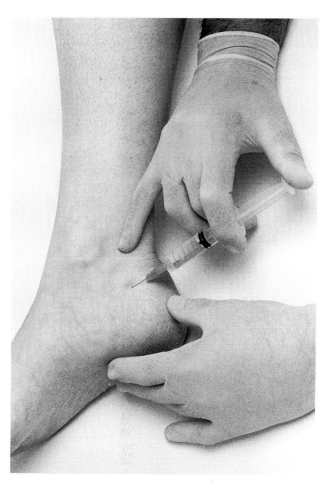

Fig. 6.23. Calcaneal nerve block.

Fig. 6.24. (LEFT) Exsanguination of the great toe with the help of a tissue. Note that the elastic band tourniquet is not tightened until the toe has been exsanguinated because this will result in venous congestion within the toe.

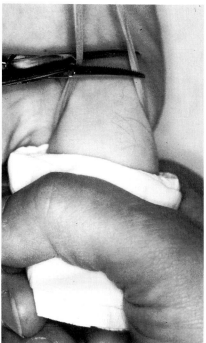

Fig. 6.25. (BELOW) Finger tourniquet.

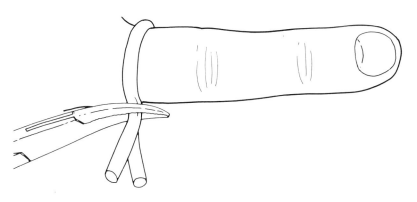

References

1. Warming lignocaine to reduce pain associated with injection. Davidson, J. A. H. & Boom, S. J. *British Medical Journal* (1992), **305**, 617–618.

2. Counter-irritation reduces pain during cutaneous needle insertion. Bourke, D. L. *Anaesthesia and Analgesia* (1985), **64**, 379.

3. Safe doses of lignocaine. *British National Formulary 1993*, pp. 484–485. British Medical Association and Royal Pharmaceutical Society of Great Britain: London.

4. Accidental injection of lignocaine with adrenaline into digits. (Personal communication). Astra Pharmaceuticals Ltd., Home Park Estate, Kings Langley, Hertfordshire, UK.

5. Utilization of epinephrine-containing anaesthetic solutions in the toes. Roth, R. D. *Journal of American Podiatrists Association* (1981), **71**, 189–199.

6. Anaphylactic shock. *British National Formulary 1990*, pp. 131–132. British Medical Association and Royal Pharmaceutical Society of Great Britain: London.

7. Treatment of anaphylaxis with sympathomimetic drugs. Fisher, M. *British Medical Journal* (1992), **305**, 1107–1108.

8. Topical anaesthesia for repair of minor lacerations. Bass, D. H., Wormald, P. J., McNally, J. & Rode, H. *Archives of Diseases in Childhood* (1990), **65**, 1272–1274.

7

Steroid injection techniques

Introduction

Injection of depot steroids may be used in the treatment of inflammatory conditions affecting tendons, aponeuroses, ligaments, joint capsules and synovial structures. Most doctors will be familiar with the injection for tennis elbow but many will be reluctant to treat other conditions. Yet many of the techniques are well within the scope of general practice. There is no reason why, given adequate instruction, general practitioners should not undertake injections for conditions such as supraspinatus tendonitis, trigger finger, or carpal tunnel syndrome. However, a condition that requires an unfamiliar technique should be referred to a specialist.

Important points to remember when injecting steroids

Things to do

Use a non-touch technique.
Use a local anaesthetic except when injecting adjacent to nerves (this may mask an intraneural injection).

Things not to do

Do not inject into tendons (this can cause rupture).
Do not inject into blood vessels (this can cause vasospasm).
Do not inject into nerves (this can cause permanent nerve damage).
Do not inject too superficially in the skin (this can cause atrophy).
Do not inject in the presence of infection.

The use of a local anaesthetic with the steroid is both kind and allows confirmation of the correct site of injection as it will result in considerable relief of the pain. The patient should be warned that once the local anaesthetic effect has worn off the pain will return after 30–60 min and in some cases for a day or two it may be more severe than previously. Treatment on limbs may need rest or splintage with bandages during this time. Generally, improvement is felt after 24–48 h and may not be maximal for 1–2 weeks. Steroid injections must not be performed in the presence of infection.

Many depot preparations are available, e.g. hydrocortisone acetate, methyl prednisolone and triamcinolone hexacetonide (Fig. 7.1). These all vary in their

Corticosteroid injections		
Preparation	Concentration (mg/ml)	Dose (mg)
Short-acting		
Hydrocortisone acetate	25	5–50
Long-acting		
Methyl prednisolone	40	5–40
Prednisolone	25	5–40
Triamcinolone	10, 20, 40	5–40

Fig. 7.1. Depot steroid preparations: triamcinolone, methyl prednisolone and hydrocortisone.

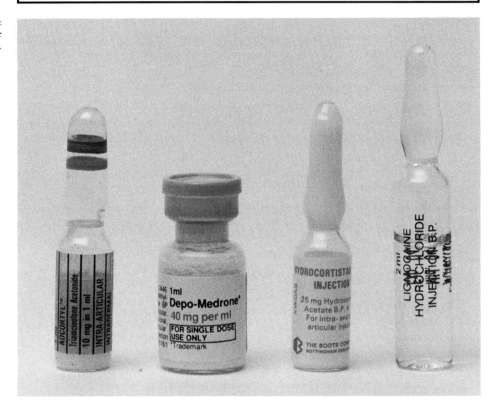

potency and duration of action. Hydrocortisone is the least potent and has the shortest duration of action. Methyl prednisolone is slightly more potent than prednisolone, is about five times more potent than hydrocortisone and can be detected up to 40 days after intra-articular injection. The very gradual reduction in plasma levels contrasts with the sharp decrease in plasma levels and withdrawal symptoms associated with the cessation of oral steroid therapy. There is no evidence of any practical difference between the stronger steroids. The dose of steroid used will depend on the soft-tissue site, or the size of a particular joint. A large joint such as the knee or ankle may require 20–80 mg of methyl prednisolone, whereas an interphalangeal joint may require only 4–10 mg. Methyl prednisolone can be obtained ready mixed with lignocaine but often it is preferable to add a specific volume of lignocaine to suit a specific case or site.

Usually a maximum of three injections are given at intervals of 2–3 weeks. However, the maximum total dose and the exact interval between injections is ill-defined. Injections should not be given prophylactically. Depot steroid preparations should not be used for intravenous or intrathecal injection.

Injections into soft tissues

With any condition, there will be tenderness at the site of the problem and in addition there may be distinct tender spots in surrounding tissues. It is found that the best results are achieved by injection of the steroid into the main site of the problem.

A number of common soft-tissue conditions are described below and the principles of treatment may be applied to many other musculo-tendonous conditions and tender areas. When local anaesthetic is used with the steroid, it is often helpful to inject a part of the total volume and assess the degree of pain relief after a few minutes. Good pain relief indicates that the injection has been placed in the correct site. Sometimes, however, the pain relief does not extend to the whole of the affected area and the patient may be able to localise a second point into which the remaining volume of steroid can be injected.

The injection should be placed around the periphery of inflamed tissue and should not be made directly into the substance of tendons or ligaments as this may lead to rupture. Injection into the substance of a nerve may result in permanent sensory or motor deficit. Care should be taken to ensure that the injection is not too superficial as this can cause atrophy of the subcutaneous fat and overlying skin.

For most injections a 23G needle with a 2 ml syringe is used. By keeping to the same needle and syringe combination, the difference between normal and abnormal injection pressures may be more readily appreciated.

Prior to injection into soft tissue, the site of maximal tenderness may be marked on the skin, which is then wiped with an alcohol swab.

Tennis elbow

Tennis elbow can occur following actions involving repeated or protracted firm gripping (where the wrist extensor muscles are essential for steadying the wrist) or following a blunt injury directly onto the lateral epicondyle. However, it is important to exclude pain referred from the neck. A tender spot is usually found on or around the tip of the lateral epicondyle or just distal to it. A tender spot is commonly found in the body of the brachioradialis but as this is of a secondary nature, injections should not be made into this site.

In order to locate the tender site, it may be helpful to ask the patient to pronate the forearm and extend the wrist against resistance. Methyl prednisolone (20–40 mg) with 1 ml of 1% lignocaine is injected into and over the tender site (Figs. 7.2, 7.3). If the injection is made in the skin only, there is a likelihood of skin atrophy and scarring as a result. The elbow should be rested for a few days and any aggravating factors avoided. Often, one injection is curative but it can be repeated after 2–3 weeks, if necessary. However, it is not uncommon to find that tennis elbow is resistant to injections of steroids. Acupuncture is a good alternative method of treatment. Transposition of the origin of the common extensor muscles is rarely necessary.

Fig. 7.2. Injection for tennis elbow.

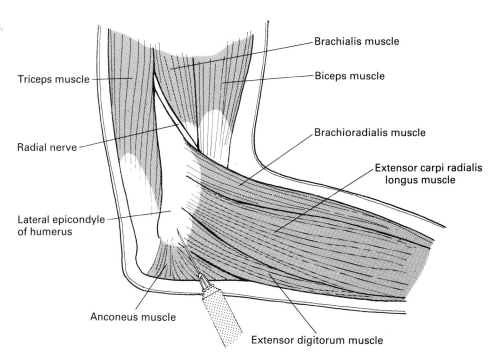

Fig. 7.3. Injection for tennis elbow.

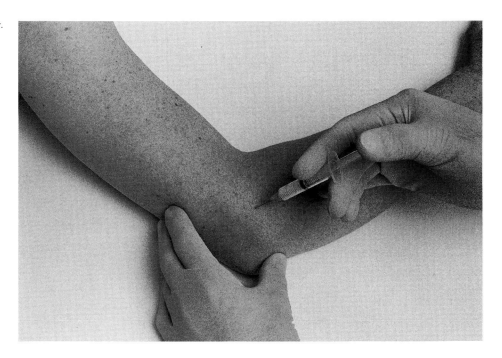

Golfer's elbow

This condition is similar to tennis elbow but affects the common flexor origin on the medial epicondyle. Methyl prednisolone (20–40 mg) with 1 ml of 1% lignocaine is injected into and over the tender site (Figs. 7.4, 7.5). Care should be taken to avoid the ulnar nerve, which is vulnerable immediately behind and distal to the medial epicondyle.

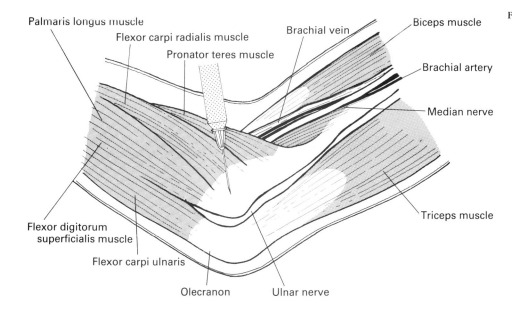

Fig. 7.4. Injection for golfer's elbow.

Palmaris longus muscle
Flexor carpi radialis muscle
Pronator teres muscle
Brachial vein
Biceps muscle
Brachial artery
Median nerve
Triceps muscle
Flexor digitorum superficialis muscle
Flexor carpi ulnaris
Olecranon
Ulnar nerve

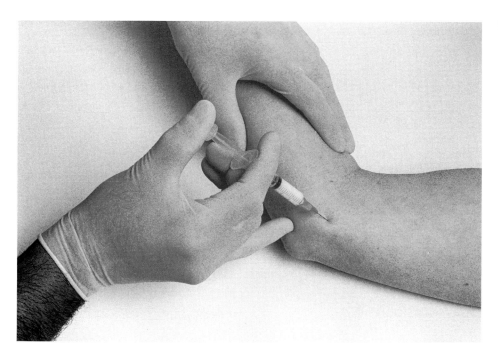

Fig. 7.5. Injection for golfer's elbow.

Tenosynovitis

Tenosynovitis usually results in marked pain associated with crepitus and swelling over the affected tendon sheaths. It can be caused by over-use, acute sprain, or follow a blunt injury directly over affected tendons.

De Quervain's tenosynovitis This is usually caused by excessive or repetitive movements of the thumb resulting in inflammation of the tendons of the extensor pollicis brevis (EPB) and abductor pollicis longus (APL) which occurs where they pass under the extensor retinaculum. It can also follow a blunt injury over the tendons themselves. In an established case there will be pain, swelling and crepitis over the radial aspect of the distal wrist. In an early case there may just be acute tenderness and pain over the tendons just distal to the distal border of the extensor retinaculum.

The tendons of EPB and APL can be identified at the palmar border of the anatomical snuffbox. Having identified the tendons, the injection is best carried out with the patient's hand supported in ulnar deviation. The needle may be bent slightly to allow an easier line of injection. The skin should be punctured about 1 cm distal to the radial styloid with the needle sliding along the tendons and avoiding the beginning of the cephalic vein, which courses over the snuffbox (Figs. 7.6, 7.7). The injection should be made into the synovial sheaths of the tendons and not subcutaneously or into the substance of the tendons themselves. Note that the radial artery passes through the anatomical snuffbox, deep to the tendons of EPB and APL and is not at risk as long as the needle is directed into the sheath along the superficial surfaces of the tendons. Actually, the synovial sheath itself cannot be felt with the needle. The needle should be inserted until the tip touches the tendon and then slightly withdrawn prior to injection. A correct

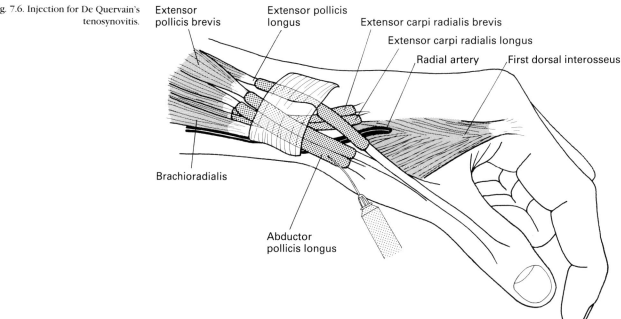

Fig. 7.6. Injection for De Quervain's tenosynovitis.

Extensor pollicis brevis

Extensor pollicis longus

Extensor carpi radialis brevis

Extensor carpi radialis longus

Radial artery

First dorsal interosseus

Brachioradialis

Abductor pollicis longus

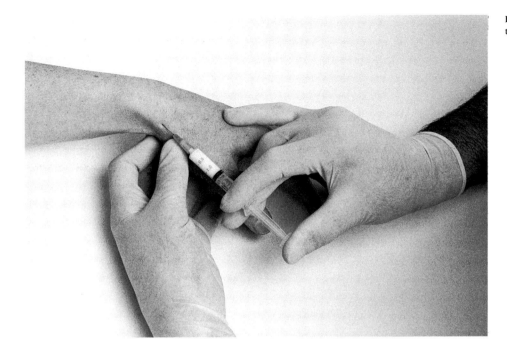

Fig. 7.7. Injection for De Quervain's tenosynovitis.

injection will result in a sausage-shaped swelling developing proximally from the injection site. A subcutaneous injection will result merely in a diffuse swelling. Methyl prednisolone (30–40 mg) with 1–2 ml of 1% lignocaine are injected. The thumb and wrist is rested in a bandage for 48 h. A further injection may be given in 2–3 weeks if necessary. There may be an incomplete resolution due to the fact that there may be more than one sheath involved. Surgical release should be considered if the condition fails to resolve.

Tenosynovitis of extensor tendons This is usually caused by excessive or repetitive movements, or blunt injury resulting in inflammation of the extensor tendons at the back of the hand or dorsum of the foot. The digital extensor tendons share a common synovial sheath, although the extensor digiti minimi has a separate sheath.

Injection of 20–40 mg of methyl prednisolone with 1–2 ml of 1% lignocaine should be made into the synovial sheaths of the affected extensor tendons (Figs. 7.8, 7.9). Although the tendons may be obscured by any swelling, the needle should be inserted so as to avoid any veins and directed so that it slides along the superficial surface of the affected tendons. The patient's hand or foot should be rested in a bandage for 48 h and elevated to reduce any throbbing. A further injection may be given in 2–3 weeks if necessary.

Tenosynovitis of the tibialis posterior This can appear spontaneously or following a sprain. Tenderness may be seen at the insertion of the tibialis posterior into the navicular and along the tendon from the navicular to the posterior aspect of the medial malleolus. The tendon can be made more prominent by asking the patient to invert the foot against resistance. Methyl prednisolone (20–40 mg) with 1–2 ml of 1% lignocaine may be injected over the insertion and into the synovial sheath (Figs. 7.10, 7.11).

Fig. 7.8. Injections around the back of the hand: Ⓐ, wrist joint; Ⓑ, extensor digitorum synovial sheath; and Ⓒ, thumb carpo-metacarpal joint.

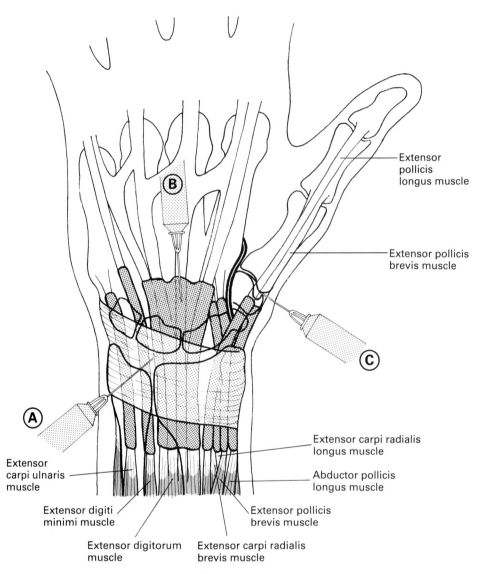

Extensor pollicis longus muscle

Extensor pollicis brevis muscle

Extensor carpi radialis longus muscle

Abductor pollicis longus muscle

Extensor pollicis brevis muscle

Extensor carpi radialis brevis muscle

Extensor carpi ulnaris muscle

Extensor digiti minimi muscle

Extensor digitorum muscle

Fig. 7.9. Injection for extensor tendon tenosynovitis.

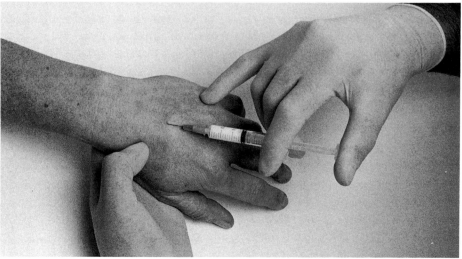

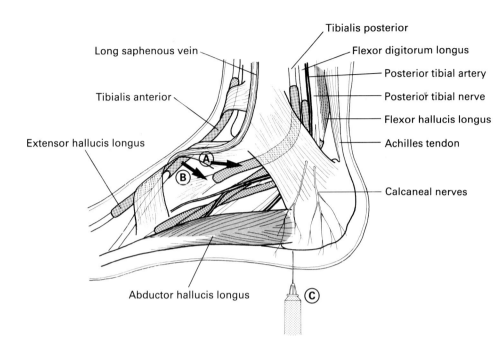

Fig. 7.10. Injections around the medial side of the foot and ankle: Ⓐ, sheath of tibialis posterior; Ⓑ, insertion of the tibialis posterior into the tuberosity of the navicular bone; and Ⓒ, injection for painful heel.

Fig. 7.11. Injection into the tibialis posterior sheath.

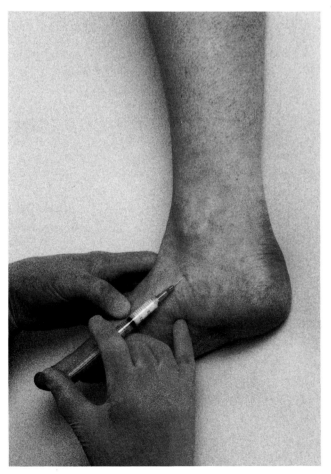

Tenosynovitis of the peroneus brevis Tenosynovitis of the peroneal tendons may follow an acute sprain or over-use. The tendon of the peroneus brevis is usually tender along its length from the base of the little metatarsal towards and around the lateral malleolus. Methyl prednisolone (20–40 mg) with 1–2 ml of 1% lignocaine may be injected over the insertion and into the synovial sheath (Figs. 7.12, 7.13).

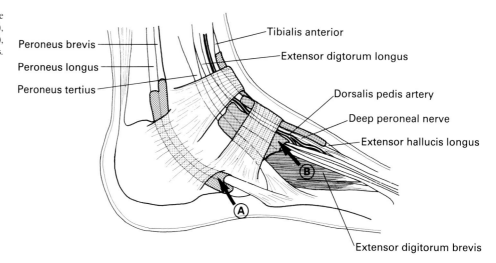

Fig. 7.12. Injections around the lateral side of the foot and ankle: Ⓐ, sheath of peroneus brevis; and Ⓑ, sheath of extensor tendons.

Peroneus brevis
Peroneus longus
Peroneus tertius
Tibialis anterior
Extensor digtorum longus
Dorsalis pedis artery
Deep peroneal nerve
Extensor hallucis longus
Extensor digitorum brevis

Fig. 7.13. Injection into the peroneus brevis sheath.

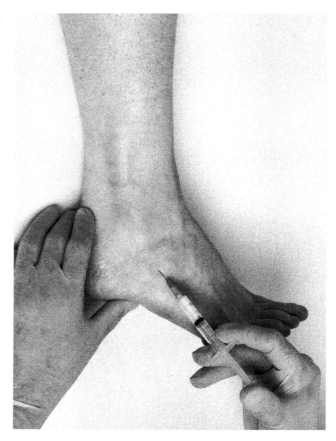

Achilles tendonitis The achilles tendon does not have a synovial sheath but can be inflamed at a site just above its insertion. It commonly occurs in athletes, may occur following friction from ill-fitting shoes, or in association with spondyloarthropathies. There may or may not be a swelling of the bursa, which lies just above and posterior to the insertion. Because of the risk of tendon rupture injection around the achilles tendon requires very careful technique and should be left to specialists.

Trigger finger/thumb

The trigger finger or thumb is caused by a bulbous swelling of the flexor tendon in association with thickening of the mouth of the fibrous flexor sheath (Fig. 7.14).

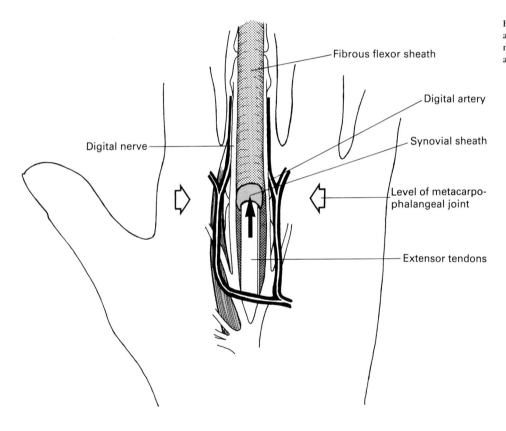

Fibrous flexor sheath

Digital artery

Digital nerve

Synovial sheath

Level of metacarpophalangeal joint

Extensor tendons

Fig. 7.14. Trigger finger, surgical anatomy (the level of the metacarpophalangeal joint is arrowed).

When the finger is flexed the swelling of the tendon moves out of the fibrous flexor sheath. When extension of the finger is attempted, movement comes to a stop when the swelling on the tendon comes against the edge of the fibrous flexor sheath. Further forced extension allows the tendon swelling to enter the fibrous flexor sheath with a 'click', the triggering (Fig. 7.15).

Fig. 7.15. Mechanism of triggering.

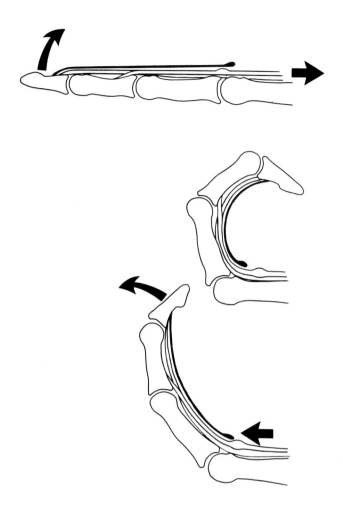

The fibrous flexor sheath entrance lies just distal to the metacarpophalangeal (MCP) joint, at the level of the mid-palmar crease and the MCP crease of the thumb. The injection can be made directly through the skin of the palm but this is not recommended as it is extremely painful. It is preferable first to anaesthetise the palmar skin with an injection of 1–2 ml of local anaesthetic through the soft dorsal skin of the web space. The needle is directed toward the proposed point of injection in the palm (Figs. 7.16, 7.17).

The patient's hand should be rested on a firm supporting surface and, once the palmar skin is anaesthetised, the steroid injection can be made through the palmar skin at the level of the MCP joint, the needle position being adjusted in a controlled painless manner (Figs. 7.18, 7.19). The synovial sheath itself cannot be felt by the needle. The technique is essentially to insert the needle at an angle of 30° down onto the flexor tendon and then to withdraw slightly prior to the injection. There should be no resistance to the injection. The injection *should not* be made into the flexor tendons themselves. Prior to injection, the patient should be asked to flex and extend the digit to confirm that the tendons are free. Provided the injection is made in the mid-line of the appropriate digit there is no risk of injury to digital arteries or nerves: 15–20 mg of methyl prednisolone is injected.

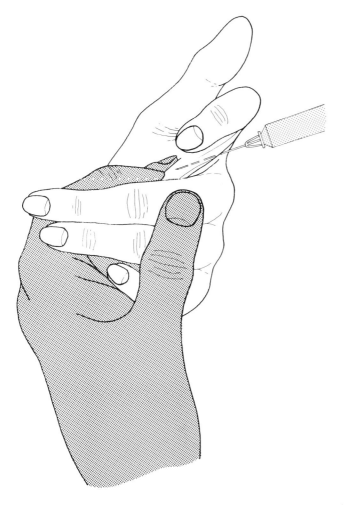

Fig. 7.16. Trigger finger, local anaesthetic.

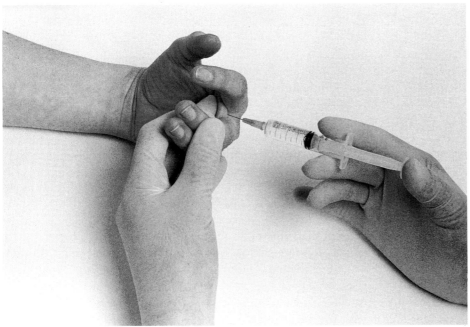

Fig. 7.17. Trigger finger, local anaesthetic.

Fig. 7.18. Injection for trigger finger.

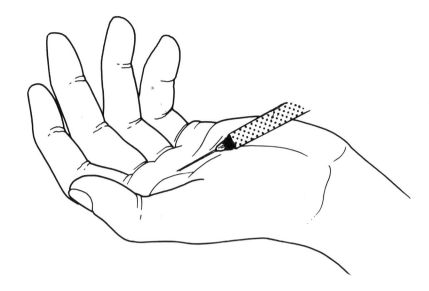

Fig. 7.19. Injection for trigger finger.

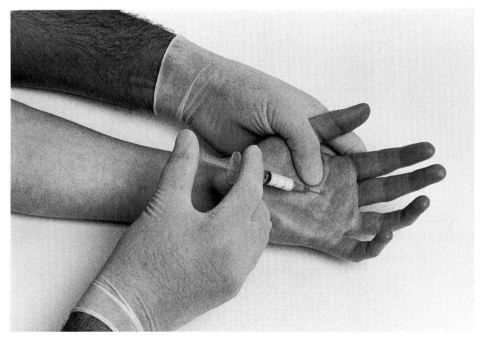

Carpal tunnel syndrome

The median nerve can be compressed in the carpal tunnel during pregnancy, in association with arthritis, following injury, or without any apparent cause. Steroid injection may be tried provided there are no objective neurological signs (blunting to pin prick, or thenar muscle wasting). The median nerve lies in the mid-line at the wrist, deep to the tendon of palmaris longus (Figs. 7.20, 7.21). It is important to note that the nerve curves deep into the hand such that although it

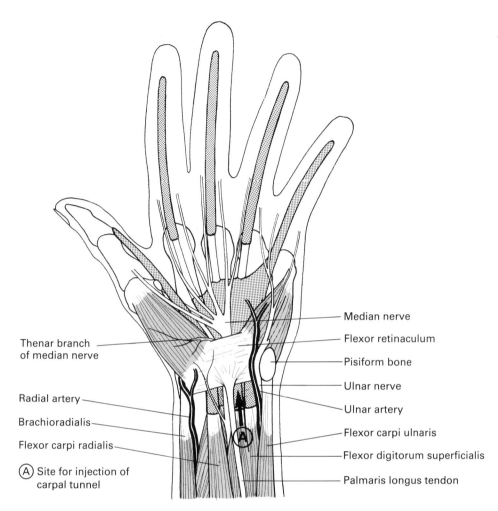

Fig. 7.20. Median nerve, anatomy (the site of injection for carpal tunnel syndrome is arrowed).

Median nerve

Flexor retinaculum

Pisiform bone

Ulnar nerve

Ulnar artery

Flexor carpi ulnaris

Flexor digitorum superficialis

Palmaris longus tendon

Thenar branch
of median nerve

Radial artery

Brachioradialis

Flexor carpi radialis

(A) Site for injection of
carpal tunnel

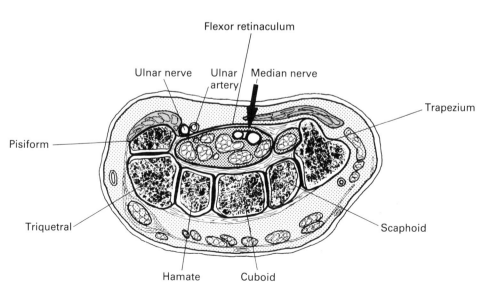

Fig. 7.21. Carpal tunnel, transverse section.

Flexor retinaculum

Ulnar nerve   Ulnar   Median nerve
               artery

Trapezium

Pisiform

Triquetral

Scaphoid

Hamate   Cuboid

may be only 5 mm below the skin at the wrist, it lies significantly deeper when in the carpal tunnel itself. Thus, the needle has to be inclined at 30° at the wrist while being directed towards the base of the middle finger.

A bleb of local anaesthetic may be injected into the skin of the wrist. It is wise to avoid deep injection of local anaesthetic so as not to disguise any paraesthesia from inadvertent intraneural injection. The patient's forearm should be rested on a firm supporting surface with the wrist in mid-extension. The skin is punctured about 1 cm proximal to the line of the wrist joint and just to the ulnar side of the palmaris longus tendon (Figs. 7.22, 7.23). If the palmaris longus tendon is absent

Fig. 7.22. Injection into carpal tunnel.

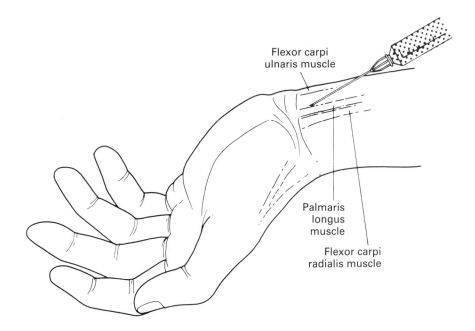

Flexor carpi ulnaris muscle

Palmaris longus muscle

Flexor carpi radialis muscle

the needle may be inserted 5 mm ulnar-wards from the mid-line. This will help to ensure that the needle passes safely above the flexor digitorum superficialis tendons and alongside the ulnar border of the nerve rather than directly over it. Methyl prednisolone (30–40 mg) is injected. The needle should slide easily into the tunnel and there should be no resistance to the injection. If paraesthesia is illicited, the needle should be withdrawn slightly. If paraesthesia persist, the procedure should be abandoned. The wrist should be rested with a splint or bandage and, if necessary, a high sling and the patient should notice some improvement within 1–3 weeks. The injection may be repeated if symptoms recur but if there is no benefit or there are objective neurological signs the nerve should be decompressed surgically.

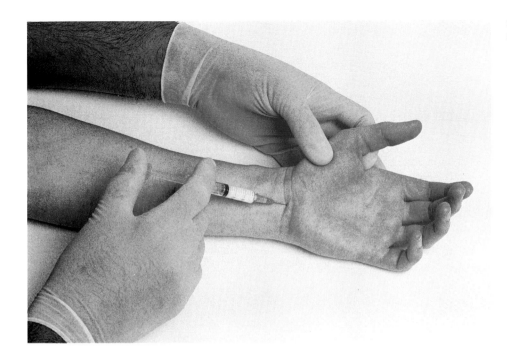

Fig. 7.23. Injection into carpal tunnel.

Bursae

Inflammation of bursae may occur after blunt trauma or friction and pressure. It is not uncommon to find a painless non-inflamed swelling of the olecranon bursa following blunt trauma. Such a swelling does not normally need treatment, as the bursa usually settles down spontaneously within 4–8 weeks. If the bursa is aspirated during this time it is likely simply to recur. Although injections can be made into troublesome non-inflamed bursa with good effect [*1*], steroid injection should normally be reserved for painful and inflamed (but non-septic) bursae.

The olecranon (Figs. 7.24, 7.25), infrapatellar (Fig. 7.26), prepatellar (Fig. 7.27) and subsartorial bursae are easily entered when they are swollen and inflamed. The trochanteric bursa may be difficult to define and the needle should be directed into the most tender spot over the upper outer part of the femur. In the obese, a long needle may be required. The Baker's (popliteal) cyst arises from deep in the popliteal fossa and is a bursa that communicates with the knee joint. It usually appears in association with osteoarthritis of the knee and a generalised knee effusion and simple aspiration is likely to result in re-accumulation of fluid within a 1–2 weeks.

The aspirates from these bursae should be clear and there should be no signs of infection. Methyl prednisolone (20–40 mg) may be injected with 2–5 ml of 1% lignocaine. The elbow or knee should be supported with a bandage for 24–48 h but gentle movements should be maintained to avoid stiffness.

Fig. 7.24. Aspiration and injection for
olecranon bursa.

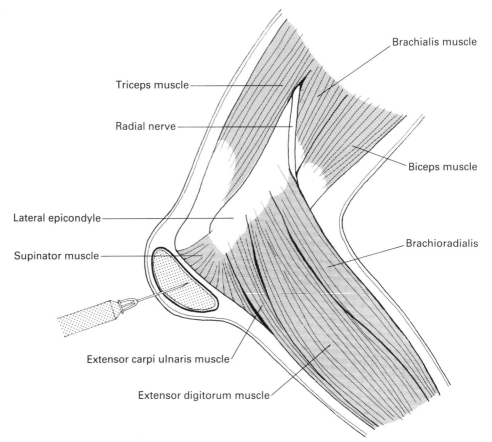

Brachialis muscle

Triceps muscle

Radial nerve

Biceps muscle

Lateral epicondyle

Supinator muscle

Brachioradialis

Extensor carpi ulnaris muscle

Extensor digitorum muscle

Fig. 7.25. Olecranon bursa.

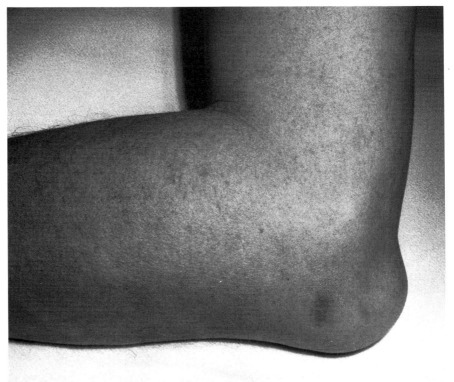

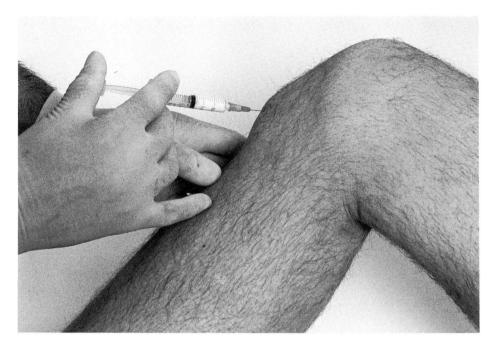

Fig. 7.26. Injection into infrapatellar bursa.

Fig. 7.27. Prepatellar bursa.

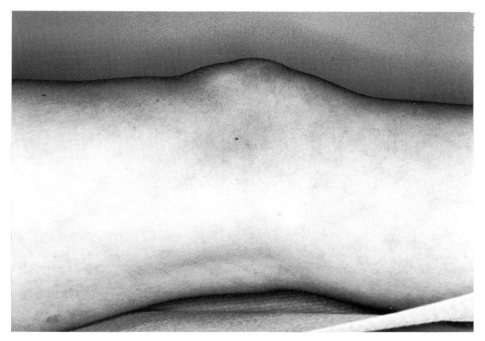

Painful ligaments

It is not uncommon to find protracted pain and tenderness following ligamentous sprains (for example, around the knee and ankle). Such cases can be significantly helped by infiltration of 10–30 mg of methyl prednisolone over the site of maximal tenderness (Figs. 7.28, 7.29). The injection should not be made into the

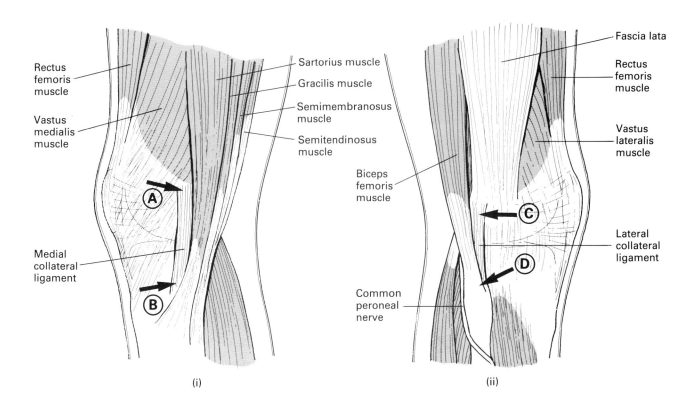

Rectus femoris muscle

Vastus medialis muscle

Medial collateral ligament

Sartorius muscle

Gracilis muscle

Semimembranosus muscle

Semitendinosus muscle

Biceps femoris muscle

Common peroneal nerve

Fascia lata

Rectus femoris muscle

Vastus lateralis muscle

Lateral collateral ligament

(i)   (ii)

Fig. 7.28. i,ii. (ABOVE) Common injection sites around the knee: A and B, upper and lower ends of medial collateral ligament; and C and D, upper and lower ends of lateral collateral ligament.

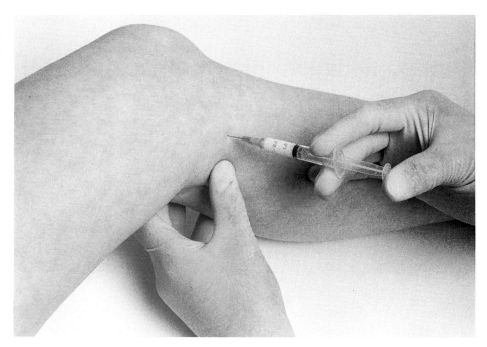

Fig. 7.29. Injection into the lower end of the medial collateral ligament of the knee.

substance of the ligament itself. A support bandage should be used for 24–48 h. In osteoarthritic joints, injections of steroids [2] or even the insertion of solid needles (acupuncture) into surrounding soft-tissue tender spots can result in significant benefit (Fig. 7.30).

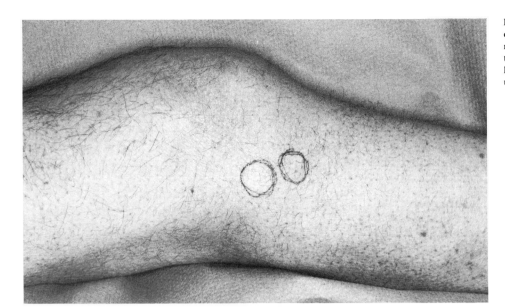

Fig. 7.30. Knee with severe degenerative changes with a soft moderate effusion. Injection into the tender spots on the medial and lateral sides of the knee resulted in useful improvement in the pain.

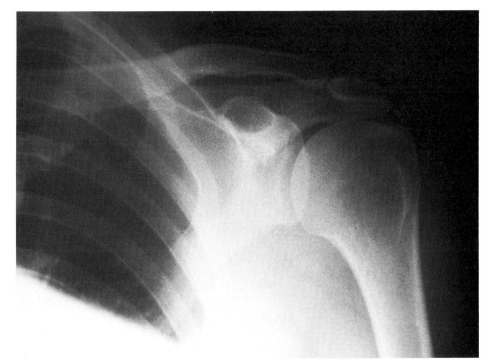

Fig. 7.31. X-ray of normal shoulder joint.

Soft tissue injections around the shoulder (Fig. 7.31)

Frozen shoulder (adhesive capsulitis) This condition may appear spontaneously or follow an injury and typically there is marked restriction in all movements of the shoulder joint. There may be no discrete tender points. Steroid injection treatment should be given in conjunction with physiotherapy and exercises. A total of 40–80 mg of methyl prednisolone may be injected over the supraspinatus tendon (see above), over the infraspinatus tendon and bursa, and into the shoulder joint itself from behind (see below). However, there is evidence to suggest that there is no significant difference in outcome between intra-bursal and intra-articular steroid injections [3].

Supraspinatus tendonitis This condition classically results in a painful arc during abduction of the shoulder. However, the pain may be difficult to localise and may be referred upwards to the trapezius and supraspinatus muscles and downwards into the upper arm. Some calcification may be present within the substance of the rotator cuff itself, or between the head of the humerus and the undersurface of the acromium. The needle is inserted lateral to and below the tip of the acromium and directed medially and slightly downwards. The injection is made fanwise around (but not into) the upper part of the rotator cuff. Methyl prednisolone (20–40 mg) is injected with 2 ml of 1% lignocaine (Figs. 7.32, 7.33, 7.34). The shoulder should be rested, but gentle movements should be maintained to avoid stiffness.

Short head of biceps The origin of the short head of biceps at the coracoid process is not uncommonly the site of protracted pain following sprains of the shoulder area. The coracoid process can be felt about 2.5 cm below the lateral end of the clavicle. Methyl prednisolone (20–30 mg) with 1 ml of 1% lignocaine is injected over the tender site (Figs. 7.32, 7.35). Care should be taken not to project the needle *below* the coracoid process where the brachial plexus and axillary vessels may be encountered.

Fig. 7.32. Injections around the shoulder girdle: Ⓐ, coracoid process; Ⓑ, acromioclavicular joint; Ⓒ, supraspinatus tendonitis; Ⓓ, long head of biceps.

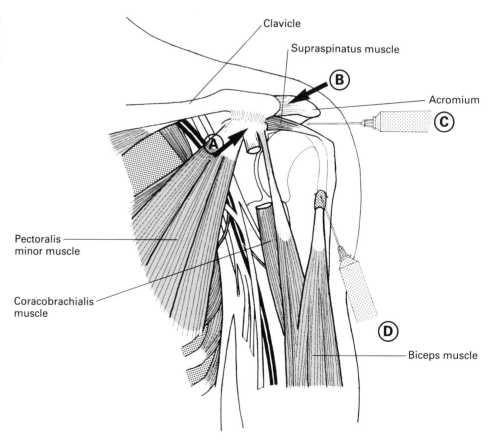

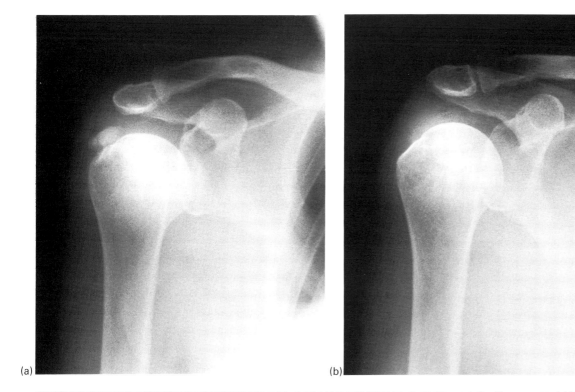

(a)   (b)

Fig. 7.33. (a) This patient presented with a painful arc. The supraspinatus calcification is clearly seen in the X-ray. (b) The second X-ray shows that the calcification has been largely absorbed 1 month after an injection of methyl prednisolone.

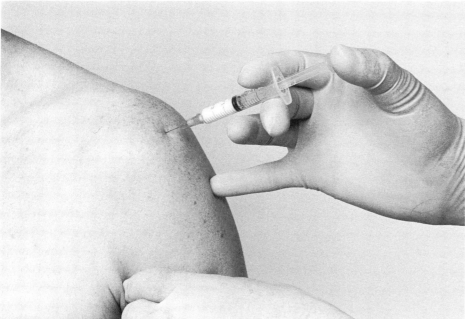

Fig. 7.34. Injection for supraspinatus tendonitis.

Long head of biceps The long head of biceps lies vertically in the mid-line of the humerus, deep to the anterior fibres of the deltoid and can be difficult to locate. It may be made more prominent if the patient is asked to flex the elbow and supinate the forearm against resistance. The needle is directed onto the tendon and then

slightly withdrawn. Methyl prednisolone (20–30 mg) with 1–2 ml of 1% lignocaine is injected (Figs. 7.32, 7.36). As the tendon has a tendency to rupture
spontaneously (especially in the elderly) the patient should be warned to avoid
lifting with the arm for a few weeks after the injection.

Fig. 7.35. Injection into the origin of
short head of biceps on the coracoid
process.

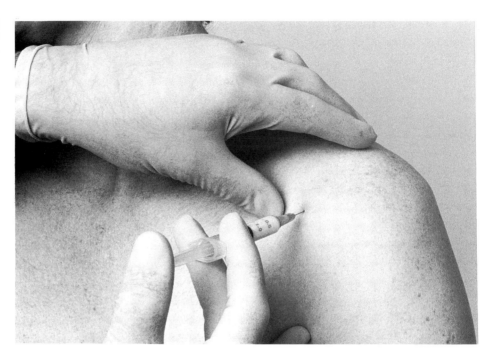

Fig. 7.36. Injection into the sheath of
the long head of biceps.

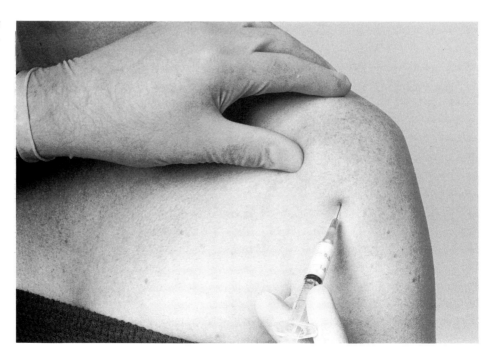

Fibromyositis

A number of non-specific conditions can present with muscle and ligamentous pains with localised areas of tenderness. These tender areas are often found, for example: around the shoulder and pelvic girdles; paravertebrally, over the sacro-iliac joints; and along the tensor fascia lata. Although it can sometimes be helpful to inject these tender spots with 10–20 mg of methyl prednisolone, good results can be obtained by the injection of local anaesthetic into the tender spots followed by stretching of the affected muscles, and also by the insertion of acupuncture (solid) needles into the tender areas.[1]

Painful heel

Often this condition appears without any apparent injury or pressure. There is no need to X-ray the foot to show a calcaneal spur as the diagnosis is clinical. The pain can occur without a spur and the treatment is symptomatic. If the discomfort is severe or prolonged then an injection into and around the site of maximal tenderness can result in rapid resolution. The site of tenderness is always localised to the middle of the heel but the pain not infrequently extends up the medial side. There are no important structures at risk during injection through the heel down to the calcaneous. Methyl predisolone (30–40 mg) with 0.5–1 ml of 1% lignocaine is injected, using a 25 mm 25G needle. The patient should be warned that the injection will be a little painful. With experience and confidence, the doctor can rapidly insert the needle through the thick skin and heel pad, down to the calcaneous in one movement (Figs. 7.37, 7.38, 7.39). Any hesitancy will result in severe pain and the risk of the patient pulling the foot away.

If the patient is very anxious or the doctor inexperienced, the heel skin can be anaesthetised prior to the steroid injection by blocking the medial calcaneal nerves below the medial malleolus (see chapter 6) (Fig. 7.40).

---

[1] Useful improvement can be gained in a variety of presentations of soft-tissue pain by inserting needles into the tender spots and leaving them for 5–20 min. This simple technique can be very effective and no reference need be made to classical Chinese acupuncture theory. Although the fine purpose-made solid needles are preferable and the least traumatic, nevertheless, 23G hypodermic needles can often be used with good effect.

Fig. 7.37. X-ray of lateral view of ankle and heel.

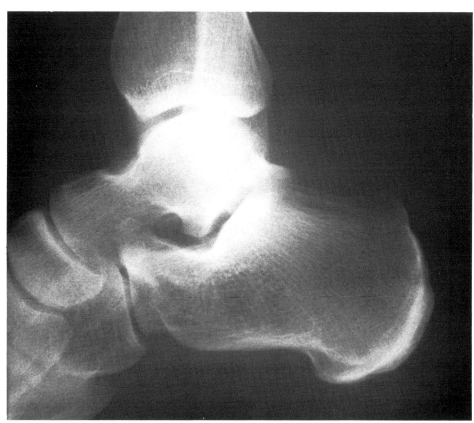

Fig. 7.38. Injection into painful heel.

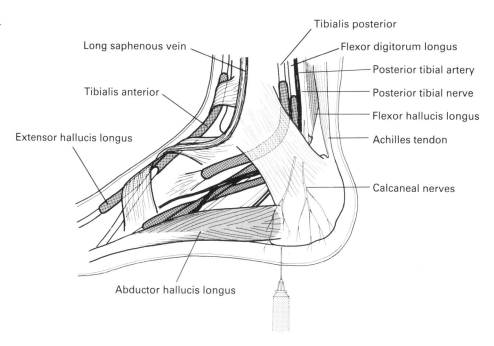

Long saphenous vein

Tibialis anterior

Extensor hallucis longus

Abductor hallucis longus

Tibialis posterior

Flexor digitorum longus

Posterior tibial artery

Posterior tibial nerve

Flexor hallucis longus

Achilles tendon

Calcaneal nerves

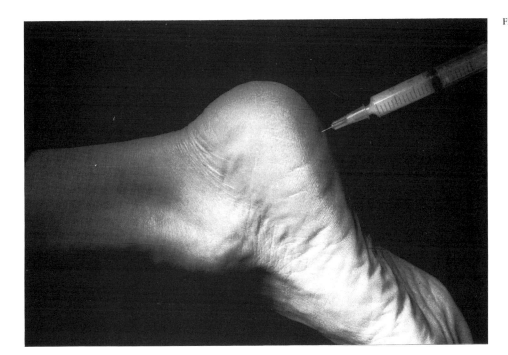

Fig. 7.39. Injection into painful heel.

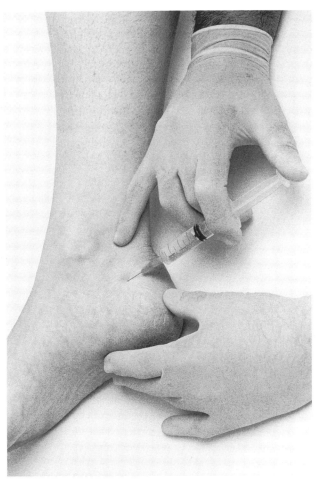

Fig. 7.40. Nerve block of the medial calcaneal nerves.

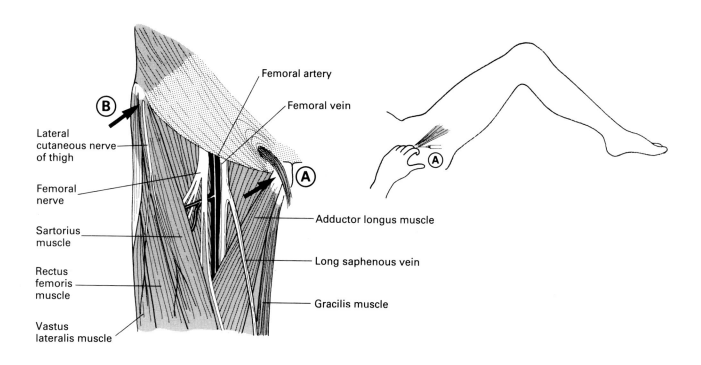

Fig. 7.41. Injection into the origin of Ⓐ, adductor longus, and Ⓑ, for meralgia paraesthetica.

Pain at the origin of the adductor longus

Pain and tenderness can be found at the origin of adductor longus after falls and abduction strains around the hip. The tendon can be made more prominent by asking the patient to abduct the hip and the tender spot is usually localised at or close to the origin on the pubic bone below the pubic tubercle. For practical purposes the tendon lies subcutaneously (Fig. 7.41, site A), and 20–30 mg of methyl prednisolone with 1–2 ml of 1% lignocaine may be injected directly over the tendon and its origin. The tender site can be awkward to palpate and identify and it may be helpful to ask the patient to pull the suprapubic skin medially and upwards while the tender spot is located with the left hand. The injection will be made easier if fingertip pressure of the left hand is kept on the tender spot during the injection.

Meralgia paraesthetica

The lateral cutaneous nerve of the thigh passes behind or through the inguinal ligament and behind or through the sartorius as it passes into the thigh, approximately 1–2 cm from the anterior superior iliac spine (Fig. 7.41, site B). There can be tenderness around this area associated with pain or paraesthesia radiating down the anterolateral side of the thigh. It is worth trying an injection of 20–40 mg of methyl prednisolone with 1–2 ml of 1% lignocaine at this site.

Joint injections

Intra-articular steroid injections are primarily indicated in the inflammatory athropathies (Fig. 7.42), although pericapsular steroid injections around painful ligaments and tendons can be of great benefit in osteoarthritis. Intra-articular injections are not usually indicated in osteoarthritis unless there is a significant inflammatory component. If there is any suspicion of a diagnosis of septic arthritis in a red, swollen joint, the joint should not be injected and the case should be urgently referred to a specialist.

With careful non-touch technique, joint injections and aspirations can be safely performed in a clean treatment room. Septic arthritis after needling a joint is very rare. A full aseptic technique is usually employed, and the skin sterilised with povidone iodine or chlorhexidine. However, some units routinely use only alcohol swabs applied for a few seconds and such experience suggests that routine full sterile aseptic skin preparation is unnecessary [4]. Whatever method is used to prepare the skin, the foundation of safe joint aspiration and injection is a strict non-touch technique. After injection or aspiration, an adhesive plaster should be placed over the puncture site and a support bandage should be applied to the joint, which should be rested for 24–48 h.

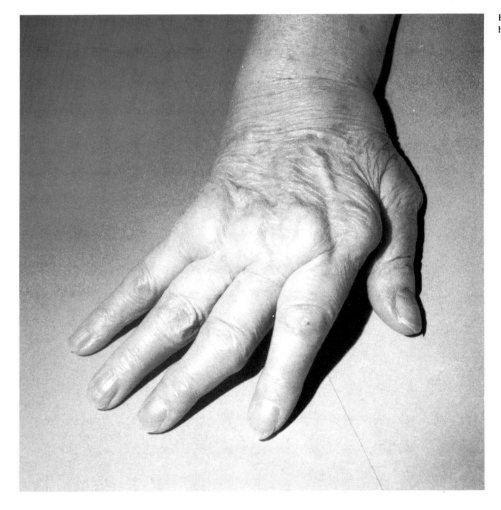

Fig. 7.42. Swelling of the joints of the hand due to rheumatoid arthritis.

Fig. 7.43. X-ray of interphalangeal
joints.

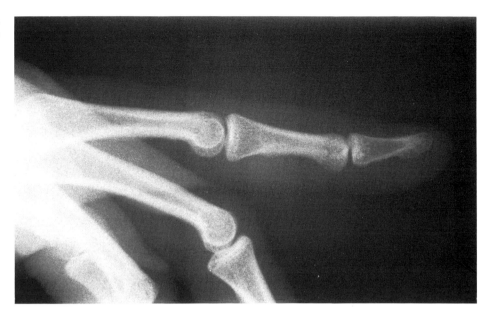

Fig. 7.44. Injection of (a)
interphalangeal and (b)
metacarpophalangeal joints (the
digital nerves and vessels run lateral
to the flexor tendons and are not
shown for clarity).

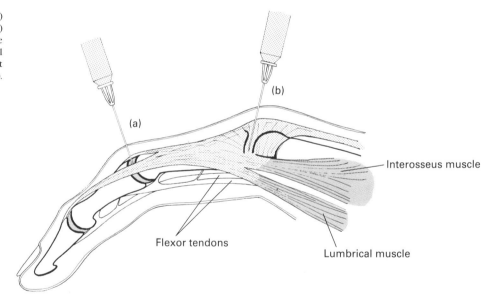

Interphalangeal and metacarpophalangeal joints

A dorsolateral approach is safe and will avoid any nerves or tendons. The joint should be flexed to open up the joint space and 2.5–10 mg of methyl prednisolone injected with or without a small quantity of 1% lignocaine. A 1 ml insulin syringe with a 30G needle is ideal for injection of these small joints (Figs. 7.43, 7.44, 7.45, 7.46).

The thumb carpometacarpal joint is often involved in osteoarthritic changes

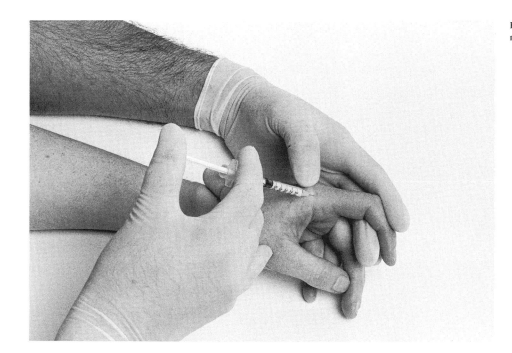

Fig. 7.45. Injection into the metacarpophalangeal joint.

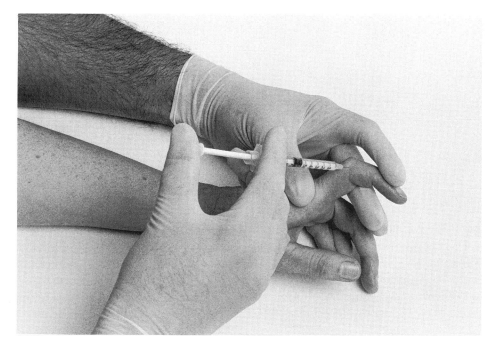

Fig. 7.46. Injection into the interphalangeal joint.

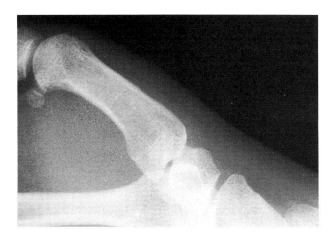

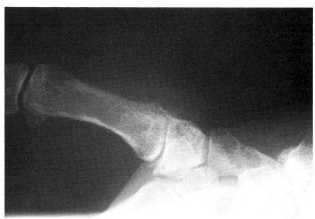

Fig. 7.47. (ABOVE) X-ray of normal thumb carpometacarpal joint.

Fig. 7.48. (ABOVE, RIGHT) X-ray of thumb carpometacarpal joint arthritis. Arthritis of the thumb carpometacarpal joint often occurs after years of repetitive movements and is usually worse in the dominant hand. This case developed after a fall.

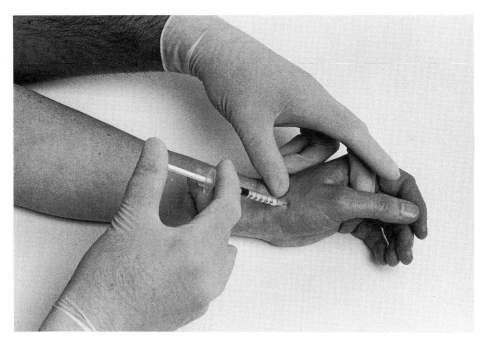

Fig. 7.49. Injection into thumb carpometacarpal joint.

and a steroid injection can sometimes provide relief (Figs. 7.47, 7.48, 7.49, 7.50). The joint is likely to be deformed and it can be helpful to identify the joint line by palpation using the thumb nail, while the patient's thumb is moved. The needle should be inserted, using a dorsolateral approach, between the thumb extensor tendons, and methyl prednisolone (2.5–10 mg) injected with or without a small quantity of 1% lignocaine.

Wrist joint

The wrist joint is best entered through the dorsal aspect. The wrist should be flexed and the needle inserted between the extensor tendons and through the site

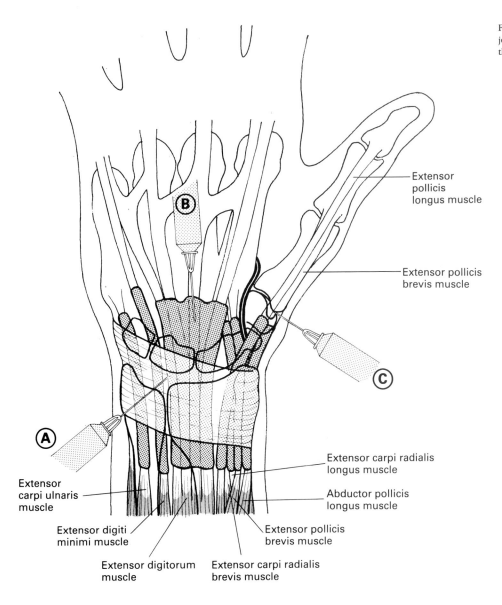

Fig. 7.50. Injection into (A), wrist joint, (B), extensor tendons, (C), thumb carpometacarpal joint.

Extensor pollicis longus muscle

Extensor pollicis brevis muscle

Extensor carpi radialis longus muscle

Abductor pollicis longus muscle

Extensor carpi ulnaris muscle

Extensor pollicis brevis muscle

Extensor digiti minimi muscle

Extensor digitorum muscle

Extensor carpi radialis brevis muscle

of maximal fluctuation (Figs. 7.50, 7.51, 7.52). Methyl prednisolone (20–40 mg) is injected with 2 ml of 1% lignocaine.

Elbow joint

The elbow joint can be entered using the posterior approach, the needle being directed horizontally lateral to the triceps tendon. Note that the ulnar nerve is vulnerable as it lies medial to the triceps tendon, behind the medial epicondyle (Figs. 7.53, 7.54, 7.55). Methyl prednisolone (40 mg) is injected with 2–5 ml of 1% lignocaine.

Fig. 7.51. X-ray of wrist joint.

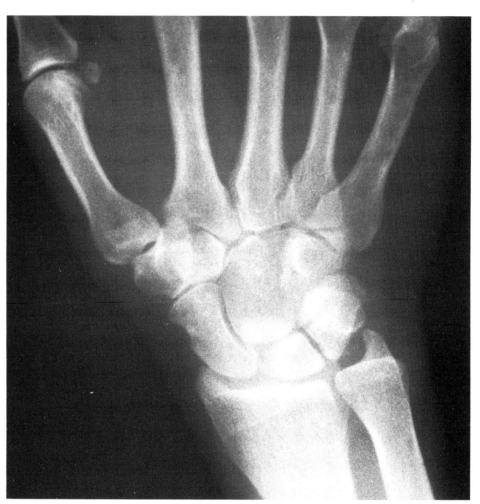

Fig. 7.52. Wrist joint injection.

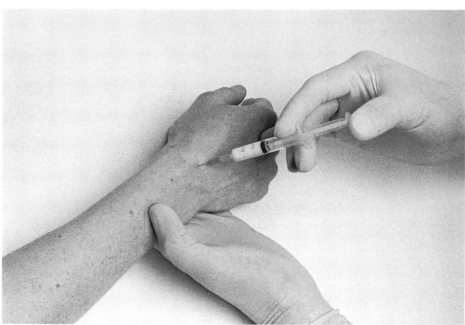

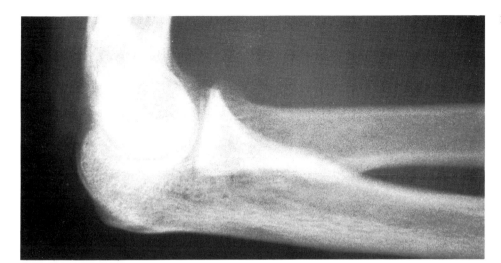

Fig. 7.53. X-ray of elbow joint.

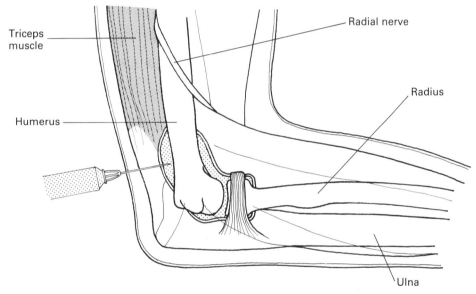

Triceps
muscle

Radial nerve

Humerus

Radius

Ulna

Fig. 7.54. Injection into elbow joint
from the lateral side of the triceps
tendon.

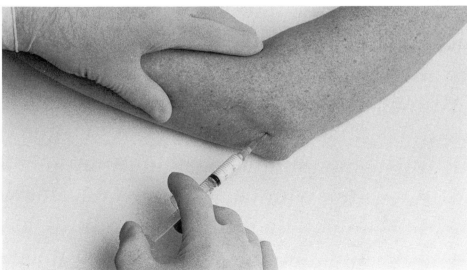

Fig. 7.55. Injection into elbow joint
from the lateral side of the triceps
tendon.

Sternoclavicular joint

The sternoclavicular joint is a synovial joint but also has a fibro-cartilage disc separating the clavicle and sternum. The needle is inserted through the site of maximal fluctuation and 20–40 mg of methyl prednisolone is injected with 1–2 ml of 1% lignocaine (Figs. 7.56, 7.57).

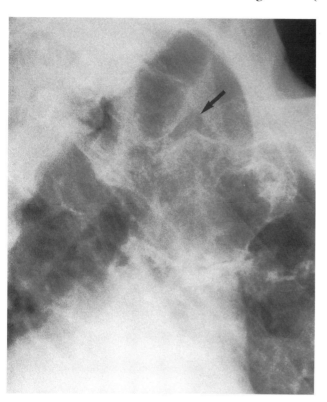

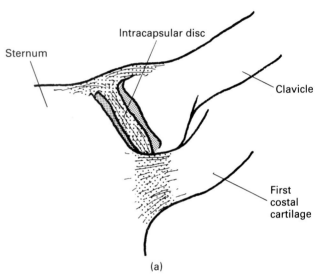

(a)

Fig. 7.56. (ABOVE) X-ray of sternoclavicular joint.

Fig. 7.57. (a). (ABOVE, RIGHT) Sternoclavicular joint anatomy.

Fig. 7.57. (b). (RIGHT) Injection into sternoclavicular joint.

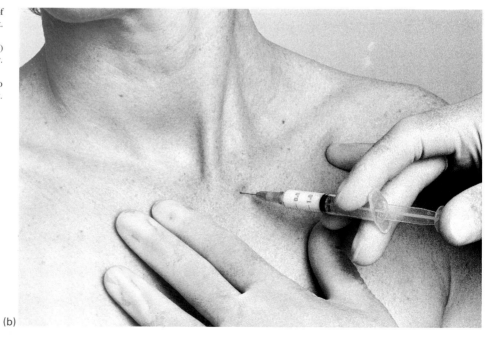

(b)

Acromioclavicular joint

The acromioclavicular joint can be entered just antero-laterally to and below the lateral end of the clavicle.

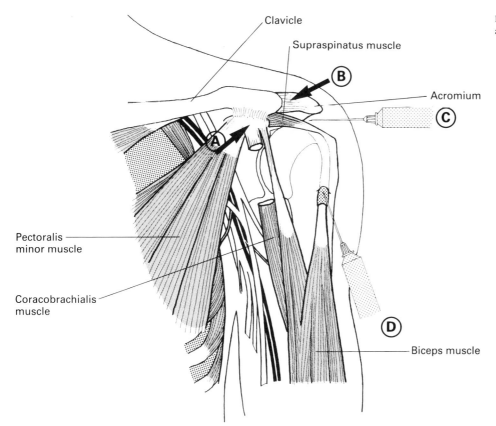

Fig. 7.58. Site of injection into acromioclavicular joint Ⓑ.

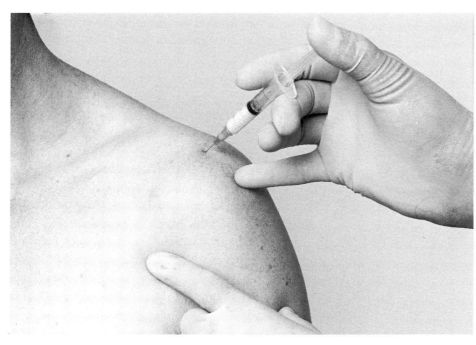

Fig. 7.59. Injection into acromioclavicular joint.

Shoulder joint

The shoulder joint is best approached from behind, where there are no important structures at risk (Figs. 7.60, 7.61, 7.62). The needle is inserted horizontally 2 cm below and 3 cm medial to the tip of the acromium, and advanced anteriorly through the infraspinatus until it is felt to have pierced the capsule and entered the joint. It is quite likely that the needle tip will touch the posterior border of the head of the humerus, but this is of no concern and indeed this confirms the position of the needle tip. Any effusion should be aspirated and 20–40 mg of methyl prednisolone is injected with 2–5 ml of 1% lignocaine.

Fig. 7.60. X-ray of shoulder joint.

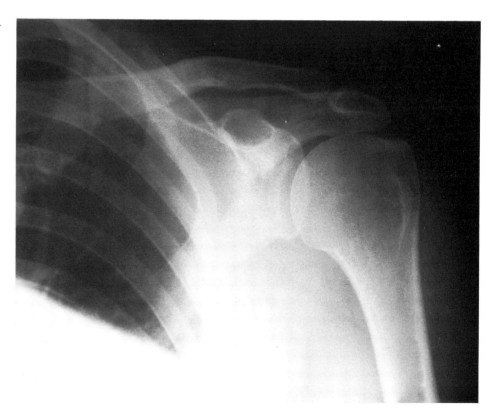

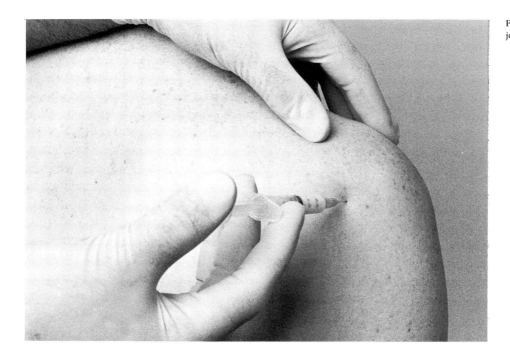

Fig. 7.61. Injection into shoulder joint: posterior approach.

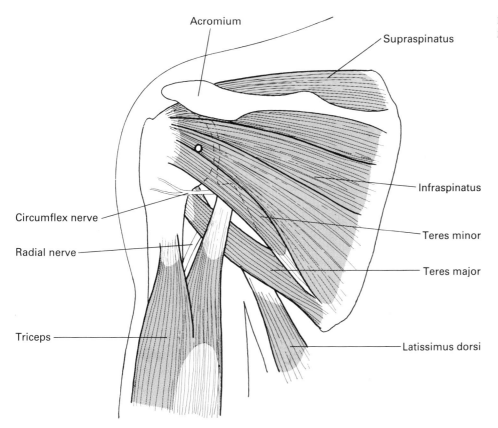

Fig. 7.62. Injection into shoulder joint: posterior approach.

Knee joint

The simplest approach to the knee joint is through the supra-patellar pouch, either medial or lateral to the rectus femoris tendon. A bleb of local anaesthetic is injected into the skin and the needle advanced down to the joint capsule where a further 5 ml of anaesthetic is placed. Following the same (anaesthetised) track down to the capsule, a 21G needle and 20 ml syringe is used to aspirate any effusion. It is not necessary to direct the needle beneath the patella itself. While aspiration is being performed the doctor's free hand should compress the knee joint so as to ease the fluid up into the supra-patellar pouch. If no fluid can be aspirated, the needle may be occluded at the tip by some synovium. This may be overcome by either reducing the suction or adjusting the needle position. The syringe is exchanged for one loaded with the steroid, and methyl prednisolone (40–80 mg) and 5 ml of 1% lignocaine is then injected (Figs. 7.63, 7.64, 7.65, 7.66, 7.67, 7.68).

Fig. 7.63. X-ray of normal knee joint.

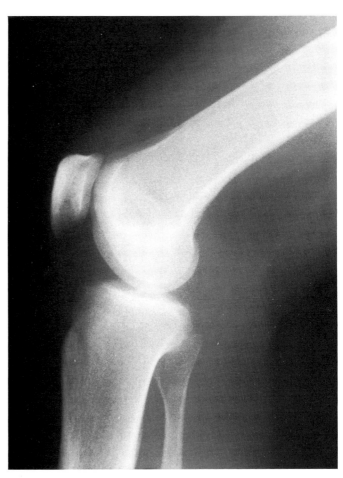

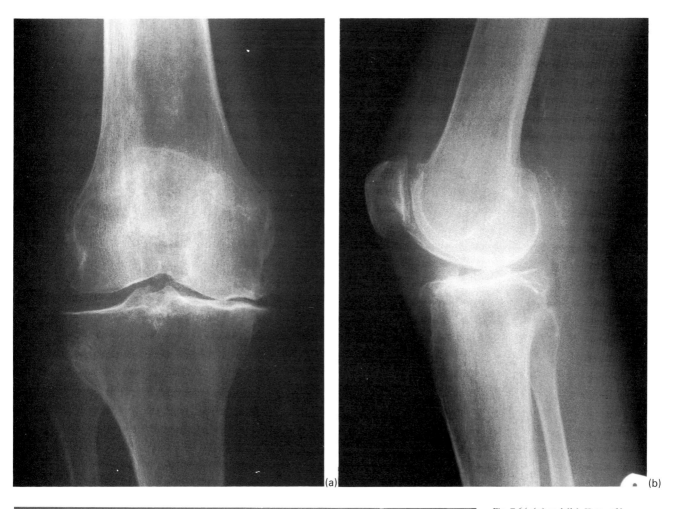

Fig. 7.64. (a) and (b). X-ray of knee joint showing degenerative changes especially in the medial compartment.

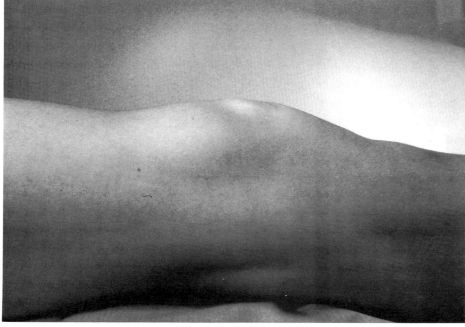

Fig. 7.65. Knee joint with effusion visible in the suprapatellar pouch.

Fig. 7.66. Swelling of the knee joint due to rheumatoid arthritis.

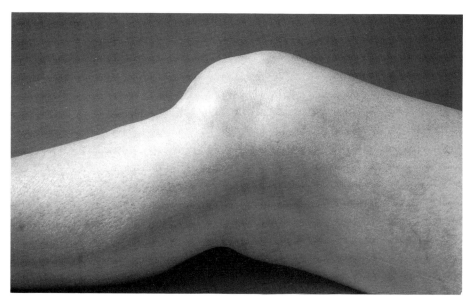

Fig. 7.67. Aspiration and injection of the knee joint through the suprapatellar pouch.

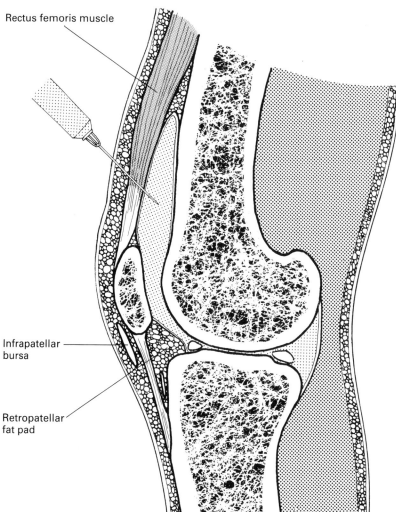

Rectus femoris muscle

Infrapatellar bursa

Retropatellar fat pad

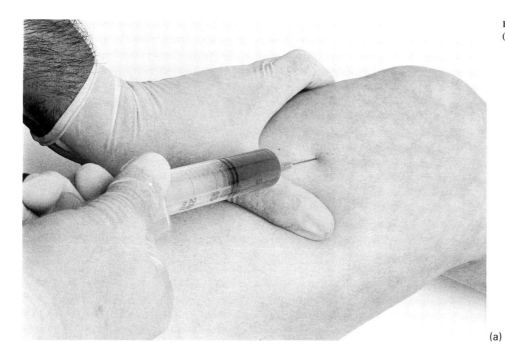

Fig. 7.68. (a) Knee joint aspiration, (b) knee joint injection.

(a)

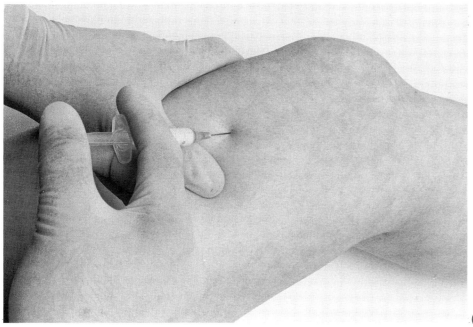

(b)

Fig. 7.69. X-ray of ankle joint.

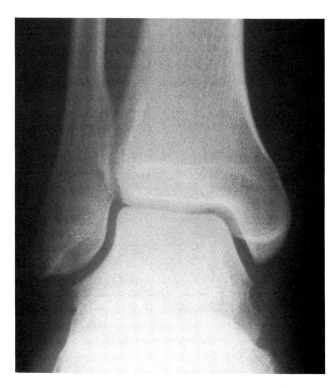

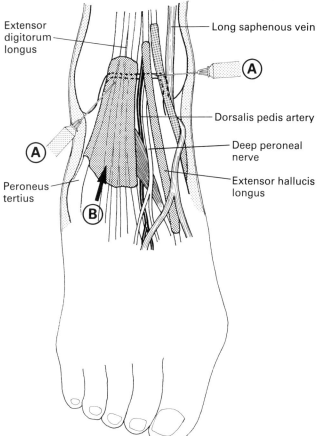

Extensor digitorum longus

Long saphenous vein

Dorsalis pedis artery

Deep peroneal nerve

Extensor hallucis longus

Peroneus tertius

Fig. 7.70. Injections into the front of the ankle: Ⓐ, ankle joint injection,
Ⓑ, injection of the sheath of the extensor digitorum longus.

Ankle joint

The ankle joint is best injected using an anterior approach with the ankle in plantar-flexion and the needle guided between any tendons at the site of maximal fluctuation (Figs. 7.69, 7.70, 7.71). The mid-line should be avoided as the dorsalis pedis artery lies there. Methyl prednisolone (20–40 mg) is injected with 2–5 ml of 1% lignocaine.

Fig. 7.71. Ankle joint injection.

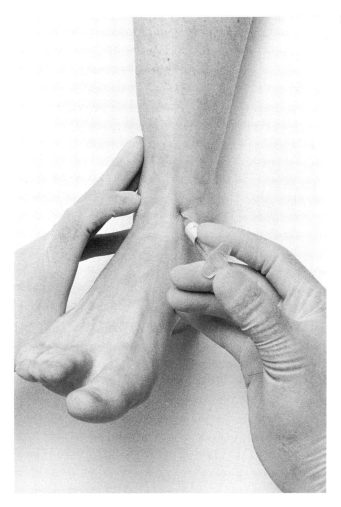

Hypertrophic and keloid scars

A side effect of depot steroid injections into the skin is atrophy. This can be used to advantage to soften and flatten small hypertrophic and keloid scars and remove the itching that can be present (Figs. 7.72, 7.73). The patient should be warned that occasionally there is a possibility of a small area of depigmentation developing at the site of the injection and also a small flare of fine telangiectatic vessels may result. The area around the scar should be infiltrated first with local anaesthetic as the injection in the dense fibrous tissue can be quite uncomfortable. A 1 ml syringe with a fine 28G needle can be used to place the steroid immediately deep to the scar and into its substance. The injection should not be made into the surrounding normal skin. It takes a few weeks to see the maximal effect of a single injection and although only one injection may be required for very small scars, a number of injections at intervals of 3–4 weeks may be required to achieve a flat, non-pruritic and soft scar.

Fig. 7.72. This patient developed a small but prominent hypertrophic scar following removal of a naevus on the chest wall. This scar is suitable for injection with a depot steroid.

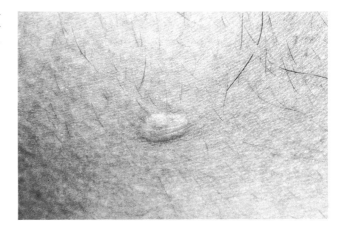

Fig. 7.73. This shows a stretched hypertrophic scar on the upper outer arm. One end of the scar was thicker and had caused persistent itching since the original surgery. A single injection of 5 mg of methyl prednisolone rapidly resolved the itching and flattened the scar.

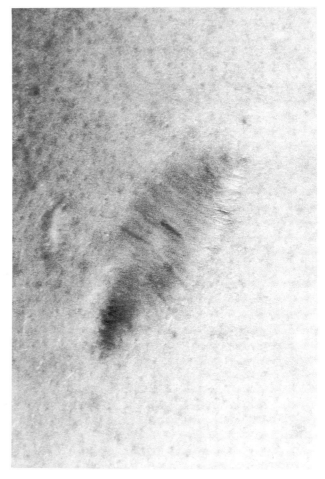

References

1. Treatment of non-septic olecranon bursitis. Smith, D. L., McAfee, J. H., Lucas, L. M., Kumar, K. L. & Romney, D. M. *Archives of Internal Medicine* (1989), **149**, 2527–2530.

2. Corticosteroid injection for osteoarthritis of the knee: peripatellar compared to intra-articular route. Sambrook, P. N., Champion, G. D., Browne, C. D., Cairns, D., Cohen, M. L. & Day, R. O. *Clinical and Experimental Rheumatology* (1989), 7, 609–613.

3. Corticosteroid injections in adhesive capsulitis: investigation of their value and site. Rizk, T. E., Pinals, R. S. & Talaiver, A. S. *Archives of Physical Medicine and Rehabilitation* (1991), **72**, 20–22.

4. A study to compare the efficacy of two methods of skin preparation prior to joint injection. Cawley, P. J. & Morris, I. M. *British Journal of Rheumatology* (1992), **31**, 847–848.

8

Aspiration and sclerosant injection techniques

Breast cyst

Although most breast cysts can be easily diagnosed as such, some can be very tense and give the impression of a solid lump. Simple needle aspiration is a safe technique [1] and can be done in the consulting room with a 21G needle and 5 ml syringe. Local anaesthetic is not required and the patient should be reassured that the procedure is no more painful than having a sample of blood taken. Aspiration of a breast cyst in the surgery avoids the worry associated with waiting for a specialist appointment and a visit to a hospital.

The patient should lie supine on the couch. The cyst can often be very mobile and it is necessary to steady it between two fingers against the chest wall (Fig. 8.1). It is a simple matter to insert the needle vertically through the skin and into the cyst but the novice may prefer to choose an approach more tangential to the chest wall. The skin should be wiped with an alcohol swab and the needle inserted through the skin and into the cyst in one smooth movement. Breast tissue is very dense and fibrous and this makes a slow and indecisive insertion both more difficult and more painful. Afterwards, the puncture wound may be covered with a

Fig. 8.1. (a) and (b) Breast cyst aspiration.

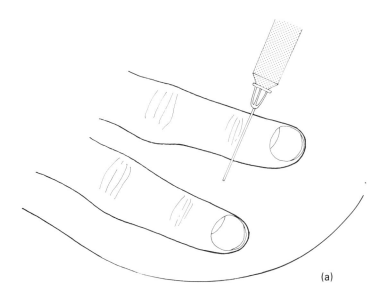

(a)

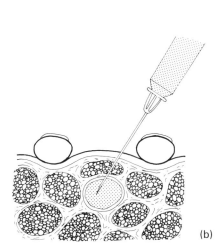

(b)

simple plaster for a short time. The aspirated fluid is usually straw-coloured or grey and is customarily sent for cytological examination but unless the fluid is blood-stained it is most unlikely to yield malignant cells.

If the aspiration fails or a lump is still palpable afterwards, the case should be urgently referred to a specialist for excision biopsy. If the lesion turns out to be a solid lump, no harm will result from the attempted aspiration (needle biopsy of breast tumours is a common procedure and does not result in seeding of the tumour). However, suction can be applied to the needle before it is withdrawn. Any aspirated material should be preserved on a microscope slide and sent for urgent cytological examination.

Ganglion

A ganglion is a cystic lesion arising from the synovium of a joint capsule or tendon sheath. Lesions on the dorsum of the wrist, dorsum of the foot and over the distal interphalangeal joints can be easily aspirated and injected with sclerosant such as sodium tetradecyl (STD 3% (w/v)). Ganglia on the ventral aspect of the wrist can be aspirated but injection should not be attempted by the inexperienced doctor, because of the risk of inadvertent extravasation around flexor tendons and the median and ulnar nerves.

The fluid inside a ganglion is thick and gelatinous and cannot be easily aspirated, hence a relatively large needle 21G is necessary along with a 10 ml syringe to

Fig. 8.2. Aspiration and injection for ganglion on dorsum of wrist using a plastic cannnula.

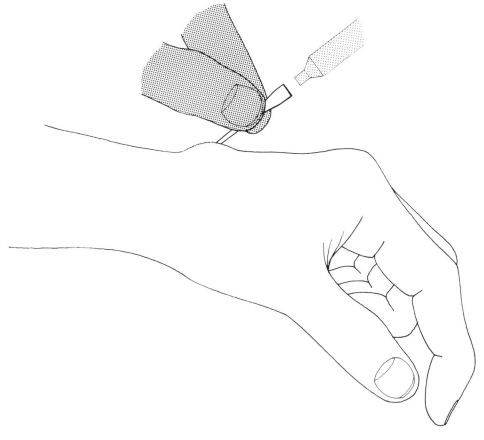

generate sufficient suction. Alternatively, an 18–21G intravenous cannula may be used to aspirate the fluid and inject the sclerosant (Fig. 8.2). The plastic cannula has the advantage that its tip is less likely to perforate the capsule while the aspirating syringe is being exchanged for the syringe containing the sclerosant.

Dorsum of the wrist and foot

This ganglion commonly occurs on the dorsal aspect of the wrist, ulnar-side of or above the extensor carpi radialis tendon. First, a bleb of local anaesthetic should be injected into the skin overlying the ganglion. A 1 ml syringe is prepared containing 0.5 ml STD. The patient's wrist should be steadied in slight flexion in order to tense the ganglion and a 10 ml syringe and a 21G needle used for aspiration. The large syringe is then removed and the 1 ml syringe connected to the needle, taking care not to withdraw the needle tip from the ganglion sac. The STD is then injected and the sac can be seen to inflate in the process. The sclerosant can be left inside the ganglion sac for 5 min and then aspirated, or it can be left *in situ*. Either method is acceptable. A wad of gauze is used to compress the site for 24 h. The procedure may be repeated if necessary in 6–8 weeks. The same technique is used for a ganglion on the dorsum of the foot (Fig. 8.3).

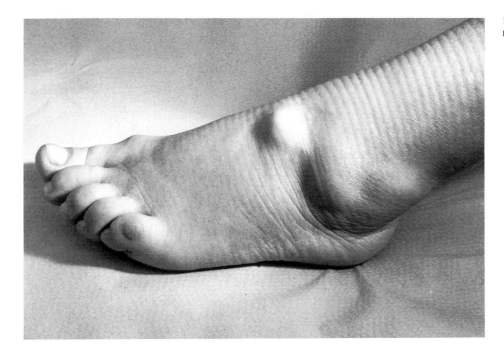

Fig. 8.3. Ganglion on dorsum of the foot.

Distal interphalangeal joint

These ganglia commonly occur in association with osteoarthritis of the distal interphalangeal joint (DIP) and are usually about 5 mm in diameter. Local anaesthetic is not usually necessary. The technique is the same as for the wrist but less than 0.25 ml of STD or phenol 80% is usually injected into the thin sac and

Fig. 8.4. Aspiration and injection for
a ganglion over the DIP joint.

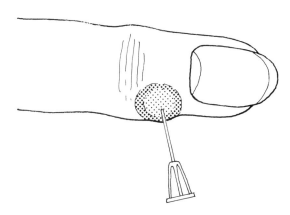

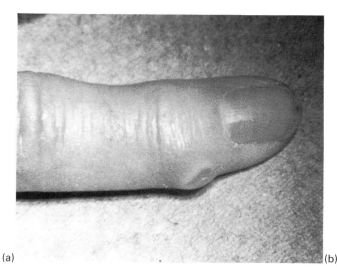

(a)

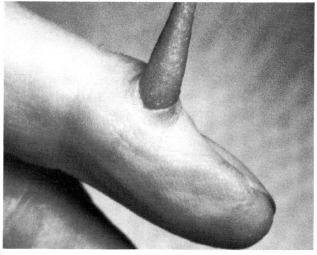

(b)

Fig. 8.5. (a) DIP joint ganglion, (b)
phenol cautery of DIP joint ganglion.

aspirated after 5 min after which a small compression dressing should be applied
for 24 h (Fig. 8.4).

An alternative technique is to slit the thin roof and cauterise the lining by using
a cotton bud dipped in phenol 80% for 3 min followed by a small compression
dressing for 24 h (Fig. 8.5). The DIP joint ganglion can also be frozen with liquid
nitrogen after the sac has been emptied (see chapter 12).

Haemorrhoids

First- and second-degree piles may be adequately treated by sclerosant injections
or rubber-band ligation. The rectum and upper half of the anal canal is supplied by
sympathetic and parasympathetic nerves and has a high pain threshold but is
sensitive to distension. Hence a rectal biopsy is painless but insufflating a sig-
moidoscope can result in discomfort. The lower half of the anal canal is supplied
by the inferior rectal branch of the pudendal nerve and is sensitive to touch, pain
and heat just like normal skin. Therefore, injection and rubber band ligation must
be performed above the pectinate line, which divides the lower and upper halves
of the anal canal and along which lie the anal sinuses (Fig. 8.6a).

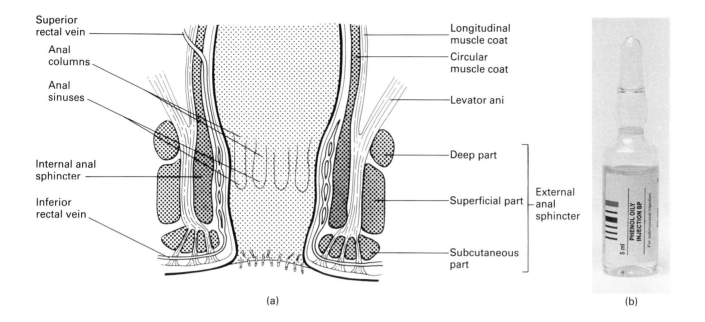

Superior rectal vein

Anal columns

Anal sinuses

Internal anal sphincter

Inferior rectal vein

Longitudinal muscle coat

Circular muscle coat

Levator ani

Deep part

Superficial part — External anal sphincter

Subcutaneous part

(a)   (b)

Sclerosant injection

The objective is to inject a small quantity of sclerosant (5 % phenol in almond oil) (Fig. 8.6b) into the submucosa just above the pile that is to be treated. This causes submucosal fibrosis, which results in shrinkage and retraction of the pile. Note that the 80 % phenol SHOULD NOT be used for injecting into haemorrhoids, as severe necrosis of the rectal wall can result.

Since the rectum (unlike the anus) is sensitive only to distension, the procedure should be quite painless, although some tenesmus may occur. The sclerosant is very viscous and has to be injected using a strong glass syringe with a special needle (Gabriel) that has a shoulder about 1 cm from its tip to help to prevent too deep an injection.

The patient lies in the left lateral position. A proctoscope is passed into the rectum and as it is slowly withdrawn, the haemorrhoids will be seen to prolapse into the top of the instrument. The piles will be seen at 3 o'clock (left lateral), 7 o'clock (right posterior), and 11 o'clock (right anterior). Approximately 5 ml of sclerosant is injected into the submucosa just above the pile to be treated (Fig. 8.7). Injection at the correct depth causes the muscosa to swell as the fluid spreads in the submucosa. Too superficial an injection results in blanching of the mucosa and this can lead to superficial necrosis. The other piles are dealt with in turn.

The patient should be encouraged to eat enough roughage to ensure loose and easy bowel movements and given laxatives if necessary. Further injections may be made for any residual piles when the patient's condition is reviewed after about 6 weeks.

Fig. 8.6a. Haemorrhoids, anatomy of anus and rectum.

Fig. 8.6b. Phenol in oil for injection into haemorrhoids.

Fig. 8.7. Injection for haemorrhoids.

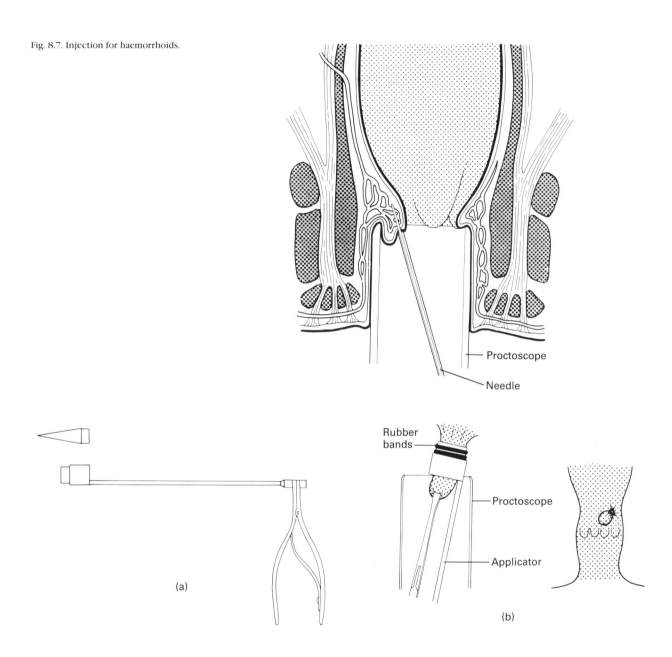

Proctoscope

Needle

(a)

Rubber bands

Proctoscope

Applicator

(b)

Fig. 8.8. (a) Rubber-band applicator, (b) rubber-band ligation of haemorrhoid.

Rubber-band ligation

Rubber-band ligation produces results as good as those obtained by injection [2] and the method is both simple and causes little disturbance to the patient. With the patient in the left lateral position a proctoscope is passed into the rectum and gradually withdrawn to allow the individual piles to prolapse into the top of the instrument. The applicator is located over the pile to be treated and the pile grasped with forceps. While traction is applied with the forceps upward pressure is applied with the applicator and the rubber band is released (Fig. 8.8). The procedure should be painless provided that the pile is ligated above the anal sinuses. Usually only one pile is treated at a time but the procedure can be repeated for two or three piles, depending on their size. The patient should be encouraged to eat plenty of roughage or be given bulk-forming agents as necessary. The patient should be warned to expect some rectal discharge as necrosis occurs and the ligated tissue will slough off in 7–10 days.

Pilonidal sinus

A pilonidal sinus is perpetuated by the presence of hairs inside the track, which create a foreign body reaction (Fig. 8.9). There are a number of methods of treating this condition and eradication of all tracks and debris is essential to prevent a recurrence. However, in practice this is notoriously difficult to achieve. Phenol (80%) injection into the sinus is worth trying if the track is short, narrow and superficial. Phenol injection should not be used in any long or deep sinus as there is a risk of producing a necrotic abscess. Such sinuses should be referred for formal excision.

The skin is shaved around the sinus and a probe directed into the cavity to assess its extent. Local anaesthetic is then infiltrated around the sinus and a fine forceps or scoop introduced to remove any hairs and debris. The surrounding skin is protected with either petroleum jelly or a gauze swab soaked in methylated spirit. The phenol is then injected down the sinus and left in place for 2–3 min. It is then expressed and the procedure repeated. A dressing is applied for a few days to mop up any seepage and healing will take 3–6 weeks to be complete.

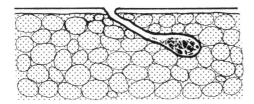

Fig. 8.9. Pilonidal sinus with a nest of hairs.

Hydrocoele

Aspiration

In the elderly or infirm, surgery is unnecessary and a hydrocoele can be quite adequately managed by repeated simple aspirations at 3–4 monthly intervals.

The scrotum is cleansed with antiseptic and exposed through a window in a paper towel. The scrotum is then tensed with the left hand and a skin wheal is raised at the proposed site of aspiration using 1% lignocaine. A 19G needle attached to a 20 ml syringe is inserted through the skin, dartos and tunica and the straw-coloured fluid aspirated (Fig. 8.10). The needle is then steadied with the left hand, the syringe disconnected, and the contents discarded, and further aspiration continued until the sac is effectively dry. Although 50 ml syringes and 3-way taps are useful, it is not necessary to keep such rarely used items in stock – a 20 ml syringe is quite adequate. Towards the end of the aspiration, care should be taken not to nick the underlying testes and cause internal bleeding as this can cause a

Fig. 8.10. Aspiration of hydrocoele.

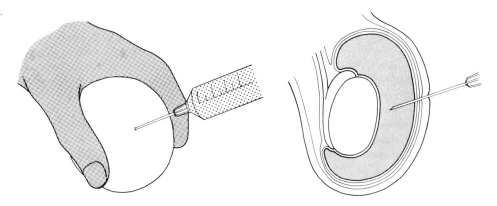

haematoma that predisposes to infection. Alternatively, an 18G plastic intra-venous cannula can be used and this minimises the risk of internal damage.

Commonly, 100–150 ml can be removed. Once the aspiration is complete, the needle or cannula is withdrawn and the testes examined to exclude any signs of abnormality. A dressing is not usually necessary but a simple gauze may be placed inside the underwear to absorb any slight bleeding.

Sclerosant injection

The treatment of hydrocoele by the injection of various sclerosing agents has been used intermittently for many centuries. Although tetracycline instillation (100–500 mg in 5 ml water) is an effective sclerosant it tends to cause moderate to severe pain [3,4] and is not recommended. Aqueous phenol (2.5%) (NOT the 80% phenol used for surface cautery) is both effective in sclerosing the sac and causes only mild pain [5].

When a sclerosant is injected into the hydrocoele sac it is advisable to use a plastic intravenous cannula as this will reduce the likelihood of trauma to the sac and is less likely to slip out during the procedure. Once the hydrocoele has been aspirated a small volume of lignocaine is injected into the sac to help to minimise any discomfort and this is followed by the 2.5% aqueous phenol (5–20 ml depending on the size of the sac). This is left *in situ*. The procedure may be repeated after 6–8 weeks if necessary. In view of the bulk of the thickened tunica vaginalis in a hydrocoele, some residual thickening is likely to remain and the patient should be warned to expect this.

Epididymal cyst

Epididymal cysts are often multiple and commonly vary in size from being a few millimetres to 10 mm in diameter. They can be left alone if asymptomatic or aspirated if tender or troublesome. Unlike a hydrocoele, it can be quite difficult to aspirate epididymal cysts because they are generally small and mobile.

Examination and firm steadying of epididymal cysts prior to aspiration can be quite painful for the patient and accidental needling of unanaesthetised cord or testes during aspiration can cause intense pain. Hence, to allow the epididymal cysts to be identified and steadied without discomfort it is useful first to anaesthetise the scrotal contents with an injection of 5 ml 1% plain lignocaine at the scrotal neck. The testis is then steadied with the left hand and a bleb of local anaesthetic injected into the scrotal skin. A fresh needle or intravenous cannula is then used to aspirate the cyst (Fig. 8.11).

Epididymal cysts may be injected with 2.5% phenol as with a hydrocoele but because of the risk of extravasation, it is unwise to attempt a sclerosant injection unless the cyst is large and easily entered.

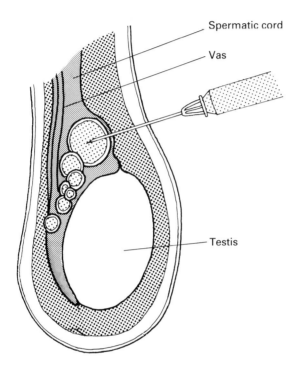

Spermatic cord

Vas

Testis

Fig. 8.11. Aspiration of epididymal cyst.

Drainage of pleural effusion

Aspiration of fluid in a terminally ill patient with recurrent pleural effusion may be performed in the surgery or in the patient's home provided the diagnosis is clear and the physical signs of dullness to percussion and reduced breath sounds are supported by a recent chest X-ray. There should be a nurse in assistance and light premedication (e.g. pethidine or diamorphine with or without diazepam) can be used if necessary. A large intravenous needle and cannula attached to a 20 or 50 ml syringe can be used to aspirate and discharge the fluid through a standard three-way tap into a receiver. The patient should be supported sitting forwards on a chair or the side of the bed.

Before proceeding, the doctor should re-examine the patient to confirm the extent of the dullness, and to select and mark the actual puncture site. This would normally be posterolaterally in the 7th or 8th interspace as insertion of a needle into the 10th or 11th interspace is likely to penetrate the diaphragm and enter the peritoneal cavity. In addition, the doctor should check and be familiar with the workings of the three-way tap. The skin is then prepared and local anaesthetic

Fig. 8.12. Drainage of pleural
effusion. The neurovascular bundle
lies immediately below the lower
border of the rib.

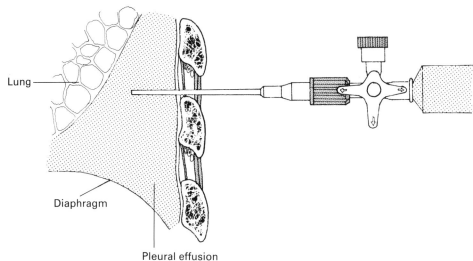

injected through the skin and down to the pleura, injecting slowly as the needle is advanced. The needle should be passed just above the chosen rib as the neurovascular bundle lies just below each rib (Fig. 8.12).

A few minutes should be allowed to ensure that the anaesthetic has worked after which the intravenous needle and cannula is inserted along the same track as the previous needle (if a large cannula is used, it is helpful first to make a small puncture in the skin with a no. 11 blade). Loss of resistance will be felt as the pleura is pierced, the needle is then withdrawn slightly and the cannula inserted further as necessary. The cannula is then connected to the three-way tap and the large aspirating syringe. The effusion is aspirated and discarded into a receiver, and care taken not to allow any air into the pleural cavity. Once enough fluid has been drained, the cannula can be removed and the puncture site covered with a small waterproof dressing.

Abdominal paracentesis

Occasionally, diuretics may fail to reduce discomfort or dyspnoea and it may be necessary to drain fluid from a terminally ill patient with gross ascites [6]. The ascites does not need to be drained completely and it may be adequate simply to remove enough fluid to alleviate symptoms. However, in some patients significant reaccumulation may appear in a few days.

Abdominal paracentesis can be done in the patient's home with the assistance of a nurse and using light premedication (e.g. pethidine or diamorphine with or without diazepam) if necessary. The procedure is simple and requires minimal equipment. Either a trocar and cannula, or a large intravenous needle and cannula (with an appropriate Luer connector) can be used to drain the fluid into a standard sterile catheter bag, which can be changed as necessary.

The patient would normally lie semi-recumbent or supine but should lie in whatever position is most comfortable as although the insertion of the cannula takes only a few minutes to perform, the fluid itself should be drained slowly over a period of time so as to avoid any acute circulatory collapse. However, contrary

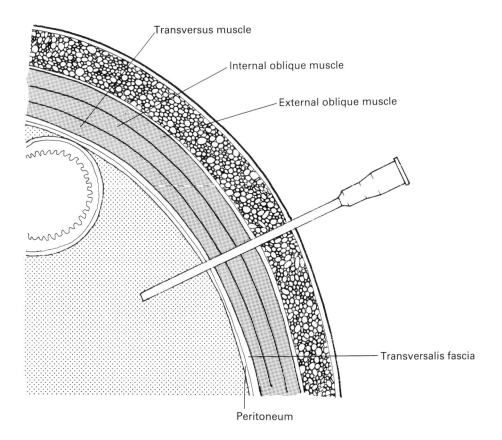

Transversus muscle

Internal oblique muscle

External oblique muscle

Transversalis fascia

Peritoneum

Fig. 8.13. Abdominal paracentesis.

to traditional reports, the likelihood of adverse haemodynamic effects resulting from the removal of up to 5 litres of fluid is small [6,7].

Before proceeding, the doctor should re-examine the patient to confirm the presence of shifting dullness, and to select and mark the actual puncture site (usually midway between the costal margin and the anterior superior iliac spine). The skin is prepared and draped with a paper towel. Local anaesthetic is then injected through the skin and down to the peritoneum, injecting slowly as the needle is advanced. A few minutes should be allowed to ensure that the anaesthetic has worked and the trocar and cannula or intravenous needle and cannula are inserted along the same track as the previous needle (if a large cannula is used, it is helpful first to make a small puncture in the skin with a no. 11 blade). Resistance will be felt as the peritoneum is approached and once the trocar or needle is felt to have pierced the peritoneum it is withdrawn slightly and the cannula inserted further as necessary (Fig. 8.13). The cannula is then connected to the drainage tubing and the rate of flow adjusted with the drainage valve. The cannula is then held in place with adhesive tapes.

Once enough fluid has been drained, the cannula can be removed and the puncture site covered with a small dressing.

References

1. Needle biopsy of breast cysts. Forrest, A. P., Kirkpatrick, J. R. & Roberts, M. M. *British Medical Journal* (1975), **3**, 30–31.

2. A randomised trial to compare rubber band ligation with phenol injection for treatment of haemorrhoids Greca, F., Hares, M. M., Nehah, E., Alexander-Williams, J. & Keighley, M. R. B. *British Journal of Surgery* (1981), **68**, 250–252.

3. Sclerotherapy for 'scrotal cysts' using tetracycline instillation. Courtney, S. P. & Wightman, J. A. K. *Journal of the Royal College of Surgeons of Edinburgh* (1991), **36**, 103.

4. Sclerotherapy for hydrocoele and epididymal cysts: a five year study. Nash, J. R. *British Medical Journal* (1984), **288**, 1652.

5. Aspiration and tetracycline scerotherapy of hydrocoele. Fuse, H., Nishikawa, Y., Shimazaki, J. & Katayama, T. *Scandinavian Journal of Urology and Nephrology* (1991), **25**, 5–7.

6. Pathophysiologic factors and management of ascites. Longmire-Cook, S. *Gynaecology and Obstetrics* (1993), **176**, 191–202.

7. Renaissance of paracentesis in the treatment of ascites. Reynolds, T. B. *Advances in Internal Medicine* (1990), **35**, 365–374.

SECTION III

9

Surgical techniques: Incisions

Incisions

A neat thin scar will only be attained by careful preparation, planning and attention to detail. Careful handling of tissues will minimise complications and allow wounds to heal as rapidly as possible. Crushing, drying and tension should be avoided.

Incision direction

The direction of the skin incision should be carefully planned so as to produce the minimal amount of scarring. In practice this is best done by pinching and corrugating the skin in different directions and noting the ease with which furrows and ridges are produced.[1] In addition, the direction of wrinkle and natural skin creases should be noted (Figs. 9.1, 9.2). Having made an examination of the site, the incision should be made parallel to the furrows, wrinkles and creases.

On the limbs, axial incisions should be avoided, especially over joints. In general, the incisions should be oblique over the long bones and transverse over the joints (Figs. 9.3, 9.4, 9.5).

Incision marking

Unless a lesion is very small it is always preferable to mark out accurately the proposed incision or excision line with a pen (*prior* to the local anaesthetic injection as this may distort the skin creases) (Fig. 9.6). The length of the skin ellipse should be approximately 2.5–3 times its width, depending on the local skin flexibility (Fig. 9.7). Too short an incision may result in undue tension or dog ears. The maximum width of the excision will be determined by the elasticity, mobility and amount of available spare skin. Extreme care must be taken not to remove too large an ellipse in areas such as the back of the hand where there is

---

[1] Langer's cadaveric lines relate to the orientation of dermal collagen. Incisions placed parallel to the dermal collagen (i.e. along Langer's lines) will heal with the collagen fibres correctly orientated and thus produce a fine scar. In practice the orientation of dermal collagen is identified by using relaxed skin tension lines (RSTLs). The RSTLs are defined by pinching the skin and noting the extent of and ease with which furrows and ridges are formed. Pinching the skin at right angles to the RSTLs will produce large furrows and ridges with relative ease.

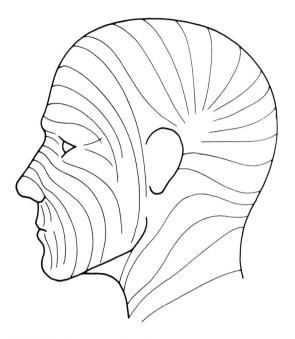

Fig. 9.1. Facial incision lines and wrinkles.

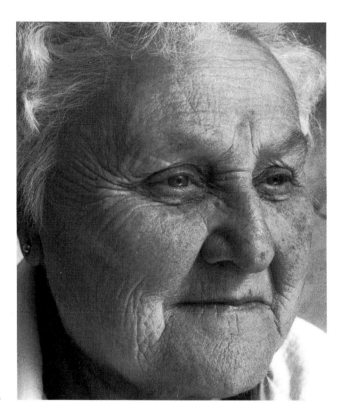

Fig. 9.2. (RIGHT) Facial skin creases.

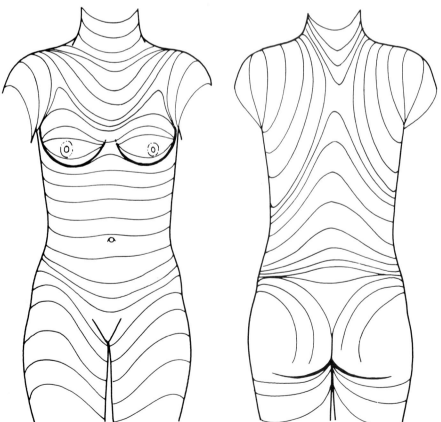

Fig. 9.3. Body and limb incision lines.

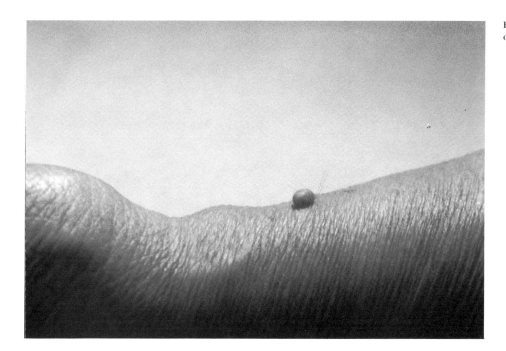

Fig. 9.4. The skin creases run obliquely on the limbs.

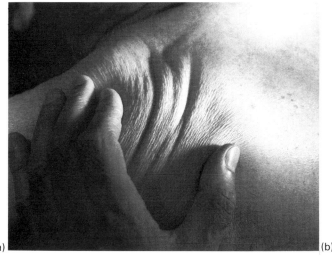

(a)

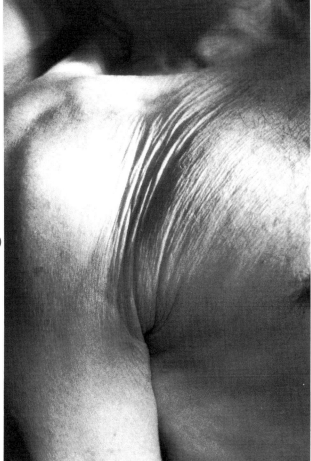

(b)

Fig. 9.5. (a) Scapular area, (b) Anterior shoulder area. The direction of the skin incision should be determined by moving nearby joints and pinching and corrugating the skin in different directions.

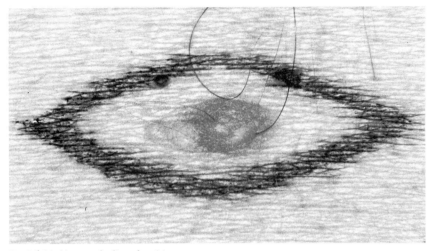

Fig. 9.6. Marking out the line of excision.

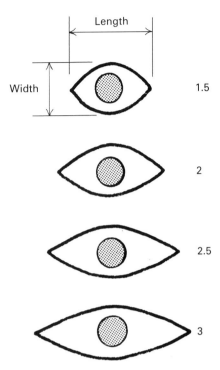

Fig. 9.7. The length of the skin ellipse should be approximately 2.5–3 times its width.

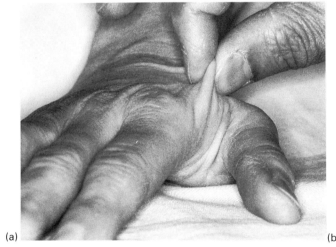

(a)

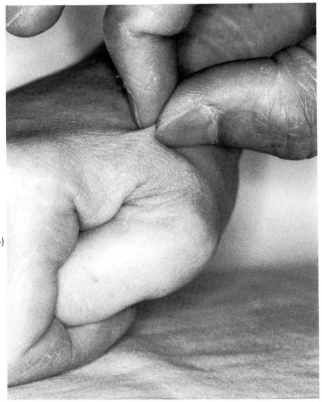

(b)

Fig. 9.8. There is very little spare skin on the back of the hand: (a) there seems to be ample spare skin when it is picked up with the thumb extended; (b) however, there is little spare skin when the thumb is flexed.

very little spare skin (Fig. 9.8). To ensure that the proposed wound edges will come together easily and without tension, it is often necessary to assess the situation by picking up the lesion and skin while flexing and extending the nearby joints.

The skin incision

The incision should be made perpendicular to the surface, as closure of an oblique incision may result in a wider scar (Fig. 9.9). The scalpel tip should cut cleanly through into the underlying fat in a single clean action while the skin is tensed with the doctor's other hand (Fig. 9.10).

A common error is to make the initial incision too shallow. This merely results in bleeding and repeated strokes of the scalpel will result in a ragged wound edge. Occasionally, and especially with small lesions, once incision of one side of an ellipse has been completed, the tension in the skin is lost, and this can cause some difficulty in making a clean and vertical incision of the other side. In such cases it

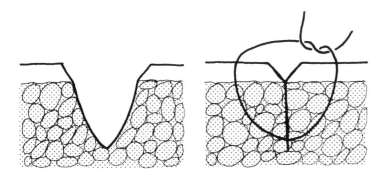

Fig. 9.9. An oblique skin incision results in a wide scar.

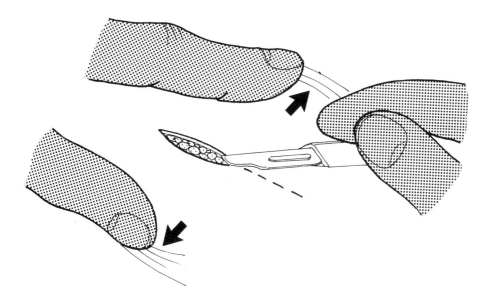

Fig. 9.10. Tensioning the skin while making the incision.

Fig. 9.11. Incision with artery clip
finger hole.

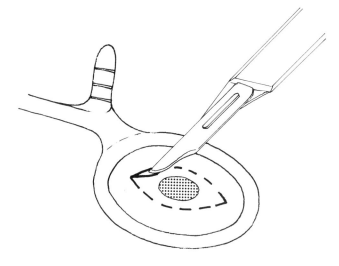

Fig. 9.12. Never cut blind as serious
damage can result.

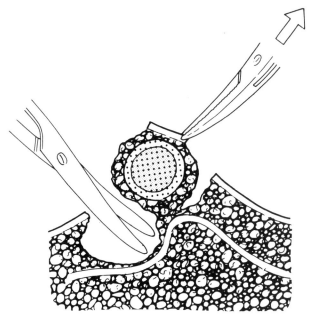

may be helpful to maintain the tension by making the incision through a finger
hole of an artery clip placed over the lesion (Fig. 9.11).

Deep dissection

Blunt dissection with scissors or an artery clip allows underlying blood vessels
and nerves to be identified and avoided, or deliberately cut and tied as necessary.
The artery clip or scissors should be inserted closed and then opened to separate
the tissue gently. Nerves are resilient structures that can withstand a certain
amount of distortion. Sharp dissection should be avoided altogether unless the
tissue being cut can be directly visualised and identified as being unimportant
(Fig. 9.12). Any long off-white structure with very fine overlying vessels and a hint

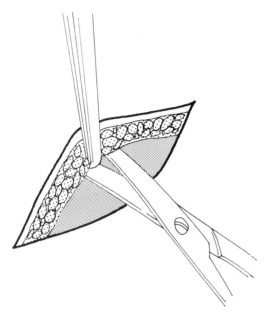

Fig. 9.13. Undermining the skin edges.

of longitudinal bundles should be considered to be a nerve and avoided. Small cutaneous nerves are unimportant and can be cut if they interfere with the dissection.

If necessary, the skin may be undermined using scissors or an artery clip to relieve any tension. The plane of the undermining should generally be between the fat layer and the deep fascia (Fig. 9.13).

Control of haemorrhage

Small blood vessels can be simply clamped with an artery clip and twisted a number of times and the clip released. Larger vessels should be tied off with a 3/0 absorbable suture. Curved artery clips are essential for easy tying and this can usually be done without an assistant by allowing the artery clip to rest tip-upwards on the patient's skin while the suture is looped around it (Fig. 9.14). If there is any

Fig. 9.14. Ligation of small blood vessel.

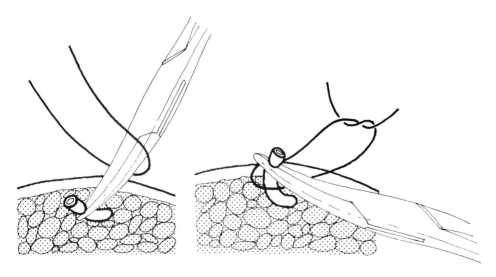

Fig. 9.15. Undersewing of inaccessible bleeding point.

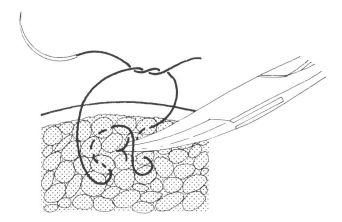

Fig. 9.16. Clipping an inaccessible bleeding point.

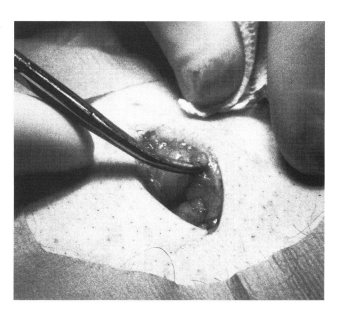

difficulty in getting an artery clip completely around a bleeding vessel, the bleeding tissue can be held with the tip of an artery clip and the vessel undersewn (Figs. 9.15, 9.16).

Incision in problem areas

It is vitally important never to cut blind or into unidentified structures. Extreme care should be taken when dissecting near any vessel that pulsates. Many important nerves and structures lie superficially in the body and a knowledge of their anatomy is essential for safe surgery (see p. 148). In particular, dissection in the posterior triangle of the neck and at the angle of the mandible should be avoided (Figs. 9.17, 9.18).

Subcutaneous lesions at the base of a finger can lie on or originate from digital nerves (Fig. 9.19). These require specialised surgical skills and anaesthetic techniques, and should be referred.

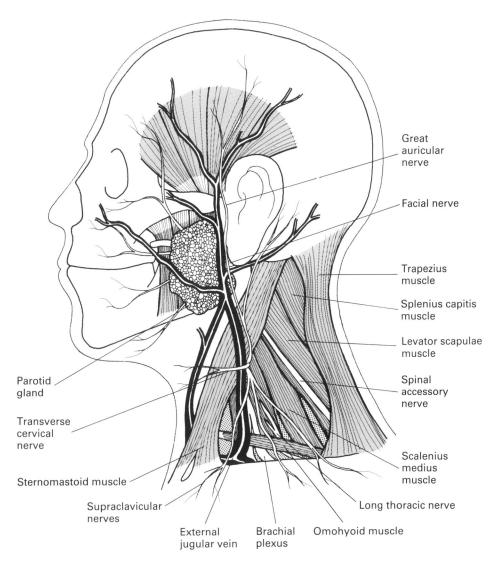

Fig. 9.17. There are many important structures to be aware of around the angle of the mandible and in the posterior triangle of the neck.

Great auricular nerve

Facial nerve

Trapezius muscle

Splenius capitis muscle

Levator scapulae muscle

Spinal accessory nerve

Scalenius medius muscle

Long thoracic nerve

Parotid gland

Transverse cervical nerve

Sternomastoid muscle

Supraclavicular nerves

External jugular vein

Brachial plexus

Omohyoid muscle

Fig. 9.18. (BELOW) These cysts should be referred to a specialist: (a) a cyst overlying the spinal accessory nerve in the posterior triangle; (b) a cyst at the angle of the mandible overlying the facial nerve; and (c) a preauricular cyst.

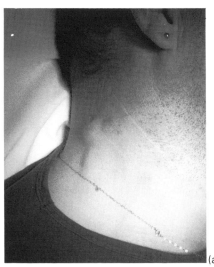

(a)

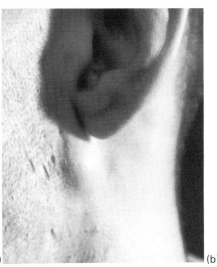

(b)

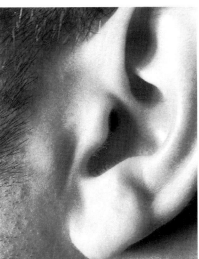

(c)

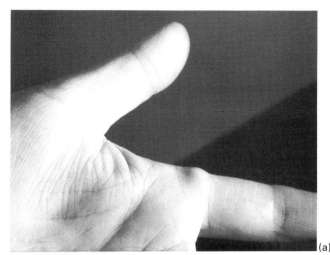 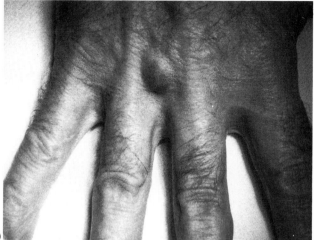

(a)   (b)

Fig. 9.19. (a) A cyst at the base of the index finger. This should be referred to a specialist. (b) In contrast to (a) this long-standing mobile inclusion dermoid can be safely removed by an experienced doctor using a simple longitudinal incision.

Important superficial nerves and structures

Vulnerable nerves
Frontal nerve above mid-eyebrow
Facial nerve at the angle of mandible
Lesser occipital nerve behind ear
Great auricular nerve over the upper part of sternomastoid
Spinal accessory nerve in posterior triangle
Brachial plexus in axilla
Radial nerve branches at wrist
Ulnar nerve behind medial epicondyle
Median nerve at wrist in mid-line
Digital nerves in finger/thumb
Femoral nerve in groin
Lateral popliteal nerve at neck of fibula
Sural nerve at back of calf

Vulnerable vessels
External jugular vein in anterior neck
Brachial artery and vein in axilla
Femoral artery and vein in groin
Long saphenous vein along the medial side of leg

Vulnerable structures
Lachrymal apparatus at medial canthus
Pleura in supraclavicular fossa

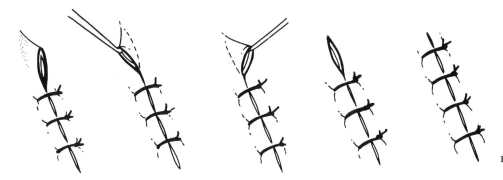

Fig. 9.20. Excision of dog ear.

Dog ears

Dog ears can arise if the excised skin ellipse is too short or the wound edges are mismatched. Dog ears if small can be flattened out by reducing the interval between the bites on the short side and increasing the interval on the longer side. Larger dog ears should be excised with a scalpel (Fig. 9.20).

10

Surgical techniques: Wound closure

Suture materials

When a suture is to be selected, consideration must be given to its physical characteristics, permanency, and likely tissue reaction.

Absorbable sutures

Catgut is made from sheep intestines, Dexon, Dexon II (polyglycolic acid), PDS (polydioxone) and Vicryl (polyglactin) are synthetic. Plain catgut loses most of its strength in a few days. Dexon retains 50% of its strength at 10 days and is dissolved completely by 90–120 days. The exact rate of absorption will depend on a number of factors, including the type of material, diameter of its fibres and the degree of inflammation. Absorption is rapid in the presence of infection.

Although synthetic absorbable sutures have a better feel and are often preferable to catgut for more involved procedures, they are usually more expensive than catgut and offer no significant advantage for the small wounds commonly seen in routine minor surgery. However, where there is a likelihood of tension in the wound, long-lasting subcutaneous or subcuticular sutures (such as undyed Dexon or Vicryl) should be used to minimise the risk of a stretched scar.

Non-absorbable sutures

Silk is the easiest material with which to tie knots but it is, for most purposes, superseded by synthetic sutures for a number of reasons. Although knot-tying with monofilament nylon may take some getting used to it causes less tissue reaction than does silk, and is more easily extricated from any crusting over a wound. In addition, monofilament nylon glides easily during removal and thereby causes less discomfort in the process. Some of the newer sutures such as Novafil (polybutester) have handling characteristics even better than those of nylon.

Braided sutures are used where monofilaments will cut through tissues or where knots must be easily tied with the minimum of turns and hence leave the minimal amount of foreign material in the wound (for example, the vas).

Fig. 10.1. Commonly used sutures
and needles.

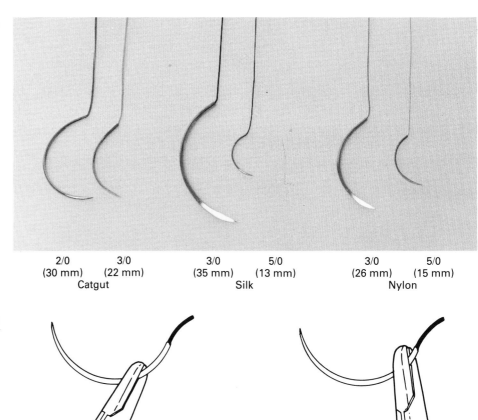

2/0	3/0	3/0	5/0	3/0	5/0
(30 mm)	(22 mm)	(35 mm)	(13 mm)	(26 mm)	(15 mm)
Catgut		Silk		Nylon	

Fig. 10.2. Needle holder gripping
needle: (a) correct, (b) incorrect.

(a)   (b)

Needles

Most modern sutures have a reverse cutting needle that has a third cutting edge
along the length of the outer curvature. This allows the needle to cut into tissue
away from the wound edges to minimise any danger of the suture cutting out
postoperatively (Fig. 10.1).

Round needles may be used to minimise trauma in delicate tissues such as the
spermatic cord.

The correct position of the needle within the jaws of the needle holder is at the
junction of the front two thirds and the back third (Fig. 10.2). If the needle is held
near the swaged end it will be liable to bend and fracture during insertion.

Skin closure

Skin suture

Suture techniques A 5/0 monofilament nylon suture is adequate for the majority
of small wounds. Larger wounds with greater tension or a subcuticular suture will
usually require 3/0 nylon sutures.

Skin sutures should simply approximate the wound edges in order to make a linear closure. They should not be used to draw the skin edges together under tension as this will just predispose to inflammation, infection and a scar with cross-markings. If there is tension in the wound, this should be first reduced by undermining the skin edges and/or the use of subcutaneous sutures.

The skin must be handled gently. If the skin is particularly delicate, dissecting forceps should be applied to the dermis of the wound edge instead of gripping the full thickness of the skin (Fig. 10.3).

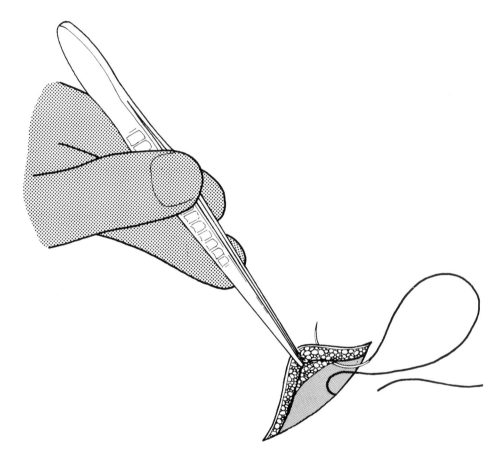

Fig. 10.3. Gripping skin edge by the dermis.

Palming a pair of scissors (Fig. 10.4) obviates the need of an assistant or for special needle holders such as the Gillies (which has inbuilt scissor blades but does not have a rachet mechanism).

The correct suture is one that just slightly everts the wound edges. The wound will gradually flatten once the sutures are removed. If the skin edges are allowed to overlap an unsightly step will result and is likely to leave a widened scar when the wound eventually flattens out (Fig. 10.5).

If the wound edge is markedly everted a broad, raw surface is exposed, which is slow to heal, is easily traumatised and adheres to dressings, making their removal both painful and difficult (Fig. 10.6a,b).

Fig. 10.4. Palming an instrument.

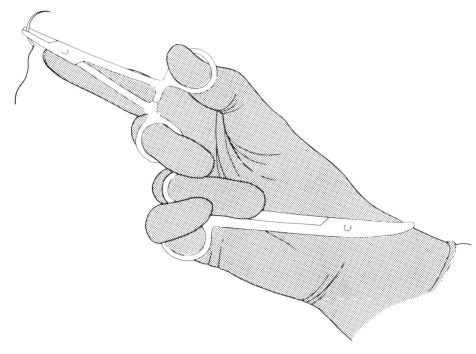

Fig. 10.5. The wound edges should
not be allowed to overlap.

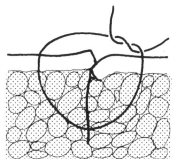

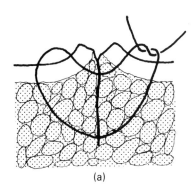

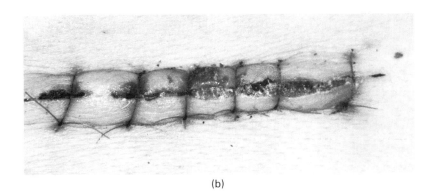

(a)   (b)

Fig. 10.6. (a) and (b). Broad raw
surface.

Simple suture The needle should approach the skin perpendicularly and be
directed through the tissues in an arc that matches the curve of the needle being
used. Too shallow a bite will result in a dead space (Fig. 10.7a).

The needle is then grasped from within the wound and an equal bite taken on
the other side of the wound. The needle should not be gripped by its tip as this is
likely to kink the needle and make it liable to breakage.

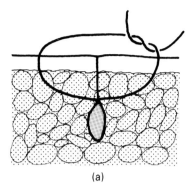

Fig. 10.7. (a) Too shallow a bite can result in a dead space.

(a)

The suture is then tied. After the first double throw, the suture is laid across the wound to allow precise tensioning of the wound. The second throw is then made and the knot locked. To avoid applying further tension on the wound, the suture should be slightly lifted up as it is tightened. The knot is then pulled to one side of the wound before the suture is cut (Fig. 10.7b,c). To avoid undue pressure, the knot should always be placed on the better vascularised side of the wound.

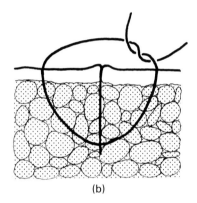

(b)

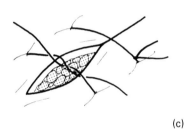 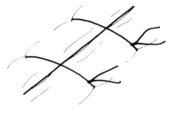

(c)

In the 'halving method' of suturing, the first suture is placed in the middle of the wound and subsequent sutures placed either side (Fig. 10.8). Further sutures are then inserted between those already in place. This technique is fine but has the disadvantage that the first (middle) suture has to be tied under relatively greater tension and the knot can slip during tying. It is preferable to place the first sutures at the ends of the wound and work towards the middle (Fig. 10.9). This minimises the tension on any individual suture and makes tying easier.

Fig. 10.7 (b) and (c) Simple suture: the suture is tied and the knot pulled to one side.

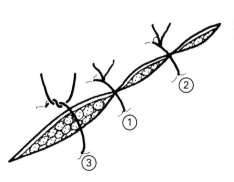

Fig. 10.8. 'Halving method' of closure.

Fig. 10.9. Suturing from each end of a wound.

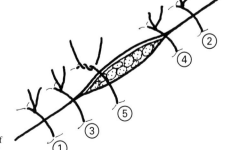

Vertical mattress suture Vertical mattress sutures may be used to correct inverting skin and step deformities (Fig. 10.10). Wounds on certain sites such as the palmar and plantar skin have a particular tendency to invert. Care should be taken to avoid uneven bites as this will lead to step deformities. It is often effective to use a combination of simple and mattress sutures. Here, a few strategic mattress sutures are placed first to evert the skin and the closure completed with simple sutures (Fig. 10.11).

Fig. 10.10. Vertical mattress suture.

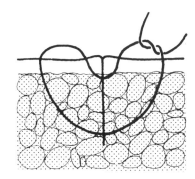

Fig. 10.11. Combination of simple and mattress suture.

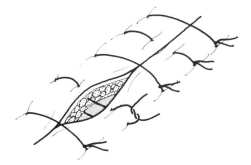

Modified Donatti suture This is a modified vertical mattress suture that can be used where the skin on one side of a wound is relatively thin and at risk. It can be inserted along the length of a wound or at the apex of a triangular flap (Fig. 10.12).

Fig. 10.12. (a) Modified Donatti suture, (b) apical suture.

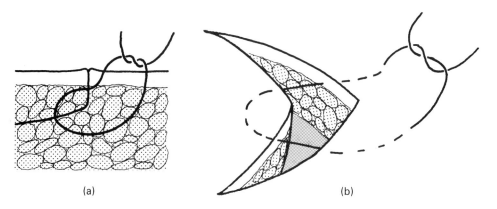

(a)   (b)

Subcuticular suture This is more correctly termed an intradermal suture. It provides a neat linear scar and avoids any cross-markings that may occur with the simple or mattress suture. A 3/0 nylon suture on a 25 mm curved needle is ideal for the majority of minor wounds (Fig. 10.13). If necessary, wound tension may be minimised by first placing a few subcutaneous sutures. For small fine wounds on the face or neck and where there is little tension, a 5/0 suture on a 15 mm curved needle is ideal. The needle is inserted into the skin about 1 cm from one end of the wound and brought out intradermally just inside the wound, about 1.5 mm below the skin surface (Fig. 10.14). The suture is pulled through the wound leaving a

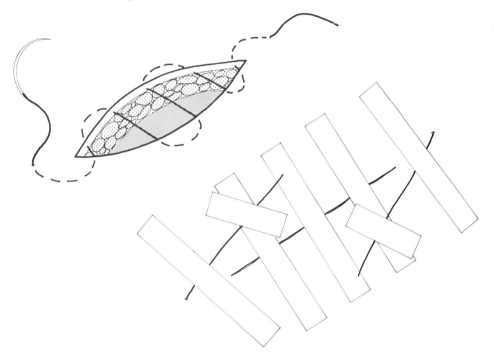

Fig. 10.13. Subcuticular suture using nylon.

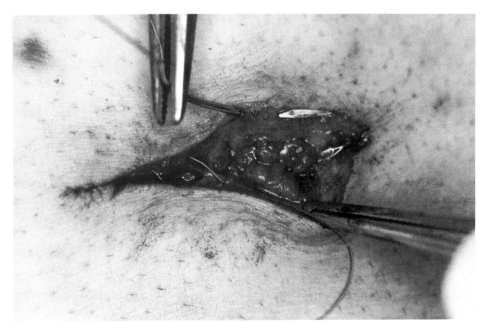

Fig. 10.14. Subcuticular suture using nylon.

5 cm length attached to an artery clip. Small equal horizontal bites are taken from each side of the wound, always remaining at the same depth. Once the suture is completed the needle is brought out through normal skin on the other end of the wound. An artery clip is applied to the suture and the needle is cut off. The suture is then gently pulled to and fro to approximate the wound edges and to confirm that it runs freely. Wrinkling of the skin should be avoided. In a well designed incision, no tension need be applied to the suture at this stage to keep the wound closed. Finally, adhesive tapes are applied along the wound to support it and approximate any slight gaps, and to hold down the ends of the suture.

In some cases an undyed absorbable subcuticular suture may be used to obviate the need for suture removal. The technique is similar but the suture is first anchored inside one end of the wound, pulled tight after each bite, and finally tied onto itself inside the other end (Fig. 10.15). This knot-tying technique requires a little practice to ensure that there is no slack in the suture (which might result in slight gaping of the wound margins) once the knot is locked.

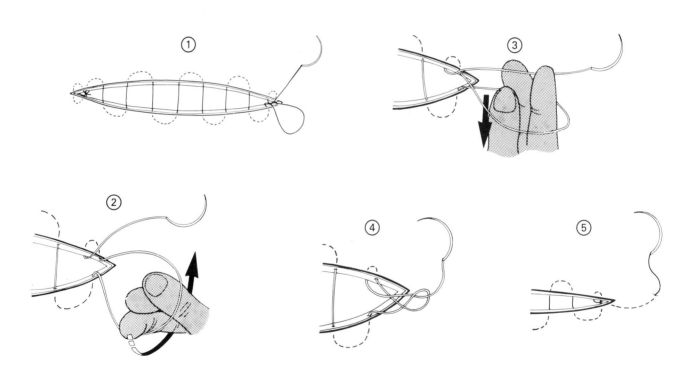

Fig. 10.15. Subcuticular absorbable suture.

Adhesive tapes

The skin should never be sutured under tension. After the wound has been closed, adhesive tapes may be used to add further support and to distribute the load over a wider area. A number of sizes of tape are available (3, 6 and 12 mm wide). The skin should be dried and the tapes applied at intervals with the finger or non-toothed forceps. The tapes should be firmly applied to one side of the wound and then gently pulled across to the other side, pulling the first wound edge against the other in the process (Fig. 10.16). If necessary, adhesion of the tapes may be improved by first dabbing Tincture Benzoin (Friar's Balsam) onto the skin. The tapes should be applied at intervals across the length of the wound and these may be further anchored with tapes parallel to the wound. Adhesive tapes can often be used to close small wounds without the use of any sutures, particularly in lacerations to the chin and forehead in children (Fig. 10.17).

It is sometimes necessary to provide additional support to a wound for a few days after removal of sutures. At this stage, non-sterile tapes such as Micropore can be used.

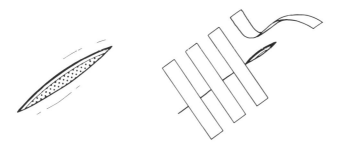

Fig. 10.16. Application of adhesive tapes.

Fig. 10.17. (a) and (b) Closure of minor laceration with adhesive tapes.

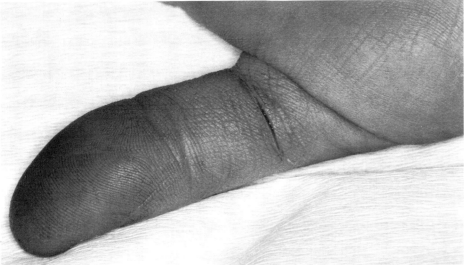

(a)

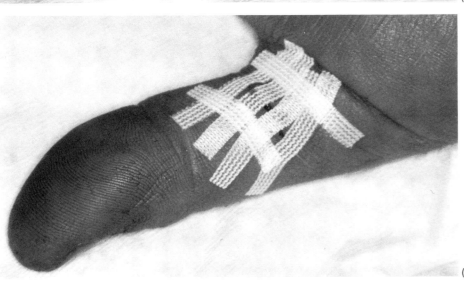

(b)

Tissue adhesive

Monomeric *n*-butyl 2-cyanoacrylate tissue adhesive (coloured blue) is available in small plastic vials and polymerises in contact with tissue fluids (Fig. 10.18). It should not be confused with proprietary 'superglues'. The material should be stored in a refrigerator when not in use. The use of tissue adhesive can result in good cosmetic results, is time-saving, and can result in cost savings, especially when factors such as dressings, local anaesthetics, suture packs, and suture removal are considered.

Tissue adhesive has been successfully used in a number of situations such as minor lacerations in children [1], management of avulsed teeth [2], scalp wounds [3], and episiotomy (see chapter 22). However, common small wounds such as on the chin are often more easily dealt with using adhesive tapes. It is designed for surface use only and should not be used inside the wound as this can delay wound healing (Fig. 10.19). Although the vials are designed for single use only, the

Fig. 10.18. Histocacryl tissue adhesive.

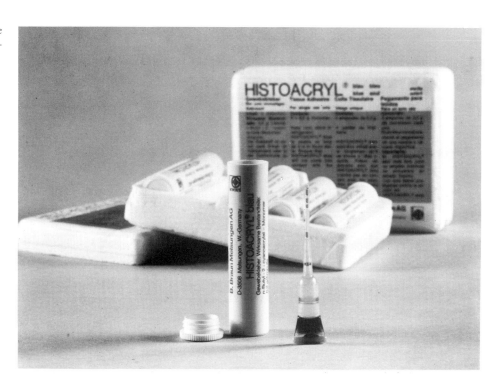

Fig. 10.19. Application of tissue adhesive. The adhesive should not be placed *inside* the wound itself.

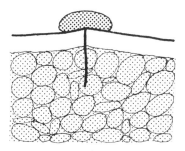

adhesive can be applied using fine capillary tubing, allowing multiple use without any contamination [*1*]. The vial end can be heat-sealed after use. Wounds larger than 3 cm or wounds subject to tension should have an additional support from sutures. Furthermore, the adhesive should not be used in isolation for deep wounds as it is difficult to obtain good cosmetic results [*4*] and any dead space will predispose to haematoma and infection.

Although with practice excellent results can be achieved, tissue adhesive can be extremely messy to use if great care is not used. The glue will harden in about 20–30 s and will stick together fingers and gloves and anything with which it comes into contact. Note that the wound edges have to be held together while the glue hardens and there is a small amount of heat generated in the polymerisation process. A disadvantage is that generally two pairs of hands are needed. One person has to dry the wound and then approximate the skin edges accurately (this may not be easy with a frightened child) and the other person has to apply small dabs of glue along the length of the wound as a thin layer (Fig. 10.20) or 'spot welds'. It is vitally important to obtain accurate apposition of the wound edges as (unlike with sutures) any subsequent fine adjustments will not be possible. The glue should be applied sparingly and not indiscriminately all over the wound.

No dressings are required, although adhesive tapes may be used as additional support if necessary. Cyanoacrylate is biodegradable but remains well after the wound has healed. The adhesive eventually separates spontaneously along with normal skin desquamation.

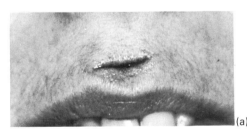 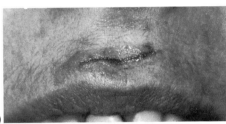

(a)   (b)

Fig. 10.20. (a) and (b) Tissue adhesive applied to a wound on the upper lip.

Skin staples

Stainless steel staples are sometimes used in casualty departments for rapid closure of scalp wounds and in more involved surgery to close long wounds. For cosmetic reasons, they should not be used on the face. Their use is governed largely by personal preference and although quick to insert, they can be rather more difficult and painful to remove (especially when encased in crust) compared with fine monofilament nylon. They have a very limited role in minor surgery, although practice nurses may be asked to remove staples from patients treated in hospital. The staples are inserted with a disposable purpose-made stapler while the skin is approximated with toothed forceps and slight tension is applied along the line of the wound. They have to be removed with a special staple-removing tool (Figs. 10.21, 10.22).

Fig. 10.21. Disposable stapler and
staple remover.

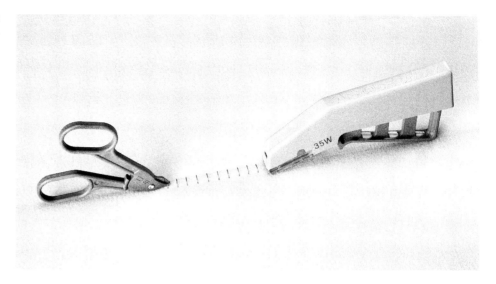

Fig. 10.22. Removal of skin staples.

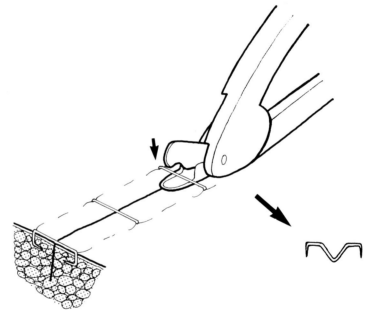

Deep sutures

As a general rule deep sutures are required whenever there is tension in the
wound. Wounds in the leg tend to gape markedly and almost always require
subcutaneous sutures. However, the subcutaneous layer is often just delicate
areolar tissue and a suture placed here is likely to cut out. A generous bite is
therefore necessary in the fat layer, preferably catching the deeper parts of the
dermis in its upper path (Fig. 10.23).

Starting and finishing the sutures in the depths of the wound allows the knot to
be buried deep in the wound (Figs. 10.24, 10.25). In order to leave the minimum
amount of foreign material behind, deep sutures should be cut as short as possible,
just above the knot.

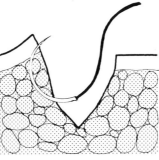

Fig. 10.23. The deep suture should take a bite of the deeper part of the dermis to prevent it cutting out.

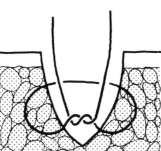

Fig. 10.24. Deep sutures with buried knot.

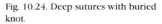

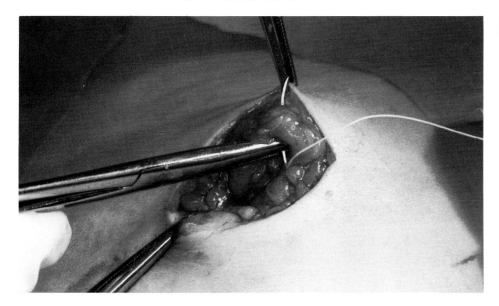

Fig. 10.25. Deep sutures with buried knot.

Suture ties

In general, two throws are quite safe for braided sutures but all monofilament sutures will require at least three throws.

Instrument tie

Having passed the suture through the wound, a short length of 3–4 cm should be left protruding through the skin. This makes it easy for the needle holder both to catch hold of the free end and to pull the free end through the coiled end. To avoid

Fig. 10.26. Instrument tie: leaving a
short end.

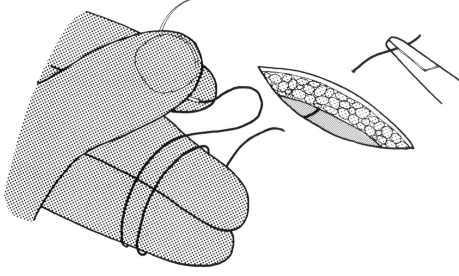

Fig. 10.27. Instrument tie.

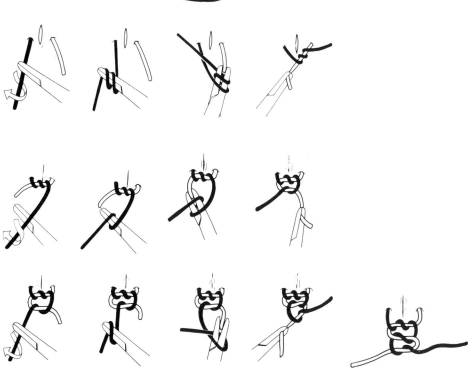

the suture being accidentally pulled right through the skin, the end of the suture
should be held with the needle holder while the needle end of the suture is
'reeled' around the left hand (Figs. 10.26, 10.27).

Hand tie

One-handed ties can be practised by using a piece of string tied to the back of a
chair or drawer handle. The illustrations (see Fig. 10.28) provided should be
scanned across the page to give an idea of motion. Both ends of the suture should

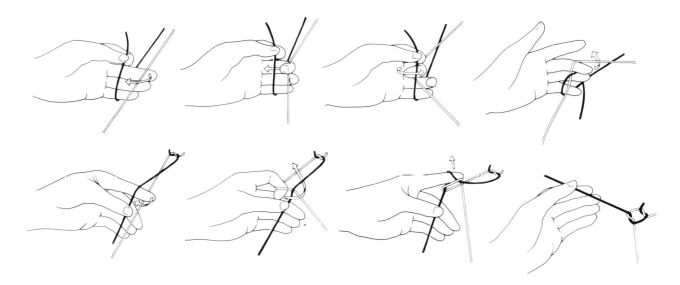

Fig. 10.28. Hand tie.

be kept taut as any slack will make things more difficult. Note that as each turn is made, the hand and suture are automatically in the correct position for the next turn to be started (Fig. 10.28).

Suture removal

Most wounds will require support with sutures for at least 7–10 days. Sutures on the face and neck can often be removed far earlier, between 3–7 days depending on the local skin tension (see Table 10.1) (Fig. 10.29).

Table 10.1. *Suture removal times postoperatively*

Suture site	Time (days)
Extensor surfaces	10–14
Flexor surfaces	5–7
Face	3–7
Scalp	7–10
Scapular area	10–14
Back	7–14

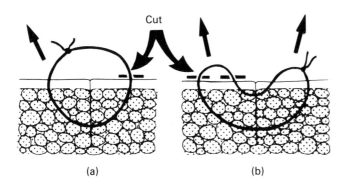

(a)   (b)

Fig. 10.29. Removal of sutures: (a) simple suture, (b) vertical mattress suture.

The longer sutures are left *in situ*, the more likely it is that residual suture track or 'ladder' markings will occur. Adhesive tapes can be extremely useful in allowing skin sutures to be removed early and thereby reducing cross-markings. It is always wise to remove a few sutures from different points along the wound to confirm that the wound has indeed healed. If at any stage during suture removal the wound edges gape, or if healing is suspect, the remaining sutures should be left in place and the wound supported with adhesive tapes for a few more days. At this stage ordinary 1 cm wide adhesive tape such as Micropore can be used as sterile adhesive tapes are not necessary.

Whenever there are tight sutures present there is an increased likelihood of wound or suture track infection. Tight sutures should be removed at the earliest opportunity (leaving any good sutures in place) and the wound supported with adhesive tapes.

When subcuticular sutures are removed, one end should be held and pulled with an artery clip in a controlled gradual way, while counter-pressure is applied to the wound with a finger. The suture should slide out easily and care should be taken if there is any resistance as the suture may break. Breakage is rare but if it does occur the suture line can often be opened up slightly at one point with the tip of a no. 11 blade and the suture grasped and removed with an artery clip.

When removing adhesive tapes if one end is lifted up and then pulled across the wound this will tend to pull the wound open (Fig. 10.30). Instead, both ends should be lifted together and towards the wound, with a finger applying counter-pressure to the wound itself.

Fig. 10.30. Removing adhesive tapes: (a) correct, (b) incorrect, this will tend to pull the wound edges apart.

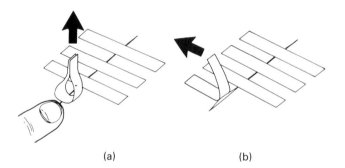

(a)   (b)

Drains and wicks

It is rarely necessary to leave a drain in a minor surgical wound. However, a plastic tube may occasionally be used for 24 h to drain the cavity after removal of a large lipoma. More commonly, a paraffin gauze wick may be used for 24–48 h in one end of a contaminated wound after removal of an infected sebaceous cyst or following drainage of an abscess.

Wound dressings

Most wounds will have sealed themselves with a crust within 24–48 h and therefore any gauze dressing may be removed at that time to allow light washing or exposure to the air. Some wounds on sites on the body such as the axilla and groin (which are prone to sweating), the buttock and sole of the foot (which are subjected to pressure), and the trunk (where clothing may be soiled) may be covered as necessary using a light gauze or simple plaster until the sutures are removed.

Most wounds can be covered with a simple fold of gauze held with an adhesive tape such as Micropore. Hypafix is a particularly useful adhesive sheet for holding down dressings as it conforms easily to different contours and is very secure. Hypafix comes in rolls and can be cut to suit the size of the dressing. For patients who are sensitive to most tapes, Dermicel tape is often well tolerated (Fig. 10.31).

Raw and granulating wounds should first be covered with a non-adherent layer such as paraffin tulle gauze, either plain or impregnated with chlorhexidine (e.g. Bactigras), or iodine impregnated rayon gauze (e.g. Inadine) (Fig. 10.32).

Bleeding surfaces such as slice wounds on the finger tip can be covered with alginate fibres (e.g. Kaltostat), which do not need to be removed but can be left to separate spontaneously.

Plastic aerosol sprays (e.g. Nobecutane) are occasionally useful for sealing wounds, for example on the scalp, where dressings would be difficult to retain.

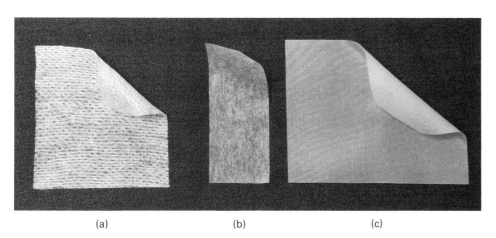

(a)   (b)   (c)

Fig. 10.31. (a) Hypafix adhesive sheet, (b) Micropore tape, (c) Dermicel adhesive sheet.

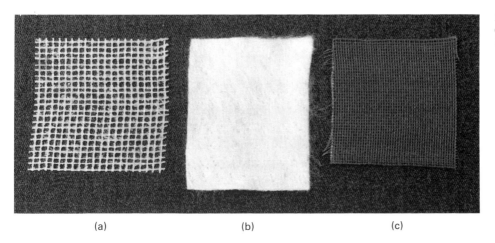

(a)   (b)   (c)

Fig. 10.32. (a) Bactigras tulle gauze, (b) Kaltostat alginate sheet, (c) Inadine rayon gauze.

References

1. Use of cyanoacrylate tissue adhesive for closing facial lacerations in children. Watson, D. P. *British Medical Journal* (1989), **299**, 1014.
2. Use of Histoacryl tissue adhesive to manage an avulsed tooth. McCabe, M. J. *British Medical Journal* (1990), **301** 20–21.
3. Use of Histoacryl tissue adhesive for primary closure of scalp wounds. Morton, R. J., Gibson, M. F. & Sloan, J. P. *Archives of Emergency Medicine* (1988), **5**, 110–112.
4. Tissue adhesive vs sutures in closure of incision wounds. A comparative study in human skin. Alhopuro, S., Rintala, A., Salo, H. & Ritsiha, V. *Annales Chirurgiae et Gynaecologiae* (1976), **65**, 308–312.

11

Surgical techniques: Cautery and curettage

Chemical cautery

Chemical cautery can be very effective in a number of clinical applications but it is most important to ensure against accidental contact and to keep children well away from storage areas and during treatment. Except in a few specific circumstances chemical cautery should not be used near the eyes or near the external urethral meatus. When chemical cautery is used on skin lesions, the surrounding skin should be protected by, for example, a layer of petroleum jelly.

Silver nitrate

Silver nitrate sticks are convenient for treating small areas such as: overgranulations after removal of splinters, or nail spicules or following surgery; raw areas after excision of skin tags; and Little's area in epistaxis, provided that bleeding has stopped. They are of little use when there is active bleeding. The patient should be warned that application causes unpleasant stinging.

A moist area can be treated by applying the silver nitrate stick directly onto the site. If the surface is dry it is necessary for the stick to be moistened first. Especially during cauterisation of Little's area, great care must be taken not to allow the silver nitrate to flow away, deeper into the nose (Fig. 11.1). It is wise to place the

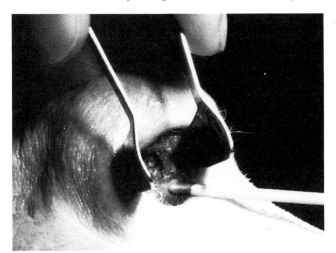

Fig. 11.1. Silver nitrate stick being used for cauterisation of Little's area.

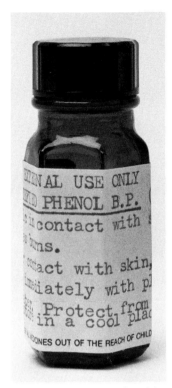

Fig. 11.2. Phenol (80%) for superficial cautery. Note that this concentration will cause tissue necrosis if inadvertently injected into the tissues.

patient's head flat to one side and to place a small pack beyond Little's area to minimise the risk.

Phenol

Chemical cautery with 80% phenol for 3–5 minutes is the treatment of choice in ingrowing toenails (Fig. 11.2a). A gauze swab soaked in methylated spirits and wrapped around the tip of the toe will effectively neutralise any excess phenol. Phenol can also be applied to a raw bed after curettage to obtain haemostasis, or pricked into viral warts or molluscum contagiosum.

Care should be taken to avoid splashing phenol while it is being poured, and to avoid spilling it onto normal skin (of patient or surgeon). Within a few seconds of contact the skin will turn white. Superficial peeling will eventually occur if contact is maintained for more than a few seconds.

The 80% phenol used for superficial chemical cautery should not be confused with the 5% phenol in oil used for injecting haemorrhoids (injection of 80% phenol into the rectal submucosa will result in severe necrosis of the rectal wall).

Trichloroacetic acid

A 33–50% solution of trichloroacetic acid can be carefully applied to areas of xanthelasma with a fine cotton bud. It can also be used to cauterise the raw surface after curettage or shave biopsy. As with salicylic acid, trichloroacetic acid can be pricked into viral warts or molluscum contagiosum with a wooden stick. The procedure results in localised swelling, erythema and tissue necrosis, and the process can be repeated after 1–2 weeks if necessary.

Aluminium chloride

Aluminium chloride (35% (w/v) in isopropyl alcohol) can be used to cauterise the raw surface after curettage or shave biopsy.

Electrocautery

Electrocautery (Fig. 11.3) is useful for treating small skin lesions, resistant solitary viral warts, and bleeding in epistaxis. It operates by passing a current through a high resistance, resulting in a heating effect. No current passes through the patient, but care needs to be taken to safeguard against accidental burns to both patient and surgeon, since the tip is hot and remains so for some time after being switched off. The cautery tips come in different sizes and shapes and these may need to be bent to a convenient angle before use. *Note that since electrocautery is a destructive technique, no unidentified lesion should be treated without histological confirmation.*

A standard wire loop or flat tip can be used for general purpose cautery such as after curettage or shave biopsy, in epistaxis, for amputating the bases of skin

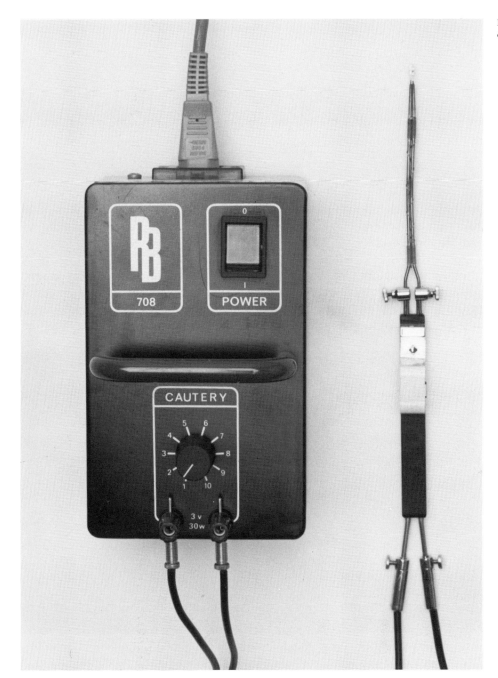

Fig. 11.3. Mains powered
electrocautery unit.

Electrocautery or diathermy *must not* be used

1. If the diagnosis is in doubt.
2. On any malignant skin tumour.
3. On any suspicious pigmented lesion.
4. To destroy any lesion, thus preventing histological confirmation.

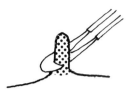

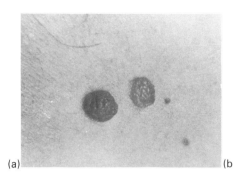

(a)

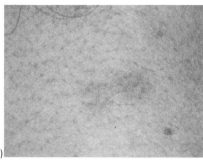

(b)

Fig. 11.4. (ABOVE) Amputation of skin tag using electrocautery.

Fig. 11.5. (ABOVE, CENTRE AND RIGHT) Electrocautery of congenital papillomata on the neck: (a) before treatment; (b) 3 months after treatment.

tags and pedunculated lesions (Figs. 11.4, 11.5), or for dealing with small haemangiomata (Fig. 11.6). A ball-ended tip, may be used for cautery of the raw bed after curettage.

Superficial electrocautery can be applied to a seborrhoeic keratosis as an alternative to cryotherapy. A pinpoint tip can be inserted into the feeding vessel of a spider naevus. To avoid accidents it is necessary to place the tip into the centre of the lesion prior to the application of the current. Care should be taken to use only a short burn to minimise any resultant pitting.

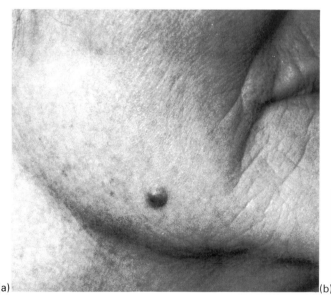

(a)

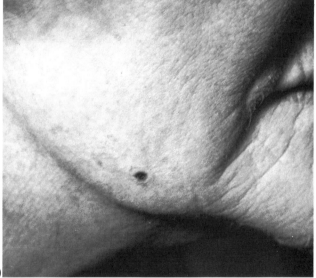

(b)

Fig. 11.6. Electrocautery to haemangioma on the face: (a) before treatment, (b) immediately after treatment.

Diathermy

For most purposes, diathermy is both a more controllable and a more versatile technique than electrocautery. The Birtcher Hyfrecator is purpose-made for minor surgery and is extremely easy to use. *Note that since diathermy is a destructive technique, no unidentified lesion should be treated without histological confirmation.*

Local infiltration or surface anaesthesia is usually necessary, although some patients may easily tolerate light diathermy to superficial lesions such as a spider naevus or tiny skin tags without any anaesthesia. When the doctor is learning to use diathermy, the power should be set low and slowly increased to achieve the desired effect. Skin preparation is not required for treating skin lesions, but, if it is used, any alcohol should be allowed to evaporate first, as it is combustible. Destruction of superficial skin lesions leaves a charred surface that usually needs no covering, heals well within 1–2 weeks and leaves little scarring.

There are two techniques in using diathermy, monopolar or bipolar.

Monopolar techniques

The monopolar (or monoterminal) technique uses a high frequency, high voltage current that discharges from one electrode to the patient. A footswitch may be used but a switching handle is often more convenient (Fig. 11.7).

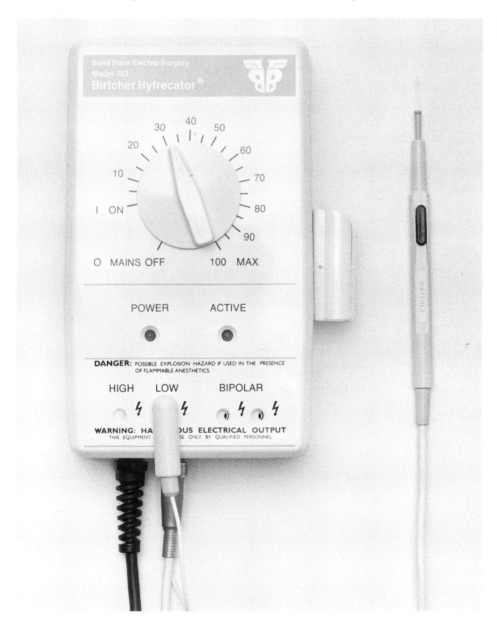

Fig. 11.7. Birtcher Hyfrecator in unipolar mode.

Desiccation The electrode is held in surface contact or inserted into the tissue. The process produces evaporation of tissue fluids followed by tissue charring. Generally, the thinner the needle, the deeper is the tissue penetration. The method can be used to good effect to treat small lesions such as spider naevi (Fig. 11.8), thread veins, molluscum contagiosum, xanthelasma, and epistaxis.

Fig. 11.8. Desiccation of a spider naevus using diathermy.

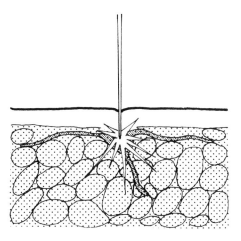

Fulgaration The electrode is held slightly out of contact with the lesion being treated, thus causing an electrical arc to the surface (Fig. 11.9). Tissue destruction is limited to the shallow area under the spark. Care should be taken to position the electrode accurately over the lesion and away from adjacent tissue or metal objects as this may divert the spark. Light fulgaration, for example, may be used to treat minor cervical erosions and superficial skin lesions such as solar keratoses.

Fig. 11.9. Fulgaration (from the Latin *fulgaratio*, to strike with lightning).

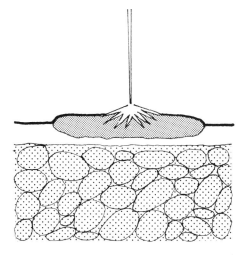

Indifferent electrode mode This involves using a large flat electrode (indifferent) in contact with the patient and applying a fine (active) electrode to the site to be coagulated (Fig. 11.10). The current is concentrated in the region of the fine electrode and creates local heat. No heat is generated at the indifferent electrode because of its large surface area. This method is commonly employed in more involved surgery and has little application in general practice.

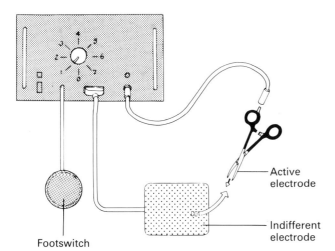

Fig. 11.10. Diathermy in indifferent electrode mode.

Active electrode

Indifferent electrode

Footswitch

Monoterminal static shock The monopolar (or monoterminal) method uses a high frequency, high voltage current that discharges from one electrode to the patient and the return path for the current is through the patient's body capacity and via garments and shoes, to ground and back to the instrument. Since the current always takes the path of least electrical resistance, any portion of the patient's body coming into contact with ground while the current is flowing may receive a burn or shock. Similarly, if the doctor touches or breaks contact with the patient during the time when the current is flowing through the patient's body, a shock may be felt by the doctor.

Thus, there are a few simple rules to follow to avoid the risk of shock: the patient should not lie on a grounded table or sit on a metal chair; the patient should not come into contact with any grounded metal objects; and, if the doctor must touch the patient, contact should be made *before* the current is switched on and contact should not be broken while current is flowing [1].

How to avoid monoterminal static shock

1. The patient should not lie on a grounded table or sit on a metal chair.
2. If necessary, touch the patient *before* the current is switched on.
3. Do not break contact with the patient while the current is flowing.

Bipolar techniques

The bipolar (or biterminal) method involves passing a high frequency current between the two insulated halves of the special bipolar forceps, which require activation with a footswitch (Figs. 11.11, 11.12, 11.13).

The use of special bipolar forceps is an excellent method for treating many skin lesions. For example, the pedicle of a pedunculated papilloma may be first crushed with an artery clip, and then coagulated and amputated by the current between the tips of the bipolar forceps; the base can be coagulated after shave

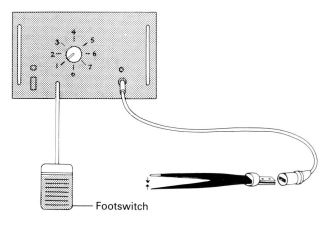

Fig. 11.11. Diathermy in bipolar mode.

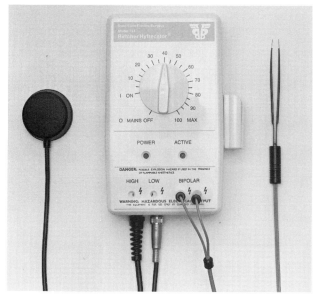

Fig. 11.12. Birtcher Hyfrecator in bipolar mode.

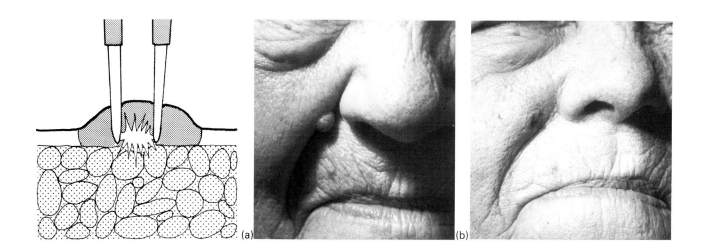

Fig. 11.13. Bipolar coagulation.

Fig. 11.14. Shave biopsy and bipolar diathermy of intradermal naevus: (a) before treatment, (b) immediately after treatment.

biopsy of an intradermal naevus until the site of the lesion is flat with the surroundings (Fig. 11.14). The final results are far superior to elliptical excision. Simple shave biopsy can result in unnecessary bleeding from the raw surface. This bleeding can be avoided by using the arc of the bipolar forceps actually to amputate the lesion flush with the skin surface. Although cryotherapy is the treatment of choice in seborrhoeic keratoses, these can be easily treated by superficial electrocautery or diathermy after local anaesthetic infiltration. The lesion will be seen to 'bubble up' under the bipolar diathermy forceps, and in so doing, separate itself from the underlying skin, which only then needs a further slight treatment to ensure complete removal.

Curettage

Curettage under local anaesthesia is a valid alternative technique for a number of skin conditions such as viral warts, seborrhoeic keratosis, actinic keratosis, keratoacanthoma and pyogenic granuloma. *In specialist hands* curettage is useful for basal cell carcinomas on areas where there is little spare or loose skin such as on the tip of the nose, ears, forehead and temple. However, it must be remembered that excision with primary suture usually takes no more time and results in a sealed wound that can be left exposed after 24–48 h. Curettage usually results in a circular wound that heals by secondary intention. Although it is sometimes surprising how neat the final result can be the method should be avoided near the eyelids, eyebrows and the mouth, as skin distortion may occur.

Obtaining a plane of cleavage is usually easy with seborrhoeic warts but it can be impossible with lesions such as viral warts. A sharp curette is essential and it is a useful technique first to encircle the edges of the lesion with an incision with a no. 11 blade prior to the curettage (Fig. 11.15).

The skin should be tensed on either side of the lesion and the lesion scraped away down to the dermis. If possible, the lesion should be removed as one piece of tissue. The dermis has a white appearance that feels 'scratchy' under the curette. The curettings should be sent for histological examination. After the curettage, the raw base should be cauterised either with diathermy or electrocautery. An alternative is to apply 80% phenol or 33–50% trichloroacetic acid to obtain haemostasis. The cauterised base is then curetted once more to ensure complete removal of the lesion and the base cauterised again to stop any bleeding. All curettings should be sent for histological examination.

Healing is by secondary intention. Curetted areas on the face can be left exposed, while those elsewhere may need to be covered with a light dry dressing. The patient should be advised that a crust will form that may take 2–3 weeks to separate off.

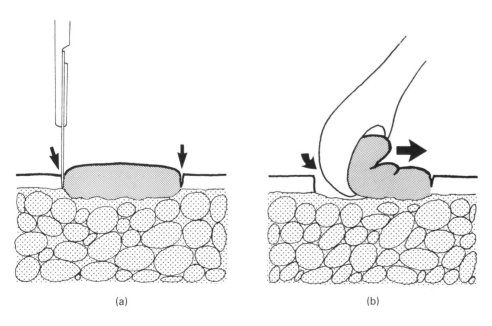

Fig. 11.15. (a) and (b) Curettage of a skin lesion.

(a)   (b)

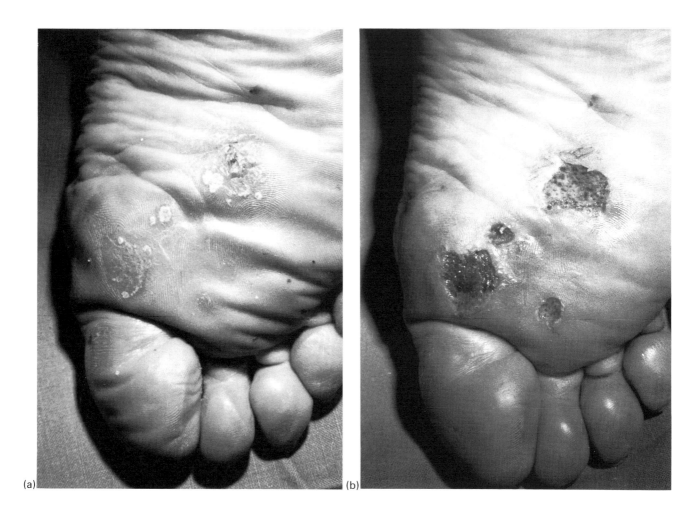

(a)   (b)

Fig. 11.16. Curettage followed by
diathermy to multiple separate viral
warts, under posterior tibial nerve
block. (a) These warts were very
painful and were resistant to topical
treatments and cryotherapy, hence
the patient elected to have the warts
curetted and was prepared to accept
the postoperative discomfort. (b)
Immediately after curettage and
diathermy. (c) Seven days after
curettage. (d) Five weeks after
curettage. Most of the areas have
only shallow crusts remaining.

Specific lesions

Viral warts Curettage of viral warts should be reserved for solitary persistent and
problematical lesions only (Fig. 11.16). It is preferable to try cryotherapy under
local anaesthesia first as recurrence can occur even after deep and careful
curettage.

Seborrhoeic keratosis Curettage of seborrhoeic keratosis need only be light as
the lesion is superficial. However, cryotherapy is faster, easier, causes no bleeding
and is the treatment of choice.

Keratoacanthoma Curettage of keratoacanthoma must be combined with a
biopsy as the tumour can be mistaken for a squamous cell carcinoma.

Pyogenic granuloma These lesions are particularly liable to bleed profusely
after curettage. Therefore, lesions on digits should be removed using a tourniquet;
adrenaline should be used with the local anaesthetic for lesions elsewhere. In
addition, firm finger pressure maintained at either side of the lesion can help
minimise bleeding during the procedure.

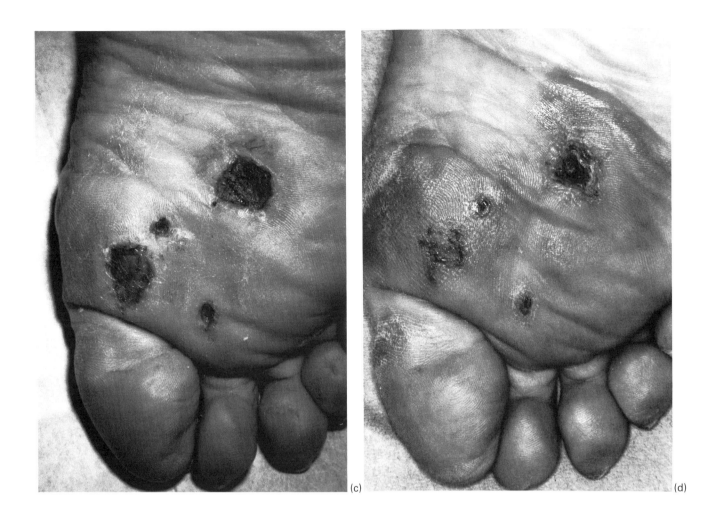

(c)

(d)

Reference

1. Monoterminal shock. *Birtcher Hyfrecator Manual* (1987). Birtcher
Corporation, 4501 N. Arden Drive, PO Box 4399, Elmonte, CA 91734, USA.

12

Surgical techniques: Cryotherapy

Introduction

Cryotherapy is an effective and well established technique and is eminently suitable for use in the general practice setting and can result in significant reductions in hospital referrals. However, *since cryotherapy is a destructive technique, no unidentified lesion should be treated without histological confirmation.*

Subjecting living tissues to low temperatures results in varying degrees of cell trauma. Cell damage is governed primarily by the rate of change in temperature (both during the freezing phase and to a greater extent, during the thawing phase) rather than by the degree of cooling achieved. Indeed, as is well known, living tissues can be preserved and remain viable at very low temperatures if the temperature is slowly reduced. The factors that cause cellular injury include the production of intracellular ice crystals, rapid electrolyte concentration changes, disruption of cell membranes and also the capillary, lymphatic and venous vessel occlusion that result in tissue anoxia. Connective tissue distortion is minimal after cryotherapy, this results in minimal residual scarring compared with other treatments such as electrocautery.

A number of cooling agents have been used in the past, for example, salt–ice mixture ($-20\,^{\circ}$C) and carbon dioxide snow ($-80\,^{\circ}$C). Liquid nitrogen ($-196\,^{\circ}$C) is both extremely effective and easy to use, either with a cotton bud or with a cryospray or cryoprobe as in the CRY-AC range of instruments.

Recently, gases such as dimethyl ether mixed with propane have been combined in convenient aerosols, for example, the Histofreezer.

When cryotherapy is applied to skin lesions, depending on the individual and the treatment site, the patient may experience a feeling varying from slight discomfort to severe pain. Therefore, when a doctor is using cryotherapy for the first time it may be helpful to experience the nature of the stinging and discomfort it causes by a short application of the cryogen to the operator's own forearm.

Treatable conditions

A wide range of conditions can be easily treated such as viral warts, skin tags, cutaneous horns, solar keratoses, molluscum contagiosum, seborrhoeic keratoses, papillomata, keratoacanthoma, benign naevi and cervical erosions.

Basal cell carcinomata, squamous cell carcinomata and suspicious pigmented lesions should be referred to a dermatologist.

It is more convenient and efficient to treat patients within a specific treatment session, although occasional patients could easily be treated as they present in the surgery.

Treatable conditions

Skin tag	Chondrodermatitis
Cutaneous horn	Keratoacanthoma
Haemangioma	Bowen's disease
Viral warts	Papilloma
Solar keratosis	Benign naevus
Molluscum contagiosum	Xanthelasma
Pyogenic granuloma	Cervical erosions
Seborrhoeic keratosis	Condylomata acuminata

(This list is not exhaustive.)

Liquid nitrogen

Liquid nitrogen is colourless, odourless, non-inflammable and inert to most chemicals. Liquid nitrogen boils at $-196\,°C$ and the skin temperature during treatment with the cryoprobe or spray may go down to $-40\,°C$. The treatment usually causes stinging and discomfort and it may be quite painful. Usually, the pain is felt once the ice-ball has formed. Sometimes, and especially in the treatment of lesions on the feet, significant pain may be felt for many hours afterwards and even over the following few days. For this reason, the treatment is generally best avoided in young children. In addition, young children might find the hissing and the spray itself particularly frightening. It is sometimes helpful for the doctor to demonstrate a touch of the cotton bud or a short burst of cryospray on his or her own or a parent's arm to reassure the young or anxious patient that treatment is quite unlike contact with steam or boiling water. In addition, a child might be reassuringly amused by a gentle flick of a cotton bud that allows a few globules of liquid nitrogen to fall onto a table surface and dart about while evaporating. An older child might be interested to know that the liquid nitrogen is so cold that if a tomato were to be put into the container and then thrown onto the floor, it would shatter like ice and then become a mushy mess once it had thawed.

Theoretically, just about any lesion could be dealt with by only one treatment. However, the degree of freezing achieved is often limited by pain and therefore a number of treatments at intervals of 1 to 3 weeks are likely to be necessary. In particular, patients with verrucae usually need to have multiple treatments. Some lesions may require the use of a local anaesthetic. Treatment of viral warts on finger tips and particularly those extending under the nails can be extremely painful and it is often kinder to use a digital nerve block. It is also sometimes wise only to treat one hand or foot at a time.

Lesions on any part of the body may be treated but the cryospray should be avoided near the eyes. Particular care should be taken to avoid vulnerable subcutaneous structures being incorporated into the ice ball. Cartilage necrosis can occur when lesions on the ear or nose are frozen. Finger joint stiffness may occur if freezing extends deep enough to involve joint capsules. Extensor tendon rupture may occur after treament over the dorsum of the hands and feet. However, if the skin is mobile, it is often possible to lift up the skin and pull the lesion away from an underlying tendon prior to freezing. Subcutaneous nerves are at risk near the medial epicondyle (ulnar nerve), sides of fingers and toes (digital nerves), and below the fibula head (common peroneal nerve).

The ice ball should extend to include a few millimetres of normal skin around the lesion (Fig. 12.1). Multiple freeze thaw cycles may be used to effect greater tissue destruction. *However, to maximize tissue destruction, it is important to allow complete thawing to occur prior to any second or subsequent freezing* [1]. For simplicity, the freezing time can be stated to start when the whole lesion is enveloped in an ice-ball and to finish when thawing starts.

No skin preparation is needed before treatment. The area can be washed normally after treatment and usually no dressings are required. Because the desired tissue damage is unrelated to the resultant inflammation, the use of a potent topical steroid cream (such as clobetasol proprinate) once or twice daily for a few days can be used to help reduce oedema and blistering [2]. Mild analgesics such as Co-proxamol may be required for a few days in some patients. A note may be made of both the freezing time and the number of freeze thaw cycles used. This may be of particular value while the doctor is building up experience in the method.

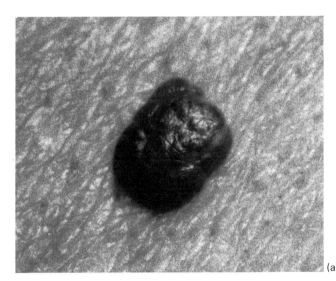
(a)

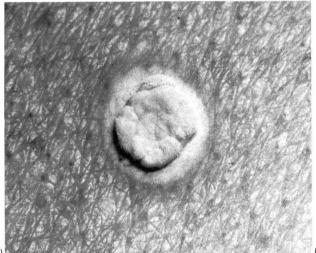
(b)

Cryobiopsy

In most circumstances where a tissue diagnosis is necessary simple excision or shave biopsy under a local anaesthetic is recommended. However, since freezing does not result in major changes in tissue architecture, a lesion can be curetted while it is frozen, allowed to thaw out and placed in formalin, as with any other tissue biopsy. Note that occasionally the raw bed can bleed after thawing, and this may require cauterisation.

Fig. 12.1. The ice ball should extend to include a few millimetres of normal skin around the lesion. (a) and (b) Treatment of a Campbell de Morgan spot (magnified).

Cotton bud

Although there are more effective techniques in cryotherapy (see below), nevertheless the cotton bud method is both inexpensive and effective for a number of superficial skin lesions. Despite being relatively slow to apply, it is a satisfactory method for use in a practice where there is a limited case-load and the cost of a cryospray is prohibitive (Fig. 12.2). Ordinary small commercial cotton buds cannot hold enough liquid nitrogen to be effective. A loose, bulky, non-compacted cotton bud is necessary and may have to be purpose-made using loose cotton wool wrapped around a small wooden stick. When dipped into liquid nitrogen and applied directly to the skin this is a cheap but rather slow method and is only generally suitable for more superficial lesions as its freezing action does not penetrate much below 2–3 mm.

A new cotton bud should be used for each patient treated as virus particles can be transferred between individuals resulting in warts in previously unaffected patients [3]. Liquid nitrogen does not kill the virus particles and infective virus can be recovered from the bottom of a totally thawed flask (but not from a full container). In theory tissue debris (which accumulates at the bottom of a container) could be picked up by a cotton bud dipped into a virtually empty flask. It is therefore recommended that cotton buds may be dipped into the main Dewar

Fig. 12.2. Liquid nitrogen flask and cotton buds.

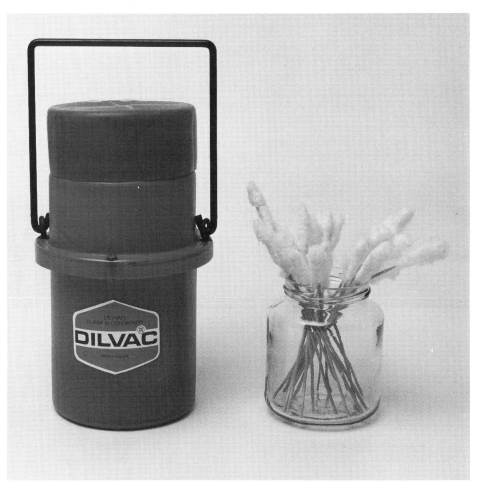

flask, provided that it is kept well filled, or alternatively the liquid nitrogen should be dispensed into a disposable vessel (such as a polystyrene cup) or a small dish which is cleaned between patients [4].

Ideally, the cotton bud should be held vertically onto the lesion to allow maximal freezing action. If the bud is held horizontally, for example when areas on the trunk are to be treated and with the patient in the sitting position, there will be a risk of the liquid nitrogen dripping and perhaps falling elsewhere on the patient (Figs. 12.3, 12.4).

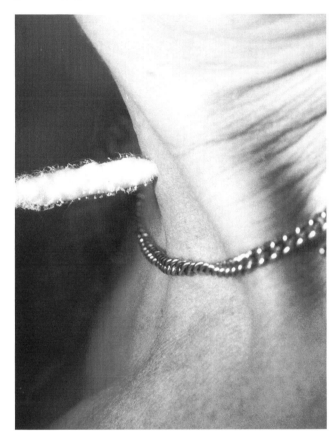

Fig. 12.3. When the cotton bud is held horizontally there is a risk of liquid nitrogen dripping elsewhere on the patient.

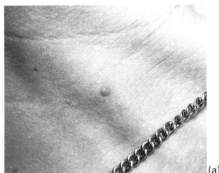 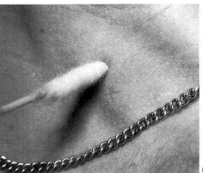 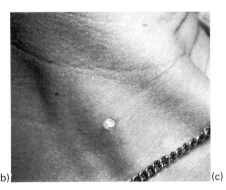

(a)   (b)   (c)

Small lesions As a good bulk of cotton wool is needed to carry enough liquid nitrogen, it is sometimes difficult to treat small lesions (e.g. skin tags) without unnecessary freezing of surrounding normal skin. Although this does not do any

Fig. 12.4. (a–c) Liquid nitrogen treatment to a papule using the cotton bud method.

real harm, nevertheless, it may give rise to wider areas of subsequent depigmentation, and consideration should be given to an alternative method of treatment, such as cautery or diathermy.

Large lesions Larger lesions, such as broad seborrhoeic keratoses on the trunk may be treated by asking the patient to lie down and the cotton bud is then held almost horizontally such that the maximal area of the bud is in contact with the lesion. In addition, a broad lesion may be treated by simply freezing in sections.

Cryospray

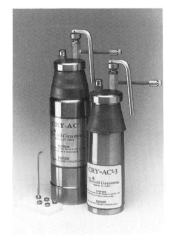

Fig. 12.5. CRY-AC Cryospray unit.

Fig. 12.6. (a) and (b) Use of cryospray to treat a seborrhoeic keratosis.

For the routine treatment of skin lesions and verrucae, the cryospray is certainly the quickest and most efficient method of using liquid nitrogen. The cryospray apparatus comprises a hand-held container with a trigger and valve system that allows the liquid nitrogen to escape as a spray through a fine nozzle (Figs. 12.5, 12.6).

The nozzle should be held approximately 5–10 cm from the lesion, and care taken not to spray near the eyes or onto normal skin. A number of different nozzle sizes can be obtained, but, with a general-purpose nozzle and a little practice, the diameter of the ice-ball can be matched to the size of the lesion by varying the distance of the nozzle from the lesion and by spraying in short bursts. Small lesions can also be treated with the use of truncated cones (or auroscope earpieces) to limit the spread of the spray. Another method of protecting adjacent normal skin is to encircle the lesion with adhesive putty (such as Blu-tack). Pedunculated lesions can be treated by first lifting the lesion away from the skin and directing the spray to the stalk (Fig. 12.7). In the treatment of lesions near the eyes, it is preferable to use an angled cryospray extension (Fig. 12.8).

Continuous use of the cryospray over many minutes (for example when treating multiple lesions) can result in the nozzle icing over. However, de-icing can be achieved by simply dipping the nozzle into a bowl of water at room-temperature.

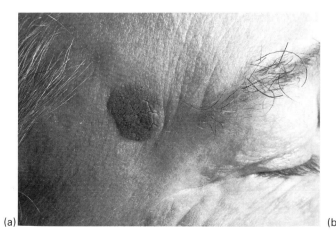

(a)

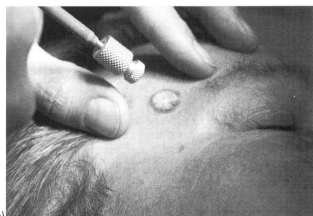

(b)

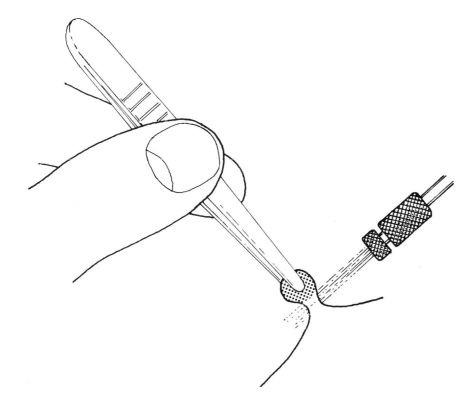

Fig. 12.7. Cryospray directed to the stalk of a pedunculated lesion.

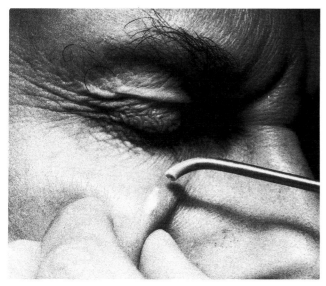

Fig. 12.8. Using an angled cryospray extension near the eyes.

Cryoprobe

The cryoprobe may be obtained either as a desk-top container connected by tubes to a hand-held trigger and metal probe (Fig. 12.9), or, more conveniently, as the cryospray hand unit but with a probe head attachment. The liquid nitrogen is allowed to escape by passing within the probe and it cools the probe in the process.

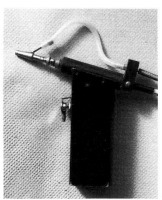

Fig. 12.9. Cryoprobe hand unit.

Only very superficial and ineffective cooling can be obtained by simply
applying the dry probe to the skin. Therefore, a dab of water-based gel has to be
applied either to the probe or to the lesion itself and the probe then placed in
contact with the lesion (Figs. 12.10, 12.11). When the liquid nitrogen is passed
through the probe, the gel freezes and causes the probe to adhere to the lesion.
Continued cooling causes the ice-ball to expand into and around the lesion.
During the freezing, the skin and probe become very firmly attached and
no attempt should be made to pull the probe free until the tissue has thawed.
Care should be taken during the treatment of lesions over tendons and joint
capsules. Once the probe has adhered to the lesion, the lesion should be lifted up
away from the underlying structures. In addition, care should be taken not to
over-freeze a lesion as defrosting may be protracted, with resultant unnecessary
tissue damage.

Use of the cryoprobe is more time-consuming than use of the cryospray and is
best for selected skin lesions near the eyes and for mucosal and cervical lesions.

Fig. 12.10. Cryoprobe and iceball.

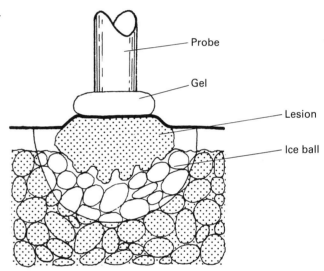

Fig. 12.11. (a) Cryoprobe with gel,
(b) cryoprobe with frozen gel, (c)
cryoprobe with iceball in tissue.

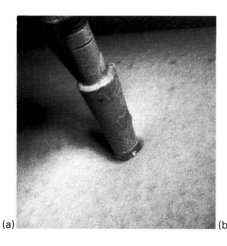 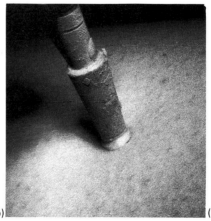 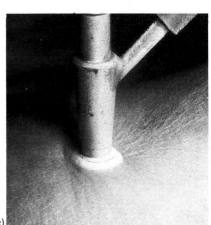

(a)   (b)   (c)

Aerosol sprays

The cost of purchasing liquid nitrogen and its delivery and storage systems can be prohibitive. Recently, however, convenient aerosols have become available e.g. the Histofreezer (Fig. 12.12) (which uses a mixture of the gases dimethyl ether and propane) and the Freon 12 (which uses dichlorodifluoromethane) [5], and these may be preferable to liquid nitrogen for many practices. The gas is allowed to escape through a hollow tube that leads to a cotton wool or foam bud. Treatment should be given in a well ventilated room as the gas used in the Histofreezer is highly inflammable, care should be taken to avoid repeated inhalation of waste gas. The bud serves as a reservoir for the coolant and can reach a temperature of −50 °C. The Histofreezer aerosols contain enough gas to treat about 40 lesions. The units can be stored for up to 3 years and are disposable after use.

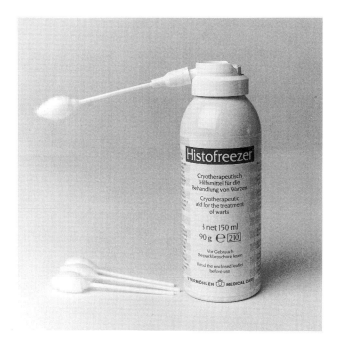

Fig. 12.12. Histofreezer.

The technique is essentially similar to that of a cotton bud with liquid nitrogen. The canister is first held upright and the gas is sprayed into the cotton or foam bud until droplets appear. The bud is then placed vertically in contact with the lesion while slight pressure is applied. If the cotton bud is topped up several times, the bud may become so saturated that ice crystals prevent aerosol function. Although aerosols are convenient to store and use, their use is limited in that freezing of only superficial lesions is possible. Since the contact of the bud with the skin results in a freeze area roughly 1 cm in diameter, it requires some practice to freeze small lesions without causing unnecessary damage to surrounding normal skin. As with liquid nitrogen, a number of treatments may be necessary at intervals of 1–3 weeks.

Clinical effects and frequency of treatment

Shortly after thawing, the lesion may show no sign whatsoever that any treatment has taken place. However, after several minutes an area of erythema may be seen surrounding the lesion. Over the next few hours the area will show signs of acute inflammation and over the next few days the lesion will either tend to shrivel or blistering will occur (Fig. 12.13).

If no change is evident within 48 h, it is probable that the treatment has been insufficient. This is particularly common after treating verrucae if the extent of freezing was limited by pain. Indeed, it is usually advisable to avoid treatment in the young or those with a low pain threshold as a short and superficial freeze of verrucae merely causes pain without any significant benefit.

The patient should be asked to return the following week for repeat treatment if there is no significant change visible. If there is some damage but no blistering or crusting (suggesting insufficient tissue destruction), the patient should be reviewed after 2 weeks for assessment and further treatment if required. If

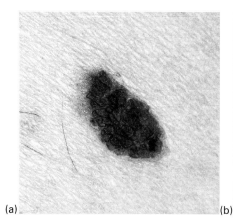
(a)

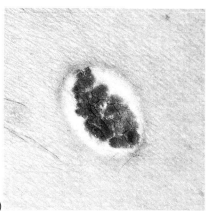
(b)

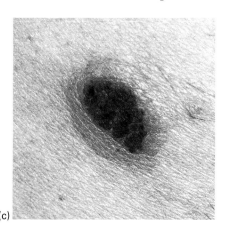
(c)

Fig. 12.13. Effect of liquid nitrogen: (a) seborrhoeic keratosis, (b) the frozen lesion, (c) early blistering is in evidence after 30 min, (d) crusting seen 2 weeks after treatment of verrucae.

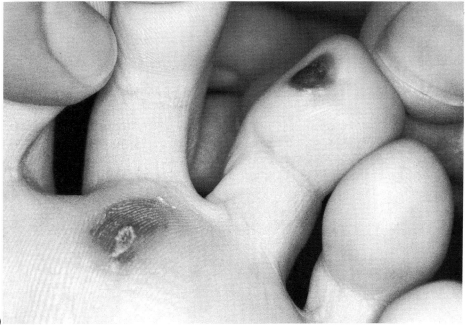
(d)

blistering does occur, review should be left for about 3 weeks to allow separation of any crust and at that time treatment may be repeated, if necessary. Simple leaflets with information regarding the nature of the treatment and what to expect are useful and may be given out for patients to read before they attend for their treatment.

Patient information leaflet
Cryotherapy treatment

Freezing with liquid nitrogen or freezing sprays destroys tissue by producing a localised area of frostbite.

Treatment usually only causes stinging, although occasionally it can be painful. Any discomfort can sometimes last for 24–48 hours. For this reason, cryotherapy is best avoided in young children.

Usually, treatment is given once every 2–3 weeks. In the treatment of warts and verrucae, it is important not to leave the intervals between treatment sessions for too long as the warts will simply grow back to their full size again and any initial benefit will be lost completely.

Immediately after the treatment it may look as if nothing has happened, but after a while some redness, swelling and blistering should appear, this is a normal response to freezing. Most skin conditions will crust over and the crust will fall off after a few weeks.

No dressings are needed after treatment and there are no restrictions concerning washing. However, if blistering is excessive or uncomfortable, the blisters can be drained and a dressing applied as necessary.

Specific lesions

Some types of lesion are more easily treated than others. For example, superficial lesions such as flat seborrhoeic keratoses and solar keratoses require a once only treatment of 5–10 s of superficial freezing. Yet many plantar warts are very resistant to multiple treatments over many weeks.

Skin tags Multiple skin tags can be frozen off, but unless great care is taken when using a cotton bud or cryospray there is always a tendency of unnecessary freezing of surrounding skin and this may cause unsightly depigmentation around the neck. Use of the cryoprobe is too time-consuming for multiple small lesions. Tissue destruction is more controlled with electrocautery or diathermy but these techniques usually require a local anaesthetic (see chapter 11).

Molluscum contagiosum The treatment of choice is masterly inactivity or simple extrusion of the core. Alternatively, these multiple lesions can be dealt with by using a short and superficial freeze. Another alternative is to prick each lesion with a pointed stick dipped in phenol.

Dermatofibroma As dermatofibroma is a deep dermal lesion, cryotherapy tends to be ineffective unless a deep freeze is created. However, since these lesions occur most frequently on the legs in women, the resultant scarring and any pitting may be worse than the appearance of the lesion. A dermatofibroma should be excised (see chapter 15).

Mucoid cysts A mucoid cyst (ganglion) over the distal interphalangeal joints can be frozen but if the lesion is near the nail bed the patient should be warned that longitudinal ridging may result with subsequent growth of the nail. Cysts on the lips can be treated using the cryoprobe, or the cryospray with an extension tube to direct the spray away from the mouth.

Viral warts Around two thirds of warts resolve spontaneously within 2 years. Nevertheless, since warts can be unsightly, painful and extensive, and can be transmitted to others, most people prefer to have their warts treated. However, since effective treatment can sometimes be extremely painful and distressing, cryotherapy is best avoided in young children and other selected cases, where alternative medical treatment with keratolytics (such as salicylic acid, glutaraldehyde and formalin preparations) should be offered as first line treatment [6]. Patients should be prepared to pare the wart down and apply the preparation daily as sporadic application is likely to fail. It should be noted that despite appropriate treatment, resistant warts are common. Warts with a long history and a large size are likely to have a poor success rate. In such cases, alternative treatments such as pricking with phenol (80%) or tricholoroacetic acid (33–50%), or curettage should be considered (see chapter 11).

HANDS Warts on the hands and extensor surfaces are often easy to eradicate and may be cured by one session of two freeze–thaw cycles with 10 s of freezing time. However, subungual and fingertip warts can be extremely resistant and extremely painful to treat. It is kinder to use a digital nerve block, after which a deep freeze treatment is given. Afterwards, analgesics such as Co-proxamol should be given (Figs. 12.14, 12.15) and it may be helpful to rest the patient's hand in a high sling afterewards to reduce throbbing.

VERRUCAE Compared to warts on the hands, plantar viral warts are more resistant to cryotherapy and mosaic warts on the heels particularly so (Figs. 12.16, 12.17). These may require a number of double freeze–thaw cycles of 20 s over 1–3 week intervals. There is no purpose in giving multiple short and superficial freezes over intervals of a few weeks. Such treatment is often less painful but the damage to the wart is minimal and (just like incomplete eradication of weeds on a lawn) the wart simply grows back to its previous state by the time the next treatment is due. A balance has to be struck between deep freezing and any pain inflicted. Keratin is a good insulator, hence, prior to freezing, large lesions should be pared down to reduce tissue bulk and hence amount of freezing required. Usually, with adequate explanation and mild analgesics such as Co-proxamol afterwards, most older children and adults prefer to accept the pain for the benefit of eradicating the warts. Occasionally, with large solitary warts it may be appropriate to use a local anaesthetic. However, injections into the thick skin of the sole of the foot are themselves extremely painful and should be avoided. Instead, injections should, if possible, be made through the softer skin of the sides of the foot or a posterior tibial nerve block used to anaesthetise the sole. If available, Entonox can be used.

Condylomata acuminata As an alternative to painting with podophyllin these can be treated as warts elsewhere, either with the cryospray or cryoprobe.

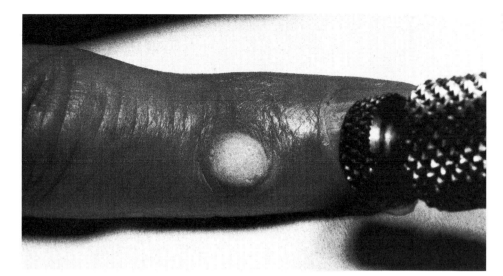

Fig. 12.14. Liquid nitrogen spray treatment to a wart on the finger.

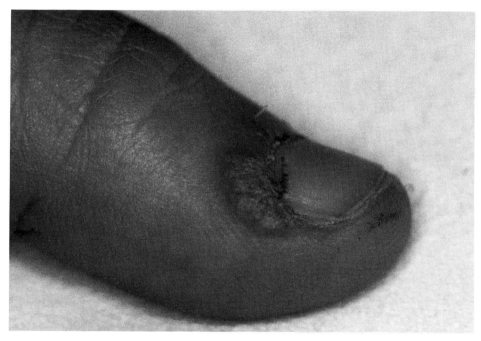

Fig. 12.15. Warts on the sides of the nail can be extremely painful to treat without a digital nerve block.

However, these cases should initially be referred to the local genito-urinary clinic for screening to exclude other sexually transmitted diseases and for contact tracing. In women, a cervical cytology report is mandatory.

Cutaneous horns Because there is always a possibility that the lesion may be a squamous cell carcinoma (particularly when there is inflammation or induration at the base) a cutaneous horn should be biopsied (see chapter 15).

Solar keratoses When small, these are extremely easy to deal with and require only a short freeze of perhaps 5 s (Fig. 12.18). Regular intermittent treatment can transform the back of the hands or the forehead and scalp of someone who has had scaly and crusting lesions for years. Extensive solar keratoses should be referred

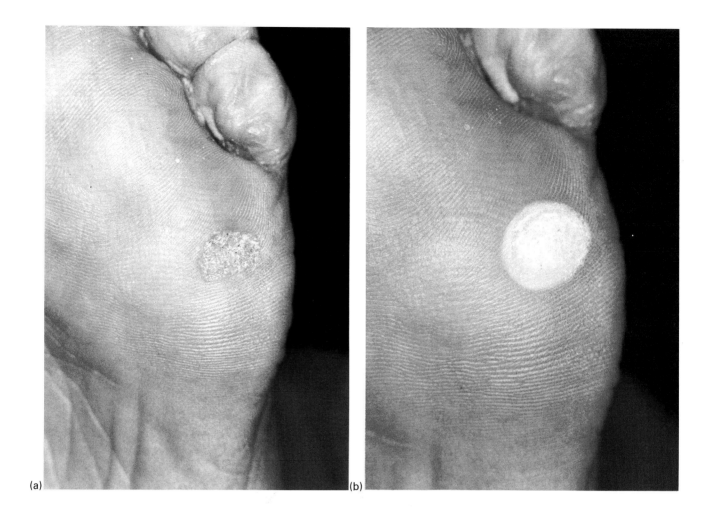

Fig. 12.16. (a) and (b) Liquid
nitrogen treatment to a verruca.

for treatment with 5-fluorouracil cream. After treatment, advice should be given regarding the avoidance of bright sunlight and use of sunscreens. A larger scaly lesion may in fact be an early squamous cell carcinoma and a biopsy should be taken if there is any doubt.

Seborrhoeic keratoses (seborrhoeic warts) These are common on the trunk in the elderly and are commonly multiple. Being superficial skin lesions they are extremely easy to treat with cryotherapy. Usually, the small and flat varieties only require a single freeze of 5–10 s. However, bulky seborrhoeic keratoses will require a number of freeze thaw cycles of 10–20 s.

Papillomata Depending on their size, papillomata can be treated with two freeze–thaw cycles of 10–20 s, repeated if necessary after 1–3 weeks. Lesions on the face and forehead are better treated by shave excision followed by cautery as this allows more accurate tissue destruction.

Keratoacanthoma These lesions should be biopsied to exclude any squamous cell carcinoma. A histologically confirmed keratoacanthoma can be treated with two freeze–thaw cycles of 10–20 s, repeated if necessary after 1–3 weeks.

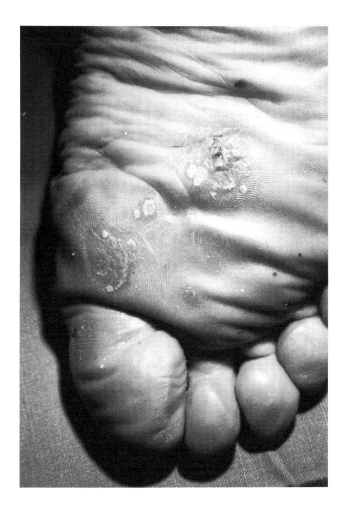

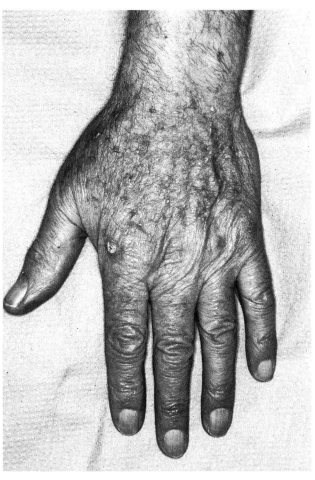

Cervical erosions A cervical smear should be taken prior to treatment. The cervix must be clearly visualised and care should be taken to avoid contact of the cryoprobe with the vaginal walls. The cone-shaped cryoprobe is placed in position before being turned on and the erosion frozen for 2 min. The patient should be warned to expect an increased discharge for 1–2 weeks afterwards. The cervix should be re-examined again after 4 weeks and a repeat treatment given if necessary (see also chapter 19).

Fig. 12.17. (ABOVE, LEFT) Extensive mosaic warts are quite unsuitable for treatment with cryotherapy.

Fig. 12.18. (ABOVE, RIGHT) Solar keratoses on the back of the hand.

Ingrowing toenail Liquid nitrogen can be used on granulations in ingrowing toenails. However, the treatment is painful and has an unacceptably high recurrence rate. It is simpler, more effective and kinder to use phenol ablation of the nail bed, which is the treatment of choice (see chapter 17).

Keloid and hypertrophic scars No single method of treating keloid and hypertrophic scars is successful in all patients. However, although many lesions will not disappear altogether, nevertheless many lesions can be satisfactorily improved using cryotherapy. Often a number of sessions are required and a progressive reduction in the scar can be seen. Hypertrophic scars and small lesions tend to respond better than keloids and larger lesions [7]. Other methods of treatment include steroid injection (see chapter 7) and excision with steroid injection (see chapter 21).

Malignant skin lesions Basal cell carcinoma, squamous cell carcinoma and suspicious pigmented lesions should not be treated but should be referred for specialist care.

Complications of cryotherapy

Blistering It is normal for blistering to occur as an effect of the treatment, but sometimes a severe response may result in haemorrhagic or infected blisters. Such blisters can be extremely painful and should be de-roofed and dressed or exposed as necessary.

Pigmentation Areas of hypopigmentation or hyperpigmentation may be left once the skin has healed after cryotherapy; although sometimes this can be permanent, improvement may occur over the following months (Fig. 12.19). This needs to be considered especially in the treatment of facial and neck lesions on dark-skinned individuals.

Infection It is rare to see an infection after cryotherapy but it is sometimes seen in large blisters. Simple deroofing is usually all that is necessary.

Ulceration This is a particular risk in the treatment of lesions on the shin. Particular care needs to be taken to avoid damage to cartilage during treatment of the ear or nose.

Fig. 12.19. Liquid nitrogen can result in areas of hyperpigmentation which can take many months to resolve. This patient has numerous seborrhoeic keratoses. The lighter patches are areas of pigmentation present 3 months after treatment with liquid nitrogen.

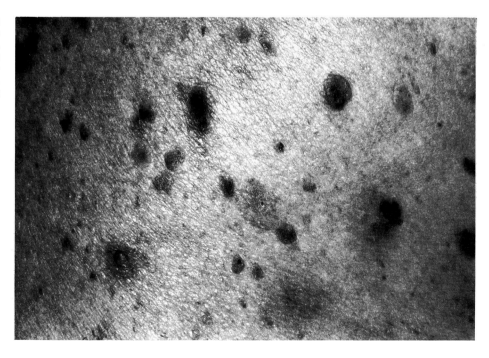

Pitting Considering the depth and extent of freezing that is often applied to various lesions, pitting is quite uncommon. However, pitting may occur with very deep skin damage.

Alopecia Patchy alopecia may occur after deep cryotherapy to lesions on the scalp.

Joint stiffness Finger joint stiffness may occur if freezing extends deep enough to involve joint capsules.

Tendon rupture Extensor tendons over the back of the hands, feet and digits are particularly at risk.

Nerve damage Subcutaneous nerves may be damaged and are particularly at risk near the medial epicondyle of the humerus (ulnar nerve), the sides of fingers (digital nerves) and below the fibula head (common peroneal nerve).

References

1. Cryosurgery – the principles and simple practice. Colver, G. B. & Dawber, R. P. R. *Clinical and Experimental Dermatology* (1989), **14**, 1–6.

2. Clobetasol proprionate ointment reduces inflammation after cryotherapy. Hindson, T. C., Spiro, J. & Scott, L. V. *British Journal of Dermatology* (1985), **112**, 599–602.

3. Transmission of papovavirus by cryotherapy applicator. Charles, C. R. & Sire, D. J. *Journal of the American Medical Association* (1971), **218**, 1435.

4. Transmission of virus particles by cryotherapy and multi-use caustic pencils: a problem to dermatologists? Jones, S. K. & Darville, J. M. *British Journal of Dermatology* (1989), **121**, 481–486.

5. The use of Freon 12 in treating verruca lesions. McDow, R. A. & Wester, M. M. *Journal of Family Practice* (1987), **25**, 73–77.

6. Nongenital warts: classification and treatment options. Bolton, R. A. *American Family Physician* (1991), **43**, 2049–2056.

7. Cryosurgical treatment of hypertrophic scars and keloids. Zouboulis, C. C. & Orfanos, C. E. *Hautarzt* (1990), **41**, 683–688.

13

Wound healing and surgical complications

Wound healing

Wounds normally heal by a continuous process that may extend for up to 1 year before full maturation has been achieved. Traumatic inflammation occurs during the first 3 days. If this inflammation is increased by the presence of foreign material then overgranulation and hypertrophic scarring may result. Some areas always seem to heal badly and hypertrophic scarring is common around the sternum and shoulder area. Keloid scarring is common in those of African origin and darker-skinned people. A reduced inflammatory response such as in debilitated patients and those on steroids will result in delayed healing. Healing occurs from the base upwards by granulation tissue and from the edges by epithelialisation. The repair process is accelerated by wound edge contraction under the influence of contractile cells known as myofibroblasts. If the wound is protected from drying out and infection, wound healing is rapid, with linear scarring. A normal surgical wound is usually sealed by a crust after 24–48 h and therefore can be washed lightly without risk and a dressing may not be necessary.

A destructive phase occurs from around days 2–5, during which time bacteria and dead tissue are digested by macrophages. This results in an increase in tissue osmolality and consequent increase in local swelling. Bruising and swelling often appears excessive in lax tissues such as the eyelids and the scrotum. Operations on hands and feet usually benefit from postoperative elevation of the limbs and ice can be very useful in reducing swelling after, for example, surgery on the eyelids or the prepuce.

The proliferative phase extends from around days 3–24 during which time collagen synthesis and deposition occurs. Collagen is laid down at essentially a fixed rate such that tissues with little collagen (e.g. intestinal wall) gain their maximal strength earlier than those with much collagen (such as tendons). The skin regains roughly 50 % of its tensile strength within 6 weeks.

The maturation phase extends from around the fourth week up to 1 year. Thus, the final appearance of any scar will not be seen until this phase is complete.

Operative complications

It is essential to have a working knowledge of the anatomical distribution of all the important superficial nerves and vulnerable major vessels (these are detailed in chapter 9). In addition, it cannot be overemphasised that *if there is any doubt about a procedure the case should be referred to a specialist*. General practitioners should only undertake what they are capable of handling *easily*. On the one hand, it is said that if you never do any surgery you will never get any complications. On the other hand, however, if you do enough surgery you will eventually come across problems, complications, an incomplete excision, or a solid tumour while dissecting out what clinically seemed to be a cyst. The unexpected *will* happen and it is essential to be prepared for such occurrences. When the unexpected does occur it is usually best to give a simple and honest explanation to the patient, discuss the possible lines of action, and ensure prompt appropriate management.

Faint

Although uncommon, it *is* possible for patients to faint and experience an hypoxic convulsion while in the supine position. Fortunately, in the case of a faint it is a simple matter to put the patient into the recovery position on the couch itself. Priority should be given to maintaining the patient's airway and avoiding the patient inhaling vomit. An artificial airway and an Ambubag should be available in case of respiratory arrest. Severe bradycardia should be treated with intravenous atropine (0.6 mg). A hypoxic convulsion is usually very short-lived but should be treated with intravenous or rectal diazepam (10–20 mg) if it does not rapidly cease.

Accidental damage to nerves and vessels

Nerves The commonest structures to be accidentally damaged are peripheral nerves. However nerves are resilient structures that can withstand a certain amount of distortion. When the doctor is working in the depths of a wound, careful blunt dissection should be used. At all times sharp dissection should be avoided unless the tissue being cut can be directly visualised and identified as being unimportant. Any long off-white structure with very fine overlying vessels should be considered to be a nerve and avoided. Small cutaneous nerves are unimportant and can be cut if they interfere with the dissection. However, accidental damage to any digital nerve or any larger nerve should be noted, the wound closed and a specialist opinion sought. Rarely, a subcutaneous lesion may turn out to be a neuroma or other solid tumour. For this reason it is advisable that all subcutaneous lesions (including what seem to be cysts) should be shelled out by blunt dissection and not incised. If a lesion is unexpectedly found to be attached to a nerve, the wound should be closed and the case referred to a specialist.

Blood vessels Main arteries always lie deeper in the tissues and should not be encountered in simple minor surgery. In general terms, if a vessel pulsates the inexperienced doctor should avoid it altogether. Almost any superficial vein may be clipped and tied off without any adverse result. Bleeding from torn small veins is usually easily controlled by packing the wound and applying pressure for 5–10 min, after which the operative field should be dry and the vessel may be clipped and tied. Uncontrollable bleeding should be extremely rare but should be treated by packing and pressure and the case referred immediately to a local accident and emergency department. Blind clipping and ties should be avoided as serious damage can result to hidden structures. If bleeding is severe an intravenous line should be established prior to transfer to hospital.

Unexpected findings

Very occasionally a subcutaneous lesion that clinically seemed to be a cyst will turn out to be a solid tumour. This should not cause undue alarm. The lesion could be benign or malignant, and either a primary or a secondary deposit. If the lesion is small and well circumscribed it should be shelled out by blunt dissection as if it were a cyst and sent for urgent histological examination. If the lesion is obviously larger or deeper or with indefinite edges, a small piece of the lesion may be taken as a biopsy, and the wound closed. The specimen should be sent for urgent histological examination and the case referred to a specialist.

Postoperative complications

Wound complications should be very uncommon in general practice minor surgery as the procedures are generally simple. If a complication does occur then both the case and the operative technique should be reviewed.

Wound pain

Wound pain usually settles within 24–48 h of surgery. Persistence of pain, throbbing or itching between 3–10 days will usually indicate tight sutures, wound haematoma or wound infection.

Suture abscess

Suture abscesses are small pockets of pus found in the suture tracks, and are usually separate from the main wound cavity itself (Fig. 13.1). They commonly

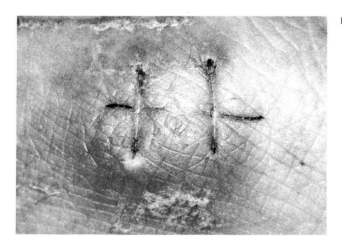

Fig. 13.1. Suture abscess.

occur if there is undue tension in the wound or the skin is of poor quality. It is usually enough just to remove the appropriate suture to allow drainage and healing. If the suture line itself has not yet healed the wound may be supported by the use of adhesive tapes.

Allergy to dressings

Occasionally patients are found to be sensitive to the adhesive tape or to the adhesive sheets used to hold down gauze dressings. A different brand should be tried (e.g. Micropore, Hypafix, Dermicel) but unfortunately patients can be sensitive to everything and anything. In certain sites, an alternative is to hold the gauze in place with a bandage, or the patient's underwear. Contact allergy can cause intense itching but this can usually be easily controlled by the use of a topical steroid cream for a few days.

Wound breakdown

Clean Sometimes a seemingly well-united wound splits open a few hours after the removal of sutures. This may have been because there had been a subcutaneous haematoma, or undue tension caused by limb or trunk movements. Such a wound is usually clean and can be repaired by either re-suture, use of adhesive tapes or tissue adhesive (Figs. 13.2, 13.3). The wound will then take another 7–14 days to unite, depending on the site.

Fig. 13.2. This clean wound in a small child broke down after the adhesive tapes loosened. It is quite acceptable to repair the wound with further adhesive tapes or tissue adhesive.

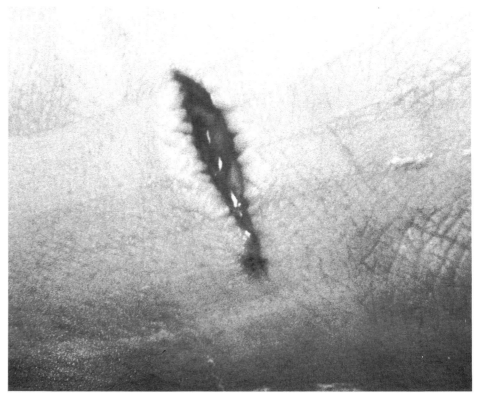

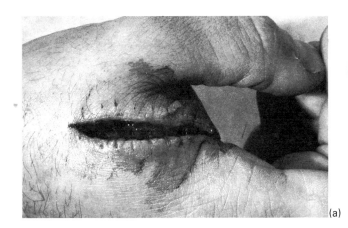 (a)

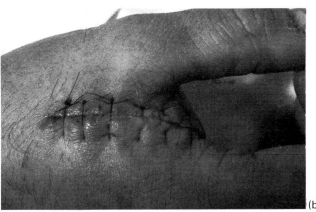 (b)

Infected Wound infection following minor surgery should be rare. Infection is more likely after surgery of crusting and inflamed skin lesions and in the presence of poor circulation or debility. It may also occur as a result of poor technique resulting in tight sutures or a haematoma. An infected wound will often break open on release of the pus. Such a wound is best left open to drain and either heal by secondary intention or by secondary suture after a period of time has elapsed to allow the granulations to be clean and free from infection. Antibiotics are generally unnecessary except in the presence of cellulitis. Any loose subcutaneous sutures are best removed as they are liable to act as a nidus for continuing infection. Sometimes, however, not all of the skin sutures need be removed as it may be possible to release pus by simply removing some key sutures and lightly packing the wound. This may avoid the need for secondary suture.

Healing by secondary intention If the broken down wound gapes such that closure is not possible without tension, it may be left to heal by secondary intention (i.e. by granulation tissue). The wound should be covered or lightly packed with a paraffin gauze and redressed once a week unless the dressings become soiled or the discharge is foul. The wound is likely to close rapidly over a few weeks and the final scar can be surprisingly small (Fig. 13.4).

Fig. 13.3. (a) This laceration broke down after removal of sutures due to a combination of a small haematoma and tension. (b) Subsequent repair with sutures.

Fig. 13.4. This patient had an infected sebaceous cyst on the side of the neck. Following excision and suture the wound became infected and broke down. (a) The granulating wound. (b) The wound had healed by secondary intention after 3 weeks, leaving a linear scar.

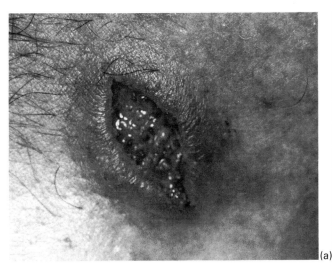 (a)

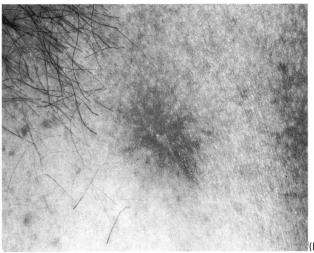 (b)

Poor scars

In Negroes and to a lesser extent in other races, hypertrophic and keloid scars (Fig. 13.5) are likely to occur after clean uncomplicated wounds over the face, shoulder and upper sternal area. In addition, all individuals are at risk of developing hypertrophic scars *in any area* if a wound becomes inflamed, infected or subject to tension. Patients should be warned of the possibility of hypertrophic scarring, and, if possible, surgery should be avoided in susceptible cases. Direct injection of depot steroids into the scars can soften and flatten small lesions (see chapter 7) and in experienced hands the scar can be excised with injection of a depot steroid into the wound edges (see chapter 17).

Flat stretched scars commonly occur in areas where they are subjected to tension and also after wound breakdown following infection or haematoma (Fig. 13.6). Thus, subcutaneous sutures and adhesive tapes should be used in association with skin sutures in any area where there is a likelihood of tension (see chapter 10).

Tiny white cysts (about 1 mm in diameter) may sometimes be found alongside the length of wounds, particularly on the face. These are unrelated to suture tracks and can be incised with the tip of a no. 11 scalpel blade and squeezed out.

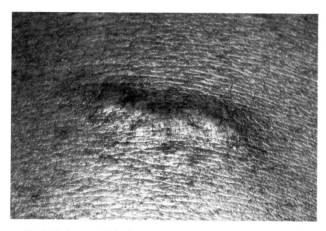

Fig. 13.5. (ABOVE) Keloid scar on the shoulder.

Fig. 13.6. (ABOVE, RIGHT) A stretched and hypertrophic scar due to tension following excision of benign lesion in lumbar area. Note that even the suture tracks are involved.

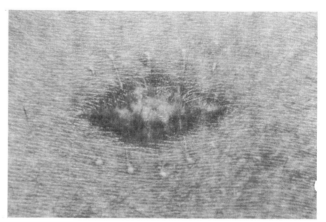

Toxic shock after minor surgery

Although toxic shock syndrome (TSS) is most commonly associated with vaginal infection following the use of tampons, it is also associated with, for example, burns, nasal packing, abscesses, and postpartum infection. The diagnosis is made when there is severe diarrhoea, rapid onset of shock, and a fine macular rash. The condition is caused by a strain of *Staphylococcus aureus* producing TSS toxin (TSST-1), but a similar toxic shock-like syndrome can be caused by other organisms such as group A haemolytic *Streptococcus* and *Escherichia coli* [1,2]. On very rare occasions toxic shock has been reported to occur after minor skin surgery [3,4]. In one fatal case the condition appeared 24 h after a minor skin operation on the back of a teenager. When the dry-looking wound was explored on the fourth day after the onset of the illness some deep necrotic debris was found from which *Staph. aureus* was isolated. Doctors should be aware of the possibility of toxic shock after minor surgery as urgent referral for aggressive resuscitation with intravenous fluids, vasoconstrictors, antibiotics, human immunoglobulin and surgical toilet is essential [5,6].

References

1. Toxic shock syndrome associated with phage group 1 staphylococci. Todd, J., Fishaut, M., Kapral, F. & Welch, T. *Lancet* (1978) **ii**, 1116–1118.
2. Toxic shock-like syndrome due to streptococcal hand infection. Craigen, M. A. C. & Wallace, W. A. *Journal of the Royal College of Surgeons of Edinburgh* (1992), **37**, 269–270.
3. Toxic shock syndrome as a complication of dermatological surgery. Huntley, A. C. & Tanube, J. L. *Journal of the American Academy of Dermatology* (1987), **16**, 227–229.
4. Toxic shock syndrome after elective minor dermatological surgery. Bosley, A. R. J., Bluett, N. H. & Sowden, G., *British Medical Journal* (1993), **306**, 386–387.
5. Toxic shock syndrome after minor surgery. Griffiths, M. J. D. & Sinclair, D. G. *British Medical Journal* (1993) **306**, 652.
6. Toxic shock syndrome after minor surgery. McAllister, R. M. R. *British Medical Journal* (1993) **306**, 652.

SECTION IV

14

Minor surgical procedures: Simple skin lesions

Vascular lesions

Campbell de Morgan spots, spider naevi and haemangiomata can all be easily treated by diathermy or fine point electrocautery after prior injection of a small bleb of local anaesthetic.

Campbell de Morgan spots

These benign lesions become more common with age and do not normally need treatment. However, they can be treated if they are unsightly or rub on clothing (Fig. 14.1).

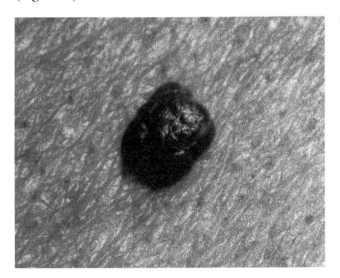

Fig. 14.1. A large Campbell de Morgan spot.

Spider naevi

These small vascular lesions can be unsightly on the face or nose. They comprise a flare of radiating vessels arising from a central feeding vessel. Pressure on the central vessel with a small probe will cause the flare to disappear. Treatment is by

Fig. 14.2. (a) Spider naevus on the cheek. (b) Immediately after diathermy to the bulky central feeding vessel.

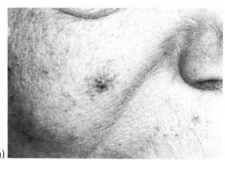

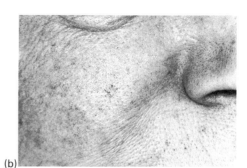

(a)   (b)

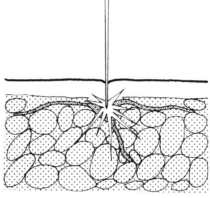

Fig. 14.3. Diathermy to spider naevus.

unipolar diathermy or fine point electrocautery to the central vessel (Figs. 14.2, 14.3).

Haemangiomata

Fig. 14.4. (a) and (b) Diathermy to a small haemangioma on the nose. The cosmetic improvement is seen immediately.

Small haemangiomatous lesions may be easily treated by multiple stepwise bipolar or monopolar diathermy burns after infiltration with local anaesthetic (Fig. 14.4). Care should be taken not to over-treat so as to avoid any resultant pitting.

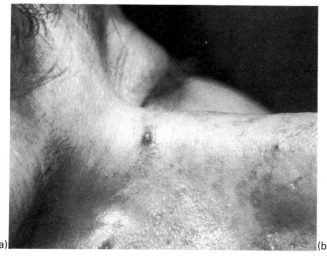

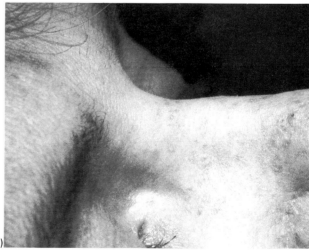

(a)   (b)

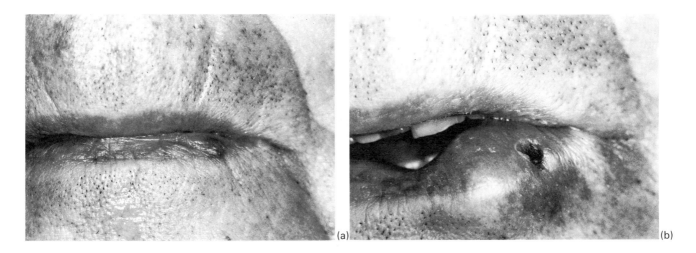

Venous lake Venous lakes are commonly found on the lips in the elderly and can be easily treated by diathermy or electrocautery.

Fig. 14.5. Venous lake on the lip, (a) before and (b) after treatment.

Pedunculated lesions

Skin tags (fibro-epithelial polyps)

These are common on the neck and in the axilla. Since they are often multiple it is reasonable to excise one or more representative examples for histology and simply tie off or cauterise the remainder (Figs. 14.6, 14.7).

Tiny tags are often found around the collar area of the neck, axilla or the eyelids. They can be held with fine forceps and swiftly amputated with a scalpel blade or

Fig. 14.6. Skin tags. (a) Multiple skin tags on the chest wall. These can be individually tied off, or removed by cautery or diathermy. (b) Skin tags on eyelid.

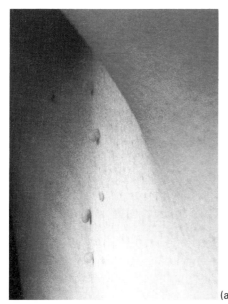

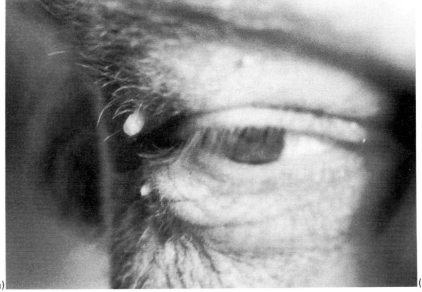

Fig. 14.7. Skin tag (fibro-epithelial polyp). This has an acanthotic epidermis with a central connective tissue stalk of loose collagen, dilated capillaries and fat cells.

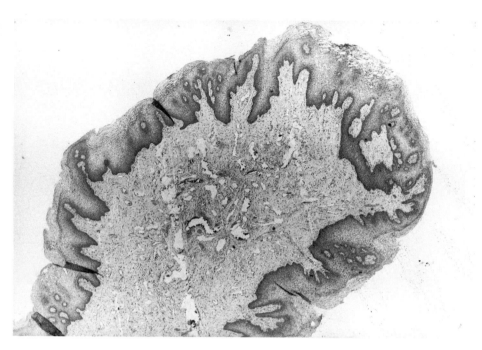

Fig. 14.8. Amputation of tiny tag.

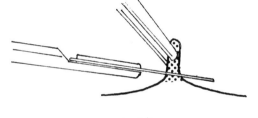

Fig. 14.9. Tie of small tag.

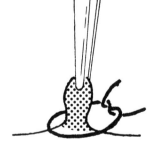

snipped with fine scissors without any local anaesthetic infiltration (Fig. 14.8). The resulting small raw sites can then be covered with small plaster dressings for 24 h to absorb any slight bleeding. Sometimes, however, a touch with a silver nitrate stick may be required to stop the bleeding. Some patients may tolerate removal of tiny tags by electrocautery or diathermy without a local anaesthetic.

Small tags can be tied off and left to separate spontaneously over a few days (Fig. 14.9). The tag should be held perpendicular to the skin with forceps while a length of thread is looped around and positioned at the base of the tag. The thread is then tightened completely. This causes only slight and momentary pain. A strong thread is needed to avoid breakage and it is unnecessary to use sterile sutures. If necessary, the bulk of the tag may be amputated distal to the tie and the site covered with a small plaster.

Pedunculated papillomata

Larger tags and pedunculated papillomata will require an injection of local anaesthetic into the base prior to treatment (Figs. 14.10, 14.11). Usually, it is possible to crush and tie the base of the lesion followed by amputation, leaving a small stump that will separate spontaneously. Occasionally, the lesion may become amputated as the thread is tightened, resulting in the tie falling free with bleeding from the raw area. In this case, the raw area should be cauterised with a silver nitrate stick. An alternative is simply to crush the base of the papilloma, amputate the lesion through the crushed area with a scalpel blade and cauterise the crushed raw area with a silver nitrate stick.

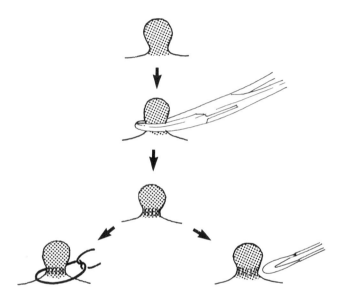

Fig. 14.10. Treatment of larger papillomata.

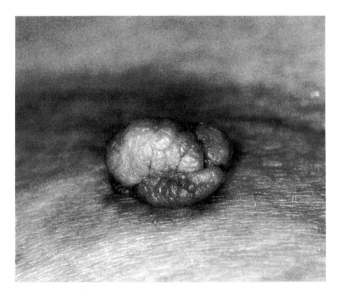

Fig. 14.11. This congenital papilloma can be easily removed by crushing the base and tying off before amputation of the lesion for histological examination.

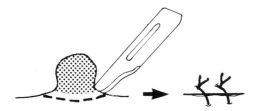

Fig. 14.12. Excision of large tag or papilloma.

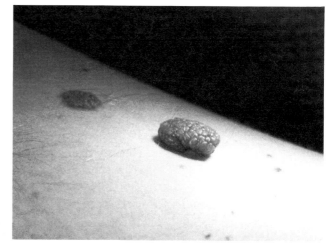

Fig. 14.13. (RIGHT) A broad-based congenital papilloma suitable for excision with a small ellipse of normal skin or by shave biopsy.

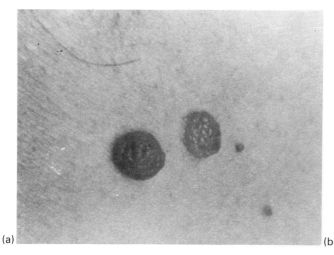

(a)

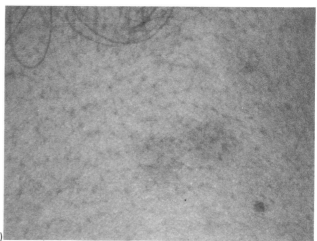

(b)

Fig. 14.14. (a) Long-standing papillomata on the back of the neck suitable for shave excision. (b) The result after 3 months.

For the bulkier lesions, it may be necessary to excise a small ellipse of skin at the base and close the defect with one or two skin sutures (Figs. 14.12, 14.13).

Another alternative for smaller tags and pedunculated papillomata is to treat with cryotherapy but this is likely to require more than one treatment (see chapter 12). Broad-based papillomata can be removed by shave excision followed by electrocautery or diathermy. The resulting flat bed develops a crust that separates after 1–2 weeks. Re-epithelialisation occurs with minimal scarring (Fig. 14.14).

15

Minor surgical procedures: Skin biopsy

As with any surgery, there are a few simple rules to follow for safe skin surgery: first, make a diagnosis; secondly, if a diagnosis is not possible decide whether the case should be best referred for treatment and management; and, thirdly, if excision is the best option, be certain that the lesion is suitable for removal in general practice.

The problem is not only of simply cutting out a lesion but also of knowing which lesions can be safely left alone. Thus, before proceeding it is important to have a working knowledge of the clinical appearances, biological behaviour and histological features of common and important skin lesions [1].

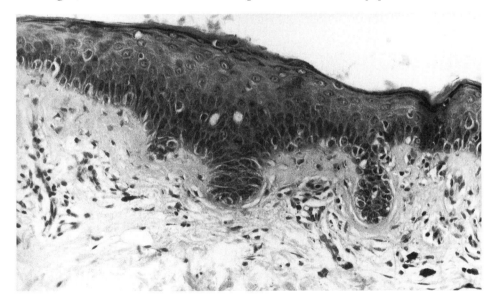

Fig. 15.1. Section through normal skin showing epidermis and upper dermis.

Benign skin lesions

Pigmented naevi

The common *freckle* is simply a flat area of increased pigmentation that tans on exposure to sunlight. The melanocytes are present in normal numbers. The *simple lentigo* is an area of pigmentation that may be flat or slightly raised, with

Fig. 15.2. Simple lentigo.

Fig. 15.3. Simple lentigo with increased dermal melanocytes and increased melanin pigment in basal keratinocytes.

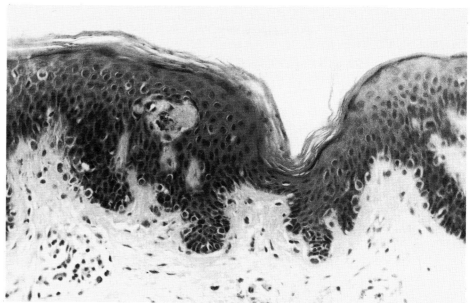

increased numbers of melanocytes in the basal layer and increased melanin pigment in the basal keratinocytes, but melanocytic activity is not increased (Figs. 15.2, 15.3). The simple lentigo does not darken on exposure to the sun.

Pigmented naevi are extremely common and in adolescents are liable to enlarge along with growth spurts. Although malignant melanoma is rare before puberty any suspicious naevus should be referred to a dermatologist, or excised and the specimen examined histologically. In addition, any asymptomatic pigmented naevus may be excised for cosmetic purposes or if it is in a site in which it cannot easily be checked by the patient.

In pigmented melanocytic naevi the melanocytes[1] of the epidermis proliferate and give rise to naevus[2] cells which may be wholly in either the epidermis or

[1] Melanocytes are the melanin pigment producing cells in the basal layer of the epidermis. They have long dendritic cytoplasmic processes which ramify between the epidermal keratinocytes and these donate melanin pigment to the keratinocytes.

[2] Naevus cells are derived from the proliferation of basal melanocytes and initially are located at the dermo-epidermal junction, from which they descend into the dermis. Naevus cells differ from melanocytes in that they lose their dendritic processes, are arranged in cell nests and are slightly larger than melanocytes. With time, naevus cell nests descend into the dermis. They become smaller, lose their pigment and may develop a neuroid appearance resembling that of Schwann cells.

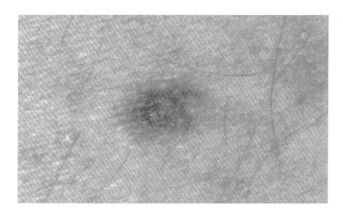

Fig. 15.4. Melanocytic junctional naevus.

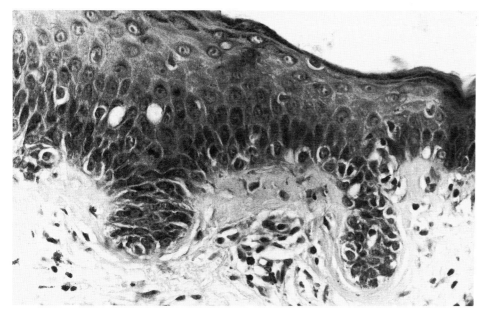

Fig. 15.5. Melanocytic junctional naevus showing nests of melanocytes at the dermo-epidermal junction and increased melanin pigment in the epidermal keratinocytes.

dermis or in both (junctional, intra-dermal or compound). The lesions may be flat, slightly raised or papular.

The *melanocytic junctional naevus* is a flat, pigmented lesion that may be indistinguishable clinically from simple lentigos (Fig. 15.4). Microscopic examination shows naevus cells in well defined nests within the lower epidermis (Fig. 15.5).

Melanocytic intradermal naevi are usually dome-shaped lesions and often bear coarse hairs. They are commonly found on the face and forehead and are usually about 3–5 mm in diameter (Fig. 15.6). They are usually pale but can be pigmented to varying degrees but show no junctional activity (Fig. 15.7). Intradermal naevi are best removed by shave excision followed by electrocautery or diathermy (Fig. 15.8). Although excision of an intradermal naevus with a skin ellipse is commonly performed, excision is often unnecessary, and is likely to leave an inferior scar with possibly permanent cross-hatch marks from the sutures.

The *melanocytic compound naevus* is usually flat or slightly raised and often contains hairs (Fig. 15.9). Characteristically, the naevus cells are seen to 'drop off' from the epidermis into the dermis (Fig. 15.10).

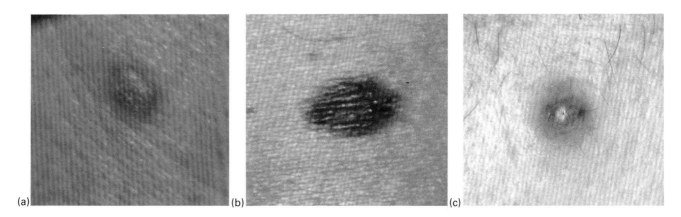

(a)   (b)   (c)

Fig. 15.6. (a–c) (ABOVE, LEFT,
CENTRE AND RIGHT) Melanocytic
intradermal naevus showing clinical
variations.

Fig. 15.7. (BELOW AND BELOW
RIGHT) Melanocytic intradermal
naevus. (a) A papillary intradermal
naevus with hyperkeratosis,
papillomatosis and nests of naevus
cells in the dermis. (b) Part of a
papillary intradermal naevus
showing naevus cells confined
within the dermis.

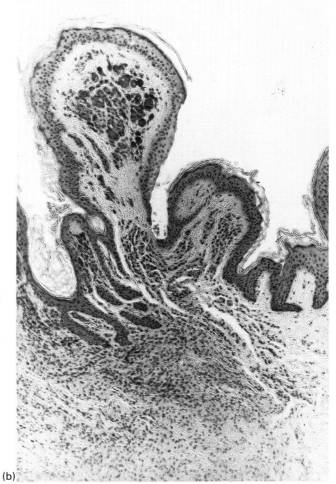

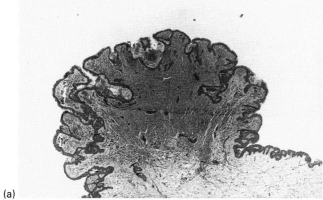

(a)   (b)

The *halo naevus* is commonly found on the trunk in children and young adults.
The central lesion is usually a compound or intradermal naevus that is surrounded
by an area of depigmentation that may take months or years to return to normal.
The halo naevus is benign and does not need excision. However, a halo of

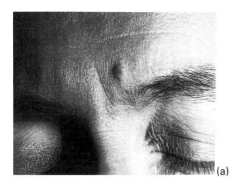 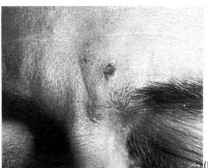 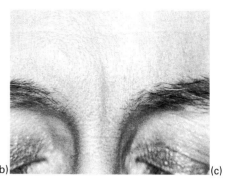

Fig. 15.8. (ABOVE, LEFT, CENTRE AND RIGHT) Shave excision and diathermy to base of intradermal naevus near eyebrow: (a) before excision, (b) immediately after removal, (c) 2 months after removal.

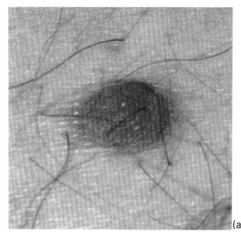 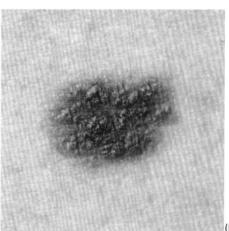

Fig. 15.9. (FAR LEFT AND LEFT) (a) and (b) Melanocytic compound naevus showing clinical variations.

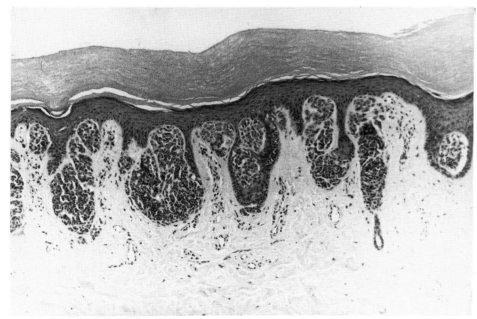

Fig. 15.10. Melanocytic compound naevus showing junctional and dermal nests of melanocytes.

depigmentation can rarely form around some other naevi, and occasionally around a malignant melanoma. If there are any atypical features (see under malignant melanoma) the patient should be referred or the lesion should be excised with a skin ellipse.

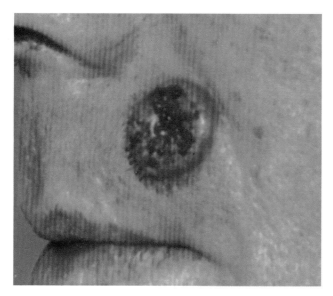

Fig. 15.11. Keratoacanthoma.

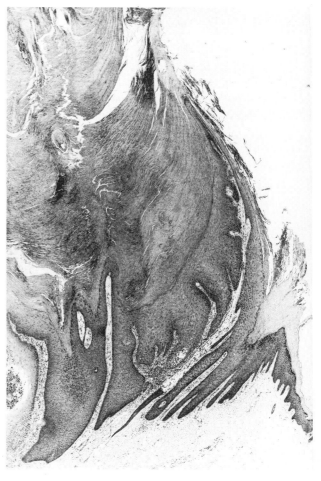

Fig. 15.12. Keratoacanthoma: the typical central keratotic plug is shown, with large islands of bland proliferating keratinocytes surrounded by attenuated epidermal 'lips' of compressed normal epidermis.

Keratoacanthoma

This benign lesion is usually diagnosed by its short history (commonly 6–12 weeks) and its central keratin plug (Fig. 15.11). However, not infrequently it can be present for a number of years and it can closely resemble a squamous cell carcinoma. Histologically, the central plug is seen with large islands of bland proliferating keratinocytes surrounded by attenuated epidermal 'lips' of compressed normal epidermis (Fig. 15.12). Keratoacanthoma can be treated by incisional biopsy followed by curettage under local anaesthetic with electrocautery or diathermy to the base. The curettings should also be sent for histological examination. However, if the lesion is small it can be excised with an ellipse of normal skin.

Seborrhoeic keratosis (basal cell papilloma)

Seborrhoeic keratoses are usually multiple, being commonly found on the trunk, neck and forehead and become increasingly common with age. The lesions vary in size and pigmentation, are greasy to touch, have a cleft surface, and appear to be

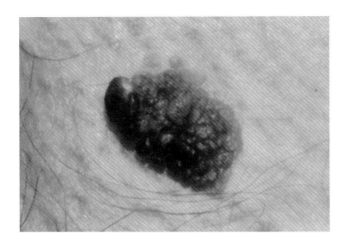

Fig. 15.13. Seborrhoeic keratosis.

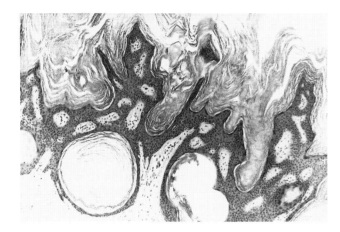

Fig. 15.14. Seborrhoeic keratosis with hyperkeratosis, papillomatosis, horn cysts and typical basaloid cells.

stuck onto the skin surface (Fig. 15.13). Microscopic examination shows hyper-keratosis, papillomatosis, horn cysts and typical basaloid cells (Fig. 15.14). The diagnosis should be confirmed by shave biopsy or curettage. However, seborrhoeic keratoses are best treated by superficial cryotherapy (see chapter 12). This allows multiple lesions to be quickly and easily dealt with without the need for local anaesthetic. Alternatively, seborrhoeic keratoses can be treated by superficial electrocautery or diathermy after local anaesthetic infiltration. When bipolar diathermy forceps are used, the lesion will be seen to 'bubble up', and in so doing, separate itself from the underlying skin, which then needs only a further light treatment to ensure complete removal. When cautery is used, the lesion will simply char. Unless the diagnosis is in doubt, *excision with a skin ellipse is unnecessary* and also results in an inferior cosmetic result.

Dermatofibroma

These benign intradermal lesions are most commonly found in women and are usually sited on the lower leg (Fig. 15.15). Dermatofibromas present as firm nodules and usually persist indefinitely. Microscopically they have an ill-defined

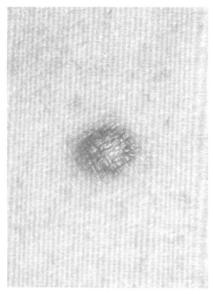
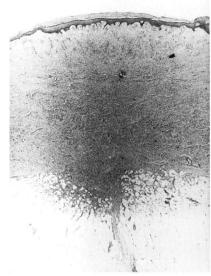
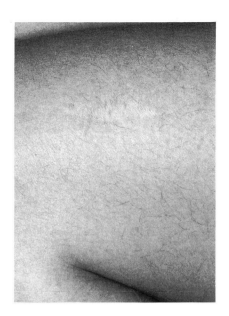

Fig. 15.15. (ABOVE)
Dermatofibroma.

Fig. 15.16. (ABOVE, CENTRE) A
dermatofibroma with a cellular
centre and ill-defined less cellular
margins in the dermis and subcutis.
The overlying epidermis shows
hyperkeratosis.

Fig. 15.17. (ABOVE, RIGHT)
Stretched scar following excision of
dermatofibroma.

margin and are composed of fibroblasts, collagen, capillaries and histiocytes (Fig. 15.16). Since the skin of the leg often gapes markedly when it is incised, dermatofibromas should be excised with the minimum margin of normal skin. However, too *short* an ellipse should be avoided as this is likely to give rise to tension in the wound, make subsequent closure difficult, and ultimately result in a stretched scar (Fig. 15.17). Particular care should be taken on the leg to ensure that the excision is in line with the skin creases. Additional wound support with adhesive tapes should be used to minimise tension and consideration should be given to the use of a long-lasting subcutaneous suture such as Dexon or Vicryl to minimise the likelihood of the scar stretching.

Premalignant lesions

Solar keratosis

Solar keratoses are commonly found as multiple, flat, scaly lesions found on sun-exposed areas such as the forehead and cheeks, ears, the bald parts of the scalp, and the back of the hands (Fig. 15.18). They are all squamous carcinomas *in situ* with keratinocytes showing pleomorphism and atypia (Fig. 15.19). The best treatment for this superficial skin lesion is light cryotherapy. Occasionally an area of keratosis may become more bulky or bleed. Such a lesion is very likely to be an overt squamous cell carcinoma or occasionally a basal cell carcinoma. Patients with these lesions should be referred.

Bowen's disease

Bowen's disease usually presents as a patch of scaly skin resembling chronic eczema or psoriasis (Fig. 15.20). Occasionally a bulky scaly lesion is seen (Fig.

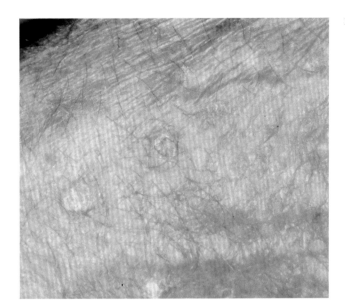

Fig. 15.18. Solar keratoses on the back of the hand.

Fig. 15.19. Solar keratosis with the epidermis showing pleomorphic keratinocytes and a column of parakeratotic keratin.

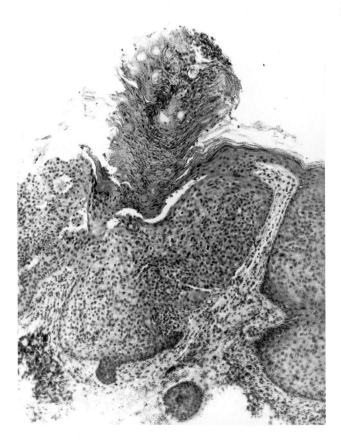

15.21). A patch of Bowen's disease is a carcinoma *in situ* and will eventually develop into a squamous cell carcinoma. The epidermis shows acanthosis and the keratinocytes are disordered and may appear highly atypical (Fig. 15.22). A small lesion can be removed completely with an ellipse of normal skin and sent for

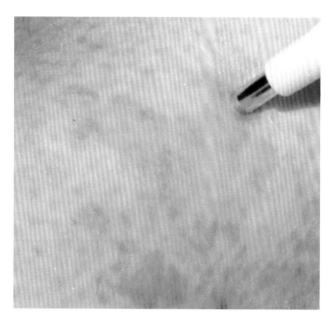

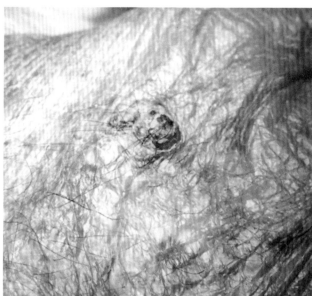

Fig. 15.20. (ABOVE) Bowen's disease presenting as a chronic scaly patch of skin (a punch biopsy is being taken).

Fig. 15.21. (ABOVE, RIGHT) Bowen's disease presenting as a bulky lesion.

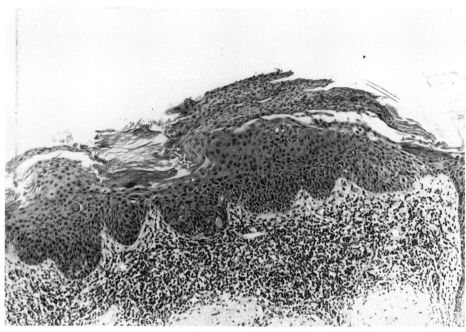

Fig. 15.22. Bowen's disease (carcinoma *in situ*) showing disordered atypical keratinocytes forming parakeratotic scale, and a chronic inflammatory reaction in the papillary dermis.

histological examination. An incisional biopsy should be taken if the lesion is larger, after which it may be treated by cryotherapy or referred to a dermatologist.

Cutaneous horn

Cutaneous horn is the clinical term for a circumscribed conical, hypertrophic lesion (Fig. 15.23). The term refers to a reaction pattern of hyperkeratosis that is associated with various different lesions. Hyperkeratotic horns are most commonly associated with solar keratosis but they can be seen with some viral

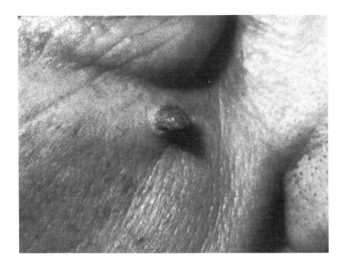

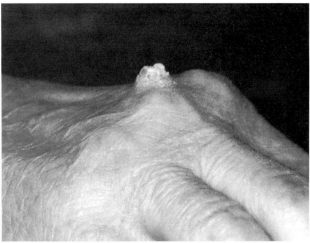

warts, basal cell papillomas (seborrhoeic keratoses), squamous cell carcinomas and rarely trichilemmomas and basal cell carcinomas. Although cutaneous horn per se is not a premalignant condition, a hyperkeratotic horn arising in a solar keratosis should be considered potentially malignant. A cutaneous horn may be treated by avulsion followed by curettage, cautery or cryotherapy of the base, but all these methods may leave damaged skin behind that itself may in time produce a new cutaneous horn. The avulsed horn and curettings should be sent for histological examination.

If there is any suggestion of inflammation or induration at the base then there is a strong possibility that the lesion may be a squamous cell carcinoma. If small, such a lesion should be treated by excision of the horn with an ellipse extending into surrounding normal skin. A larger lesion should have an incisional biopsy taken of its base, or be referred to a dermatologist (Fig. 15.24).

Fig. 15.23. (ABOVE, LEFT) Cutaneous horn on the cheek.

Fig. 15.24. (ABOVE, RIGHT) This cutaneous horn should not be excised by the inexperienced doctor as there is very little spare skin on the back of the hand. An incisional biopsy of the base of the lesion should be done to exclude a squamous cell carcinoma, following which the lesion may be excised, or the base cauterised or treated by cryotherapy.

Malignant lesions

Only very small basal cell carcinomas that are in sites with plenty of spare skin should be excised in the doctor's surgery. Larger basal cell carcinomas, squamous cell carcinomas and suspicious pigmented lesions, should all be referred to a dermatologist or surgeon.

Basal cell carcinoma

This is the commonest malignant skin tumour and can usually be identified by the pearly rim with its fine blood vessels (Fig. 15.25). There are cystic, morphoeic, pigmented and superficial multifocal variants (Fig. 15.26). An ulcerated lesion may be difficult or impossible to distinguish from a squamous cell carcinoma. The characteristic cells have a large oval nucleus and little cytoplasm and the connective tissue stroma proliferates with the tumour cells, which often show a peripheral pallisaded arrangement (Fig. 15.27).

As an alternative to excision, a small lesion may be curetted, followed by

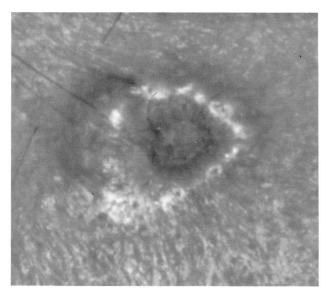

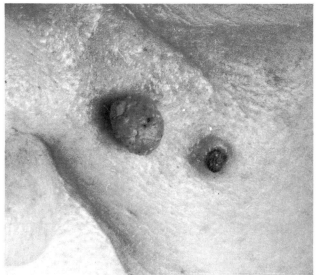

Fig. 15.25. (ABOVE) Basal cell
carcinoma.

Fig. 15.26. (ABOVE, RIGHT) Both of
these lesions on the cheek were
basal cell carcinomas.

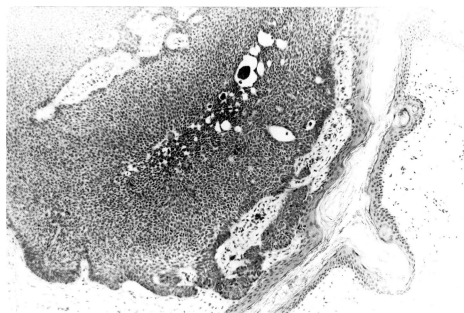

Fig. 15.27. A nest of basal cell
carcinoma in the dermis, showing
pigmentation and a characteristic
peripheral pallisade.

cautery to the base, or treated by cryotherapy. All curettings should be sent for histological examination.

Squamous cell carcinoma

Squamous cell carcinoma (Fig. 15.28) can occur on any part of the skin and can also arise from within an area of solar keratosis, Bowen's disease, or chronic ulceration (Marjolin's ulcer). Squamous cell carcinoma has a progressive course that can result in metastatic spread, leading to death. The tumours are asymmetric, endo-exophytic lesions that invade the dermis and consist of keratinocytes showing severe polymorphism and atypia (Fig. 15.29).

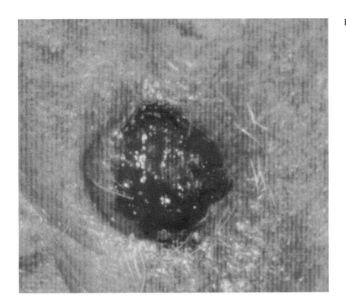

Fig. 15.28. Squamous cell carcinoma.

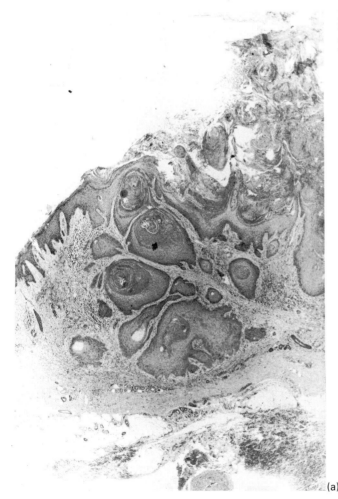

(a)

Fig. 15.29. (a) Low power, (b) high power. A well differentiated keratinising squamous cell carcinoma with nests of atypical squamous cells invading the dermis, which shows an inflammatory reaction to the tumour.

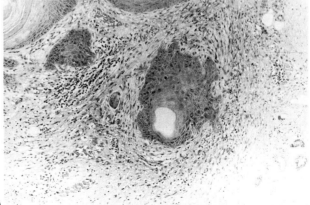

(b)

Malignant melanoma

The doctor should always be alert to the possibility of a pigmented lesion being a malignant melanoma. The incidence of malignant melanoma is on the increase and there are a number of signs and symptoms that should arouse suspicion. A seven-point checklist is divided into major and minor features. Any patient with a lesion showing any of the three major signs (growth, irregularity in shape, irregularity in colour) should be referred to a dermatologist. Lesions showing any of the minor features add weight to this decision [2].

Malignant melanoma

Suspicion should be aroused if the following signs and symptoms are present in a pigmented lesion.

Major features
1. Enlargement in previously static lesion.
2. Irregular outline.
3. Irregular pigmentation.

Minor features
4. Larger than 7 mm diameter.
5. Itching.
6. Oozing, crusting or bleeding.
7. Inflammation.

Malignant melanoma occurs in all age groups, although it is uncommon before puberty. It can present in a variety of forms but all malignant melanomas originate at the dermo-epidermal junction. Typically there is irregular junctional proliferation and downward streaming of the round (epithelioid) or spindle-shaped melanoma cells into the dermis. The tumour cells possess atypical nuclei and show variable pigmentation.

Superficial spreading melanoma is the commonest type and is typically a slightly raised irregular pigmented lesion (Figs. 15.30, 15.31). It is commonly

Fig. 15.30. Superficial spreading malignant melanoma.

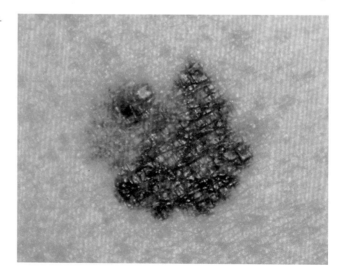

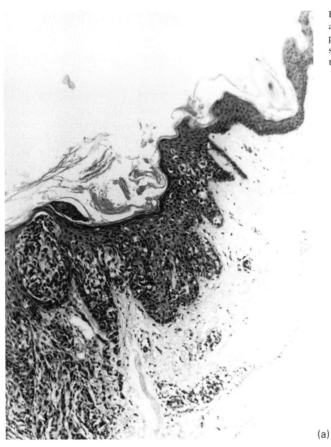

Fig. 15.31. (a) Superficial spreading malignant melanoma with invasion of all layers of the epidermis at one edge and invasive growth into the papillary dermis nearer the centre of the lesion. (b) Predominantly *in situ* superficial malignant melanoma with most of the melanoma cells invading the epidermis.

(a)

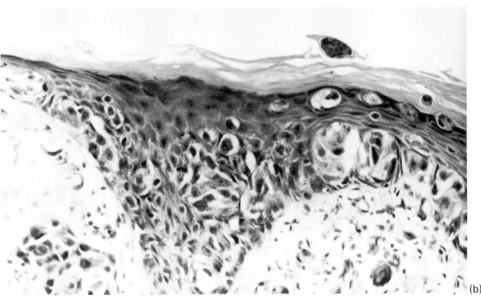

(b)

found on the trunk in men and on the legs in women and develops from a superficial spreading malignant melanoma *in situ*. The prognosis depends largely upon the stage of the disease and the depth of downward invasion.

Nodular melanoma is the most malignant type and is usually markedly raised and very dark (Figs. 15.32, 15.33). On occasion it may lack pigment and may be mistaken for a pyogenic granuloma, or the result of an insect bite.

Lentigo maligna is usually found in the elderly and is often seen as a relatively large slow growing irregular flat pigmented lesion on chronically sun-exposed

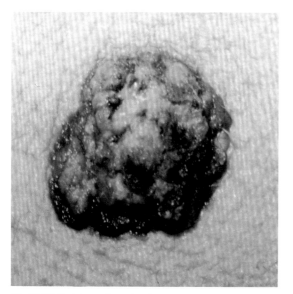

Fig. 15.32. Nodular malignant melanoma.

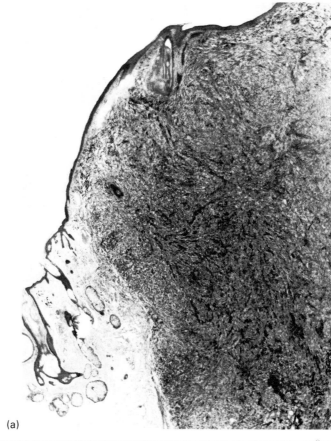

(a)

Fig. 15.33. (a) Nodular malignant melanoma with heavy pigmentation invading the dermis. (b) Nodular malignant melanoma with prominent nucleoli and variable cytoplasmic pigmentation, nuclei and mitotic figures.

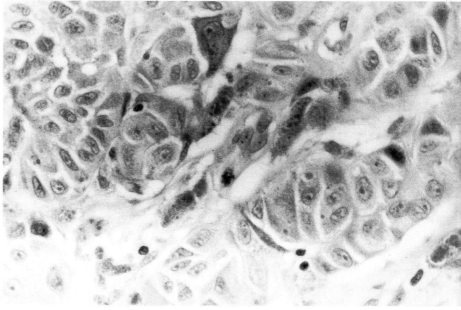

(b)

sites. The lesion typically is completely smooth with a dull non-reflecting surface (Fig. 15.34a). Histologically, the lentigo maligna is a malignant melanoma *in situ* with an increase in basal melanocytes, which have atypical nuclei (Fig. 15.35). The tumours are slow to metastasise and carry a good prognosis. The change from radially spreading lentigo maligna to vertically invasive lentigo maligna melanoma is indicated by the development of increased or patchy pigmentation, or of an elevated nodule within the area of pigmentation (Fig. 15.34b).

Acral lentiginous melanomas are usually found on the palms or soles of the feet. In the United Kingdom, subungual melanoma is usually found on the great toe. Acral melanoma may occasionally be inadvertently treated as a pigmented plantar wart or an ingrowing toenail [3].

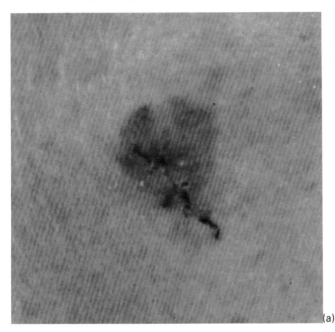
(a)

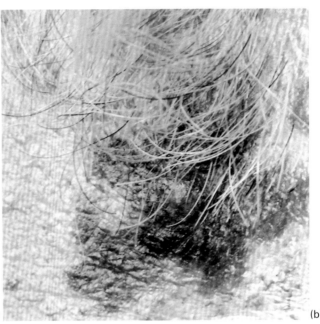
(b)

Fig. 15.34. (ABOVE, LEFT AND RIGHT) (a) Lentigo maligna (an incisional biopsy has been taken). (b) Lentigo maligna melanoma appearing as thickening and increased pigmentation within a long-standing patch of lentigo maligna.

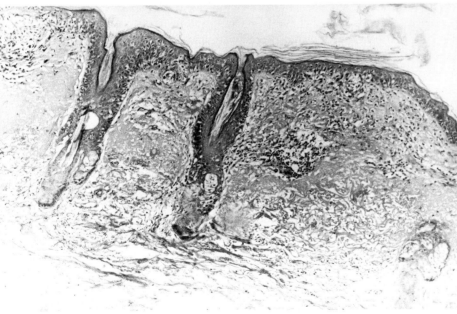

Fig. 15.35. Lentigo maligna showing a continuous proliferation of atypical melanocytes at the dermo-epidermal junction extending into hair follicles. The upper dermis shows solar elastosis and a mild chronic inflammatory reaction.

It has been known for some time that adults who have had a renal transplant have an increased risk of developing skin cancer, and malignant melanoma is three times as common in the patients as in the normal population. Recently it has been found that children who have had renal transplants have an increased incidence of melanocytic naevi and this is correlated with the length of the immunosuppression. Of particular concern is the tendency for melanocytic naevi to appear on the palms and soles, since these naevi may carry a increased risk of malignant change [4].

Incompletely excised lesions

Despite a clinical impression of a complete excision with a margin of normal skin, a pathological report may occasionally state that an excised lesion extends near to or up to one of the cut margins. Although this is technically termed an *incomplete* excision it is not necessarily *negligent* surgery.

Benign lesions

Incomplete excision of benign papillomata and naevi should cause no concern. The patient should be informed of the situation and should be forewarned that recurrence may occur. It is a simple matter to excise any remnant but if there is minimal lesion visible clinically, then, since the lesion has been shown to be benign, further excision may be considered unnecessary. Recurrent lesions may sometimes have unusual histological appearances. However, if the pathologist is informed that the lesion is a recurrence and given the previous histological diagnosis, any unusual features can be anticipated and over-diagnosis can be avoided.

Malignant lesions

Basal cell carcinoma If there is an incomplete excision of a small basal cell carcinoma then provided that there is adequate spare skin and the doctor has appropriate surgical experience, the wound itself may be excised with a margin of about 3 mm, resutured, and the wound specimen sent for histological examination. Interestingly, when this is done the sections of the second biopsy sometimes fail to reveal any remaining tumour, and basal cell carcinomas recur in only about a third of cases when tumour is reported to be present at or near the surgical resection margin [5,6] (note that this *does not* apply to squamous cell carcinoma or malignant melanoma). Where there is little spare skin or the doctor is inexperienced, the case should be referred to a specialist.

Squamous cell carcinoma and malignant melanoma If on histological examination an excised lesion unexpectedly turns out to be a squamous cell carcinoma or a malignant melanoma and the margin of clearance is inadequate, the case should be urgently referred to a specialist. There should be no cause for undue alarm as the specimen in this case is essentially an incisional biopsy. At the present time there is no compelling evidence to suggest that incisional biopsy of malignant melanoma followed by definitive resection within 30 days increases the likelihood of metastases [7,8]. However, this should not be regarded as an argument for a casual approach to malignant melanoma. Current recommendations are that incisional biopsies should be avoided if possible [9]. Nevertheless, in specialist hands an incisional biopsy *is* appropriate in selected uncertain cases and in areas such as the face and digits [10], in order to avoid an unnecessarily extensive resection.

Biopsy techniques

Whenever possible, a skin lesion should be removed completely (excision biopsy) with an appropriate margin of normal tissue. However, it is sometimes appropriate to remove only a part of the lesion (incisional biopsy), and with obviously benign lesions a shave biopsy is sometimes the treatment of choice. Punch biopsy has little place in general practice.

Shave biopsy

This method should be confined to obviously benign exophytic lesions such as papillomata and seborrhoeic keratoses. The technique involves the use of a scalpel blade to slice off a skin lesion almost flat with the surrounding skin under a local anaesthetic (Figs. 15.36, 15.37). The resulting raw surface can then be

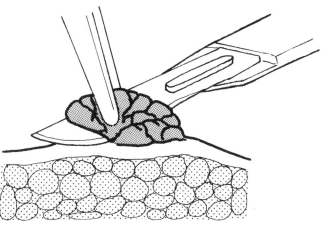

Fig. 15.36. Shave biopsy technique.

Fig. 15.37. (a–c) Shave biopsy of intradermal naevus.

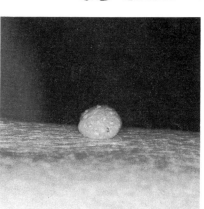
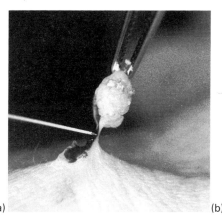
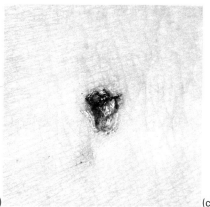

(a)   (b)   (c)

cauterised flat by electrocautery or diathermy. It is advisable to use adrenaline with the local anaesthetic so as to minimise any bleeding. However, for more bulky lesions it is preferable to perform the amputation by cutting with an electrocautery tip or using bipolar forceps as this virtually eliminates bleeding altogether.

Flattening the biopsy specimen onto a piece of blotting paper allows better orientation for fixation and sectioning.

Incisional biopsy

If excision and direct closure of a lesion would be difficult because of its size or location (e.g. nose, face or the hand), part of the lesion may be removed as an incisional biopsy for histological examination (Fig. 15.38). Once the diagnosis has been established definitive treatment (curettage, cryotherapy, cautery, diathermy or excision) can be planned.

The site of the biopsy must be selected to provide a representative sample of the lesion (Fig. 15.39). If necessary, more than one site should be biopsied. The

Fig. 15.38. Incisional biopsy.

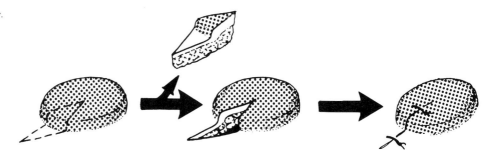

Fig. 15.39. Incisional biopsy confirmed a diagnosis of pyoderma gangrenosum in this large ulcer on the leg of a patient with rheumatoid arthritis.

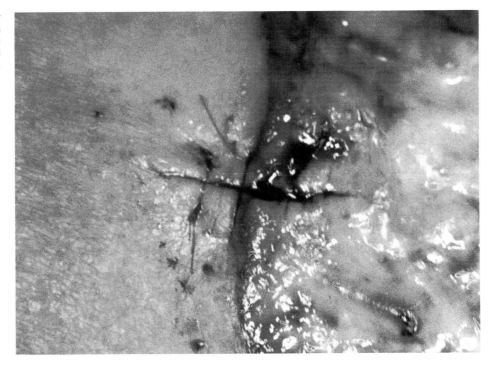

long axis of the biopsy must be carefully planned both for cosmesis and for its possible incorporation within any subsequent definitive excision. In order to define the surface extent and depth of the lesion, the excision should extend out into normal skin and deep into normal subcutaneous fat.

A small elliptical incision is made, taking care that the width of the excised ellipse is not so great as to prevent easy closure. The edge of the normal skin is picked up with forceps and the excision is completed without damaging the lesional part of the specimen. The wound is closed with simple interrupted nylon sutures.

Excisional biopsy

The majority of benign lesions and simple small basal cell carcinomas can be easily removed in the doctor's surgery. However, unless the doctor is experienced, lesions on areas where there is little spare skin (such as the head, face, ears and hands) should be referred to a specialist. Larger basal cell carcinomas, squamous cell carcinomas and all suspicious pigmented lesions should be referred for specialist treatment.

Fig. 15.40. Specimen being placed into a pot containing formalin.

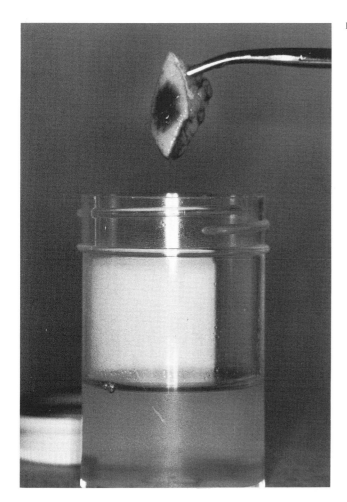

The margin of clearance The margin of clearance depends on the nature of the lesion. For benign lesions the full thickness of the skin is excised with a minimum margin of 1–2 mm of normal skin, depending on the site of the lesion. At least 4 mm clearance should be allowed for basal cell carcinomas [11] that are less than 2 cm in diameter. The excision should extend well into the superficial fat. No excision should be attempted if there is doubt about the ability to close the wound, and the resection margin should not be compromised in order to allow closure. Anything other than small simple lesions should be referred to a specialist.

All excised lesions should be sent for histological examination.

Skin preparation Routine skin preparation is appropriate for most lesions but excision of an ulcerated lesion with weeping and crusting is quite liable to result in either postoperative wound infection or break-down. The risk of this happening can be reduced by asking the patient to paint the lesion with povidone iodine or chlorhexidine for 24 h prior to surgery and, in addition, leaving a cotton ball soaked in the antiseptic skin preparation solution directly on the lesion for 5–10 min prior to excision.

Skin excision Most skin lesions can be removed by a simple elliptical incision. The ellipse should be planned to lie with its long axis aligned with natural skin creases or wrinkle lines. The proposed skin ellipse should be marked out prior to injection of the local anaesthetic as the volume of the anaesthetic can stiffen the tissues and disguise the natural skin creases. Ideally, the length of the ellipse should be about $2\frac{1}{2}$ to 3 times its width (Fig. 15.41).

The specimen is dissected free from the deep layer either with scissors or a scalpel, and removed (Figs. 15.42, 15.43). It is usual to have at least some bleeding from the wound edges at this point and so it may be helpful to plug the wound with a gauze swab while the lesion is transferred into a specimen container and preparation made for suturing the wound.

If necessary, the skin may be undermined to relieve any tension. Deep sutures are rarely required for the majority of small lesions. However, a 3/0 absorbable suture may be used to tie off any blood vessels and to approximate the fat layer if necessary. The skin may be closed with simple interrupted sutures or a subcuti-

Fig. 15.41. Skin ellipse.

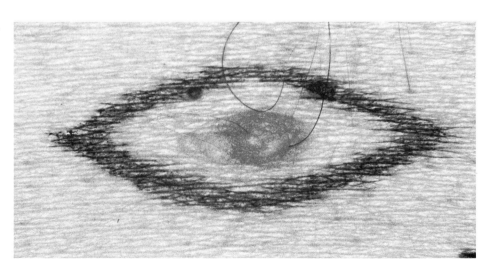

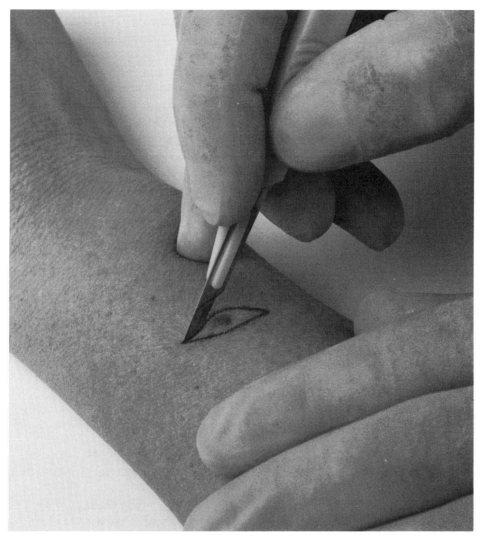

Fig. 15.42. Making the skin incision.

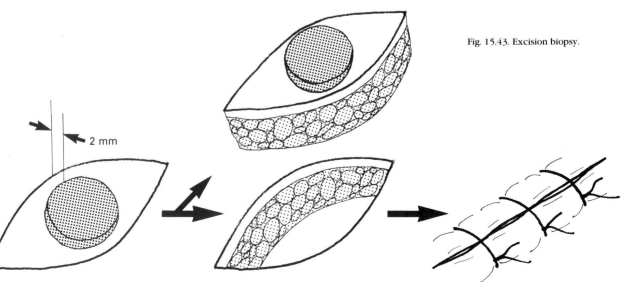

Fig. 15.43. Excision biopsy.

2 mm

cular suture supported with adhesive tapes. A 5/0 monofilament nylon suture is adequate for the majority of small wounds. Larger wounds with greater tension will require 3/0 nylon sutures and it is extremely rare for a thicker suture than this to be required.

Most wounds will have sealed themselves with a crust within 24 h and therefore any light gauze dressing may be removed at that time and the wound exposed to the air. The patient may shower but not soak in a bath. However, some wounds on sites on the body such as the axilla and groin (which are prone to sweating) and the buttock and sole of the foot (which are subjected to pressure) may be best left covered until the sutures are removed.

References

1. *Textbook of Dermatology*. 4th edn. Rook, R., Wilkinson, D. S., Ebling, F. J. G., Champion, R. H. & Burton, J. L. (eds.). Blackwell Scientific Publications: Edinburgh.

2. Application of 7 point checklist in assessment of benign pigmented lesions. Higgins, E. M., Hall, P., Todd, P. *et al. Clinical and Experimental Dermatology* (1992), **17**, 313–315.

3. Malignant melanoma. Mackie, R. & McHenry, P. *Practitioner* (1992), **236**, 760–766.

4. Excess melanocytic naevi in children with renal allografts. Smith, C. H., McGregor, J. M. & Barker, J. N. W. N. *Journal of the American Academy of Dermatology* (1992), **28**, 51–55.

5. Significance of marginal extension in excised basal cell carcinoma. Gooding, C. A., White, G. & Yatsuhashi, M. *New England Journal of Medicine* (1965), **273**, 923–924.

6. Prognosis of 'incompletely-excised' vs 'completely-excised' basal cell carcinoma. Pascal, R. R., Hubby, L. H., Lattes, R. & Crickelair, G. *Plastic and Reconstructive Surgery* (1968), **41**, 328–332.

7. Does biopsy type influence survival in clinical stage 1 cutaneous melanoma? Lederman, J. & Sober, A. J. *Journal of the American Academy of Dermatology* (1985), **13**, 983–987.

8. Excision biopsy of malignant melanoma by general practitioners in South East Scotland 1981–91. Herd, R. M., Hunter, J. A. A., McLaren, K. M., Chetty, U., Watson, A. C. H. & Gollock, J. M. *British Medical Journal* Vol 305: 12 December (1992), **305**, 1476–1478.

9. Excisional biopsy as the first therapeutic procedure versus primary wide excision of malignant melanoma. Landhaler, M., Braun-Palco, O., Leitl, A., Konz, B. & Hölzel, D. *Cancer* (1989), **64**, 1612–1616.

10. Primary management of melanoma. Rampen, F. H. J., Kint, A., Hunter, J. A. A. & Hulsebosch, H. J. *British Journal of Dermatology* (1984), **111**, 431–436.

11. Surgical margins for basal cell carcinoma. Wolf, D. J. & Zitelli, J. A. *Archives of Dermatology* (1987), **123**, 340–344.

16

Minor surgical procedures: Subcutaneous lesions

Temporal artery biopsy

The anterior branches of the superficial temporal artery are readily accessible and easily biopsied in suspected cases of temporal arteritis. The artery lies *above the deep fascia*, on the surface of the temporalis muscle; the vessel is easily located by palpation and indeed it can often be seen (Fig. 16.1).

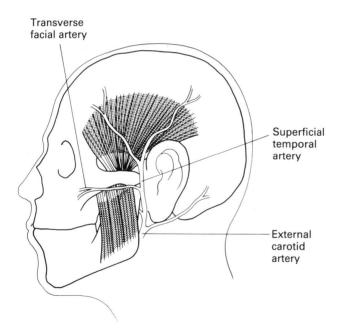

Transverse
facial artery

Superficial
temporal
artery

External
carotid
artery

Fig. 16.1. Superficial temporal artery: surgical anatomy.

Once located, the line of the artery should be marked on the skin prior to the injection of local anaesthetic and a vertical incision is planned to lie within the skin creases and if possible, within the hairline. The incision is made through the skin and into the subcutaneous fat, taking care not to cut the artery itself, and 2 cm of the artery is exposed by blunt dissection with an artery clip or scissors. Tying the artery ends prior to transection (instead of clipping the ends) minimises any chance of bleeding from the cut ends. By means of an artery clip, a length of 3/0 absorbable suture is passed behind the artery and one end is tied off and the procedure is repeated on the other end of the vessel. The segment of the artery is lifted with fine forceps and 1 cm excised with scissors (Fig. 16.2).

If necessary, absorbable subcutaneous sutures may be used to approximate the skin edges before the skin is closed with 5/0 nylon. A light dressing may be applied for 24 h after which the wound may be left exposed. Skin sutures may be removed at 5–7 days.

Fig. 16.2. Temporal artery: incision and biopsy.

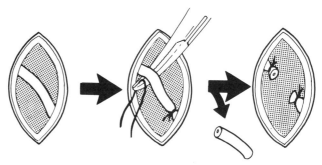

Lymph node biopsy

In general terms, lymph nodes in the neck, supraclavicular fossa, axilla or groin should be biopsied under a general anaesthetic. However, if they are very easily defined and the doctor experienced, superficial lymph nodes may be excised using local anaesthetic infiltration.

The incision should be made in the line of the skin creases over the swelling and should be at least twice the size of the node to be biopsied to ensure that the whole dissection is carried out under direct vision. The fat and superficial fascia should be incised in the line of the wound and the lymph node or group of nodes exposed using blunt dissection. If necessary, a small self-retaining retractor may be inserted to aid the dissection. The tissue that tethers the deep surface of the node will contain small blood vessels and lymphatic channels. An artery clip is placed across this pedicle, which is then ligated and divided, leaving the clip attached to the specimen (Fig. 16.3). The capsule of the node should not be grasped, since this may distort the histological features. The wound is closed with subcutaneous absorbable sutures and 3/0 nylon to the skin.

Fig. 16.3. Ligation of lymph node stalk.

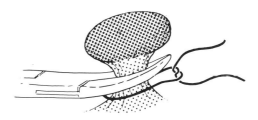

Skin cysts

Milia

These very small epithelial cysts are commonly found on the cheeks in adults and are distinct from the very fine milia in babies, which require no treatment. The

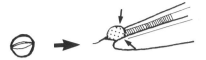

Fig. 16.4. Incision and extrusion of milia.

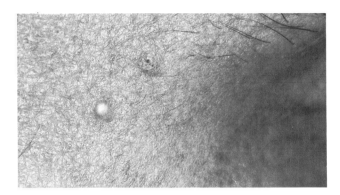

Fig. 16.5. Milia in an adult.

overlying skin can be easily nicked with a no. 11 blade without local anaesthetic and the whole cyst can then be gently squeezed out with non-toothed forceps (Figs. 16.4, 16.5).

Sebaceous cyst

Sebaceous cysts (Fig. 16.6) are essentially of two basic histological types, although the distinction has no significant practical relevance. Those arising from hair follicle cells are more properly called pilar cysts and occur on hair-bearing areas such as the scalp. Epidermoid cysts arise from non-hair-bearing areas such as the palms and soles.

Fig. 16.6. Sebaceous cyst.

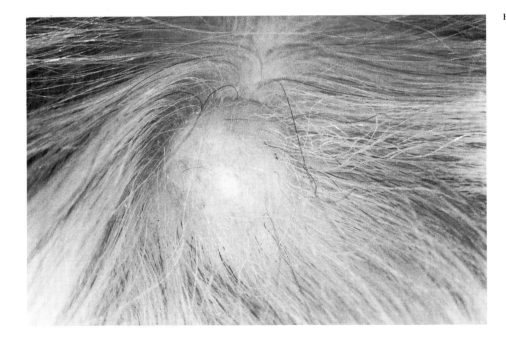

Although usually simple to diagnose, nevertheless a sebaceous cyst can sometimes be mistaken for other lesions such as: a thyroglosal cyst in the midline at the front of the neck; a branchial cyst anterior to the sternomastoid at the junction of its upper third and lower two thirds; a parotid tumour at the angle of the mandible; a congenital dermoid cyst at lines of embryonic fusion; a lymph node; or an osteoma of the skull (Fig. 16.7). Rarely, a solid subcutaneous tumour (such as a secondary deposit of a malignant melanoma) may be mistaken for a sebaceous cyst and the diagnosis made only during the dissection (see chapter 13 for management of unexpected findings). Very rarely a cyst may have an early carcinoma growing in its wall. Thus, all excised cysts should be sent for histological confirmation.

Cysts in some sites of the body can cause great difficulty in their removal. Unless the doctor is experienced, cysts on the face (Fig. 16.8), overlying the posterior

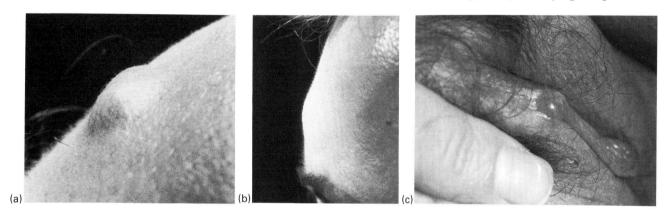

(a)   (b)   (c)

Fig. 16.7. (ABOVE, LEFT, CENTRE AND RIGHT) (a) Sebaceous cyst on the forehead, (b) an osteoma of the skull, (c) this longstanding labial lesion turned out to be a benign hidradenoma.

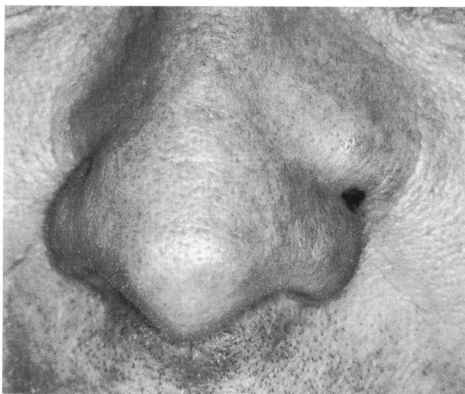

Fig. 16.8. Sebaceous cyst on the face.

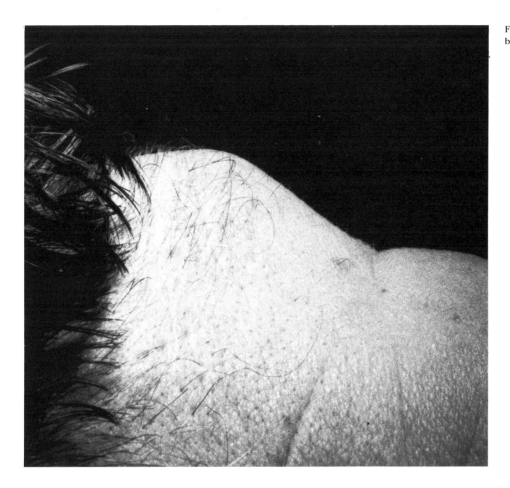

Fig. 16.9. Sebaceous cyst over the back of the neck.

triangle of the neck or behind the angle of the mandible should be referred because of the risk of damage to the spinal accessory and facial nerves.

Removal of cysts on the back of the neck may be more difficult and more bloody than expected because the skin there is often thick and firm (Fig. 16.9). If possible, the cyst should be removed whole. The cyst wall is often (but not always) attached to the deep layer of the overlying dermis. If any remnant of the cyst wall is left behind the cyst is likely to recur. For this reason, incision and squeezing out the contents is not recommended (except when infected). Although puncturing and emptying the cyst can allow the deflated cyst wall to be removed through a smaller incision and is an acceptable technique, the method can be both messy and tiresome, particularly if there is bleeding.

When removing small cysts in the scalp it is often enough to trim hair immediately over the cyst itself and then to hold the rest of the hair out of the way with adhesive tapes (Fig. 16.10).

Small cyst Small cysts can often be quickly removed by blunt dissection with an artery clip or scissors after simple incision over the dome (Fig. 16.11).

Large cyst Except when small, the cyst should be removed in continuity with a small skin ellipse to avoid any redundant skin and dead space (Fig. 16.12). An elliptical incision should be centred on the punctum, with care taken not to

Fig. 16.10. Exposing cyst on scalp
using adhesive tapes.

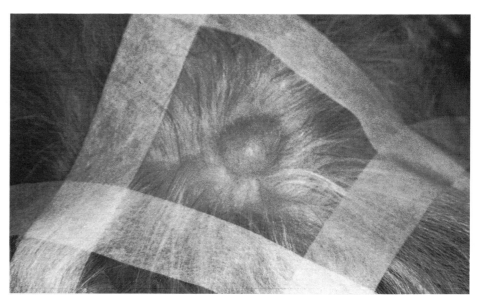

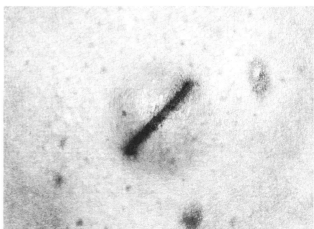

Fig. 16.11. Excision of a small sebaceous cyst by simple incision over the
dome.

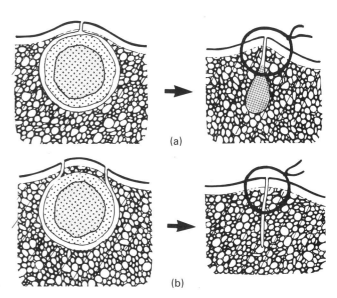

Fig. 16.12. Excision of a sebaceous cyst, avoiding dead space.

Skin cysts

245

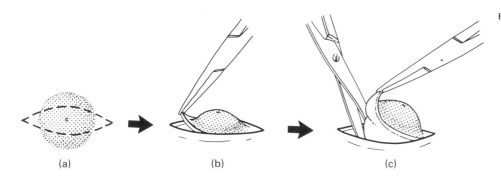

Fig. 16.13. Sebaceous cyst, excision.

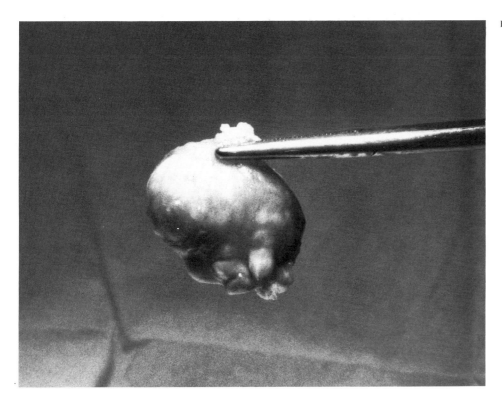

Fig. 16.14. Sebaceous cyst specimen.

puncture the cyst. Starting at one end the incision is carefully deepened by sharp dissection until the plane between the cyst and the subcutaneous fat is identified. Once this plane has been entered the cyst may be easily shelled out by blunt dissection with an artery clip or curved dissecting scissors (Fig. 16.13, 16.14). It may be helpful to retract one end of the skin ellipse with an artery clip. Special care should be taken when dissecting in the neck or face to avoid accidental damage to any underlying vessels or nerves, particularly when applying traction (Fig. 16.15).

If the cyst is accidentally incised during the initial skin incision or during the excision, subsequent dissection may be difficult and messy. In these circumstances it may be helpful simply to make a fresh, slightly more lateral skin incision, allowing the dissection to proceed further away from the cyst wall and minimising spillage of cyst contents into the wound (Fig. 16.16). Any spillage should be mopped up with a wet swab.

Fig. 16.15. Care should be taken to avoid accidental damage to underlying vessels or nerves, especially when applying traction.

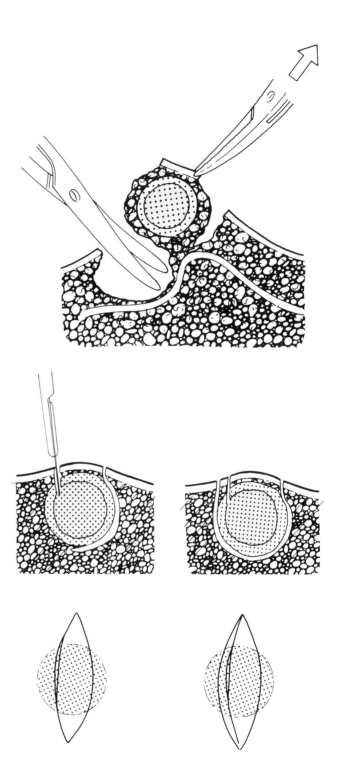

Fig. 16.16. Sebaceous cyst, secondary incision.

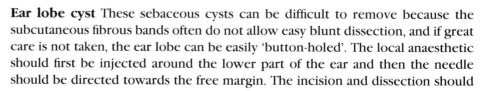

Ear lobe cyst These sebaceous cysts can be difficult to remove because the subcutaneous fibrous bands often do not allow easy blunt dissection, and if great care is not taken, the ear lobe can be easily 'button-holed'. The local anaesthetic should first be injected around the lower part of the ear and then the needle should be directed towards the free margin. The incision and dissection should preferably be on the posterior side with the ear pulled and held forwards by adhesive tapes. Note the small hypertrophic scars that appear secondary to ear piercing and may be mistaken for a sebaceous cyst (Fig. 16.17). Simple excision of such lesions is likely to result in a recurrence (see chapter 21).

Inflamed sebaceous cyst If the cyst is red and painful but the overlying skin is not too angry and indurated, then it is often kinder to excise the cyst followed by primary suture as above rather than subject the patient to incision and drainage followed by later excision (Fig. 16.18). The local anaesthetic always takes longer to work when there is inflammation and excision of the inflamed cyst will always give rise to more bleeding during the procedure. However, if adequate time is left for the adrenaline to work then any bleeding will be minimised.

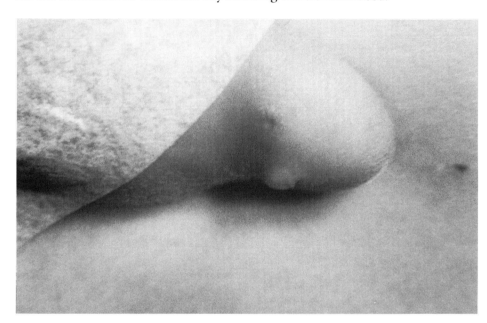

Fig. 16.17. This may look like a sebaceous cyst in the ear lobe but is in fact a hypertrophic scar secondary to ear piercing.

Fig. 16.18. (BELOW, LEFT AND RIGHT) (a) and (b) Excision of infected sebaceous cyst in scalp.

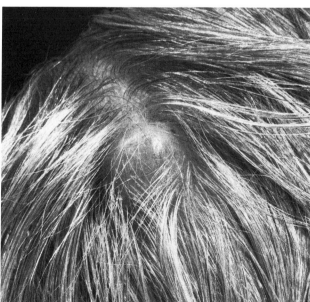

(a)

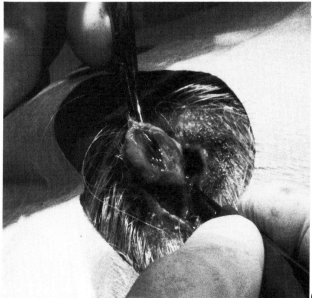

(b)

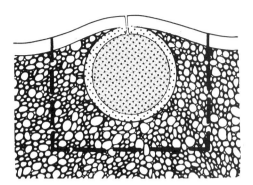

Fig. 16.19. Excision of previously infected sebaceous cyst.

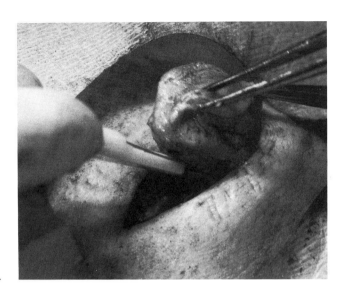

Fig. 16.20. Sharp dissection of previously infected sebaceous cyst.

Previously infected sebaceous cyst The elective excision of a previously infected cyst may be quite difficult and bloody because dense fibrous tissue forms and destroys the tissue planes. In such circumstances it may be impossible to 'shell out' the cyst. Instead, the cyst should be excised by sharp dissection in continuity with a block of subcutaneous tissue (Figs. 16.19, 16.20). Because of the inevitable bleeding it is often necessary to plug one side of the wound with a gauze swab while dissecting on the other side. Some curved artery clips should be at hand to clamp any bleeding vessels and it is advisable to load a needle holder with a 3/0 suture prior to the procedure so that the first suture can be placed immediately as the gauze swab is removed.

Inclusion dermoid

An inclusion dermoid is commonly found in the terminal pulp spaces of a finger and is easy to dissect out as there are no deep structures at risk distal to the insertion of the flexor tendon. Lesions of the fingers proximal to the distal interphalangeal joint, and those commonly found just distal to the transverse palmar crease, should be referred for specialist treatment, since they may encroach on the digital nerves, vessels and flexor tendons.

Before proceeding it is helpful to mark out the position of the cyst with a circle. The patient's finger should be anaesthetised with a digital nerve block and exsanguinated prior to application of a rubber band tourniquet. A longitudinal incision should be made over the most prominent point and the cyst excised by blunt dissection.

Meibomian cyst (Chalazion)

The meibomian glands lie within the tarsal plate, behind the orbicularis oculi muscle, and drain through the conjunctival surface of the eyelid. A meibomian cyst (Fig. 16.21) is not a true cyst but a granuloma of a meibomian gland. Usually

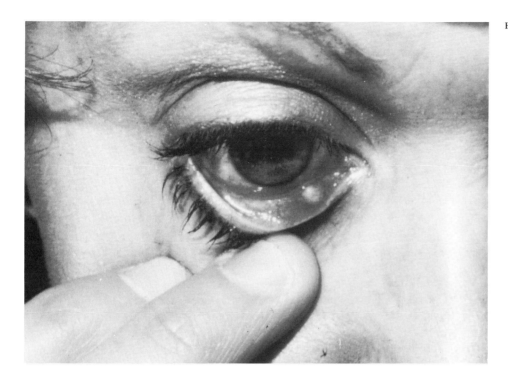

Fig. 16.21. Meibomian cyst.

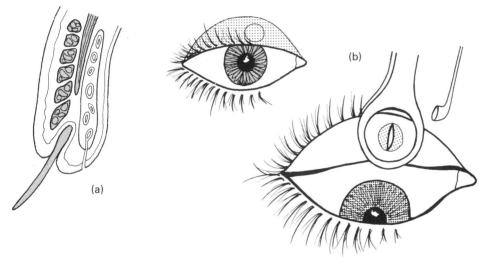

Fig. 16.22. (a) Cross-section through upper eyelid. (b) Curettage of meibomian cyst.

(a)

(b)

the lump appears gradually and without acute inflammatory symptoms or signs. If the eyelid is everted, the conjunctiva may initially be red or purple over the nodule, and later it becomes greyish due to the granulation tissue. Spontaneous resolution is uncommon or slow. Treatment consists of incision and curettage through the palpebral conjunctiva (Fig. 16.22). Very occasionally a meibomian cyst can present as a small acute abscess and this should be simply drained through an incision in the palpebral conjunctiva without any need for curettage.

The eyelid should be infiltrated with a small quantity of lignocaine and a few drops of amethocaine instilled in the eye. The lid is then everted and a chalazion ring clamp applied. This holds the lid steady and reduces the amount of bleeding. Without the clamp even a few drops of blood will obscure the operative field and make the procedure tedious. A vertical incision is made into the cyst and the granuloma scraped out with a small curette.

An eye pad is used for a few hours until the anaesthetic has worn off and an antibiotic ointment is applied for several days postoperatively. The patient should be warned that after the curettage the cavity fills with blood and therefore a 'lump' may persist for many days after the operation.

Lipoma

Small superficial lipomata are easily diagnosed and 'shelled out' under local anaesthesia. However, largely because of the thickness of the skin and underlying fat, lipomata on the back or over the scapulae may be much deeper than expected. Occasionally the lesion may be subfascial, that is deep to the deep fascia. For this reason, the inexperienced practitioner should refer larger and deep lipomata for excision in hospital.

The fat lobules of a lipoma are usually larger than and are easily distinguished from those of normal subcutaneous fat. The tumour is usually well defined with a very thin capsule and can be either dissected out or removed using the 'squeeze' technique.

In the dissection method, an incision is made over the swelling and deepened until the lipoma is identified. The incision need only be perhaps two thirds of the length of the lesion. Once the plane is found between the lipoma and the subcutaneous fat, the lipoma is shelled out by blunt dissection using scissors or a finger (Figs. 16.23, 16.24, 16.25). Occasionally there are some tethering vessels

Fig. 16.23. (a–c) Lipoma dissection.

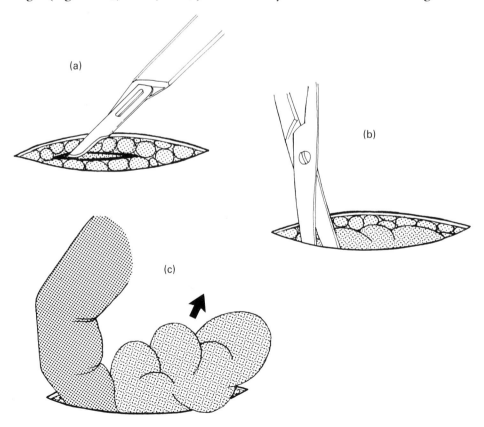

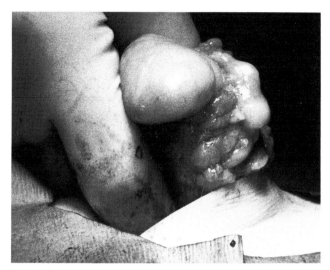

Fig. 16.24. Dissection of lipoma with the finger.

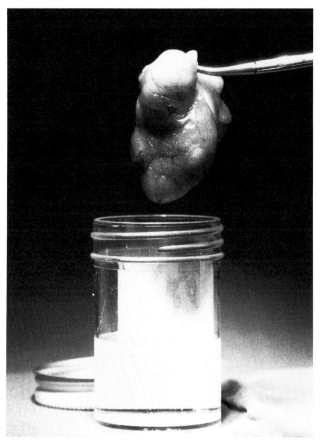

Fig. 16.25. Lipoma specimen.

on the deep surface of the lipoma and these should be ligated with absorbable suture unless they are very fine. The wound should be closed taking care to avoid any dead space.

In the 'squeeze' method, a smaller incision is made and traction is applied to the lipoma while digital pressure is applied around the lesion circumference to squeeze it out of the wound (Fig. 16.26). Since the wound is deliberately small, its cavity cannot be easily inspected. Therefore, particular care should be made to ligate any sizable tethering vessels to ensure against any bleeding inside the wound.

Injection site granuloma

Commonly found in the buttocks long after irritant injections such as intramuscular iron, these granulomata are felt as hard (they are often calcified) subcutaneous nodules which may or may not have some overlying skin tethering and dimpling.

If the skin is tethered to the underlying granuloma it may be removed as a narrow ellipse in continuity with lesion.

Fig. 16.26. Lipoma 'squeeze' method.

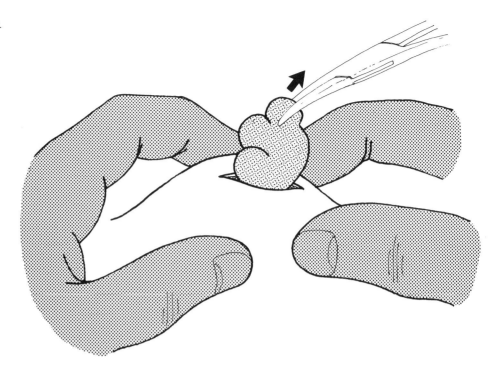

Rheumatoid nodules

These lesions are commonly found over the olecranon and if uncomfortable or obtrusive they may be excised in much the same way as a large sebaceous cyst. However, they have to be removed by sharp dissection as they are likely to be tethered in fibrous tissue and do not 'shell out'.

17

Minor surgical procedures: Toenail surgery

Ingrowing toenails

An ingrowing toe nail is caused by the edge of the nail digging into the nail wall resulting in inflammation of the tissues around the nail. Ingrowing toenails have little to do with ill-fitting shoes. The condition is commonly found in individuals who have bulky nail walls such that the edge of the growing nail is obliged to dig into the surrounding tissue instead of sitting well clear (Fig. 17.1).

Patients with ingrowing toenails are often inadequately treated and in-

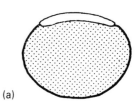

(a)

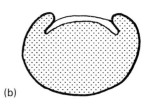

(b)

Fig. 17.1. End view of (a) normal toe, (b) toe with bulky nail walls.

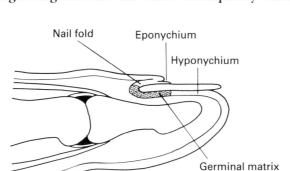

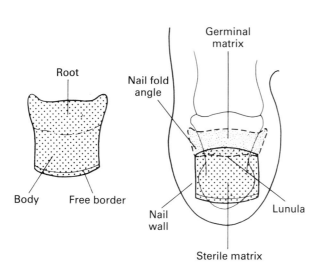

Fig. 17.2. Toenail anatomy.

appropriately given antibiotics when simple quick minor surgery is effective in producing relief resolution within 24 h. Ingrowing toenails can be extremely painful and problematical for the patient and, since the inflammatory process is initiated and maintained by the nail edge digging into the nail wall there is no reason not to treat the condition energetically and at the earliest opportunity, as for any foreign body or splinter.

Non-inflamed ingrowing toenail

Simply cutting down the side of the nail adjacent to the nail wall can be done in selected cases where there is painful ingrowing of the nail without inflammation. The side of the nail can often easily be trimmed away from the nail wall in a gentle curve. The patient should be instructed to trim and file the nail regularly in the same manner and may in so doing avoid any further trouble. It is a fallacy that cutting the nails straight and allowing the nails to grow long prevents ingrowing. It does not (see Fig. 17.4c).

Inflamed ingrowing toenail

When inflammation is present, cutting down the side of the nail is often unsatisfactory and is likely to leave nail spicules, leading to further inflammation. If the nail is already elevated and surrounded by granulation tissue, the nail edge may sometimes be taken off with scissors without local anaesthetic and with minimal discomfort to the patient (Fig. 17.3).

However, in most cases it is necessary to remove a nail segment under a local anaesthetic. For simple ingrowing toenails it is never necessary to remove the whole nail and antibiotics are rarely required. Since the problem is essentially due to mechanical pressure, the treatment is surgical. Antibiotics are required only if there is cellulitis but even this will rapidly resolve after removal of a nail segment (Fig. 17.4).

Fig. 17.3. (a) and (b) When the nail has already lifted it can sometimes be trimmed away from the nail wall without using a local anaesthetic.

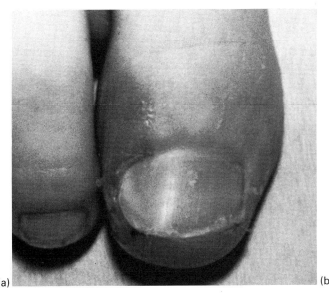
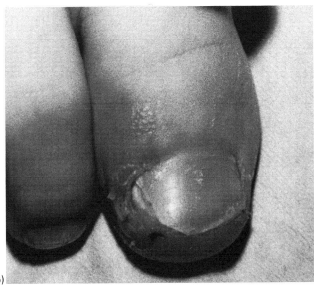

(a)

(b)

Treatment for inflamed ingrowing toenails

1. Treat as soon as possible as for any foreign body reaction.
2. Antibiotics are usually *unnecessary*.
3. Recurrence rate is high after simple nail avulsion.
4. It is rarely necessary to remove the whole nail.
5. Segmental nail bed phenolisation is treatment of choice.
6. Gross inflammation is not usually a contraindication to phenolisation.

There is always the possibility to keep in mind that a subungual lesion or ulceration around the nail may be a malignant melanoma or squamous cell carcinoma, although rare (Fig. 17.5).

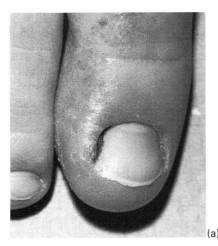 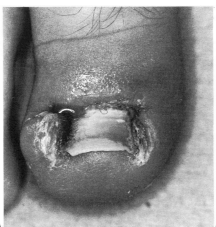 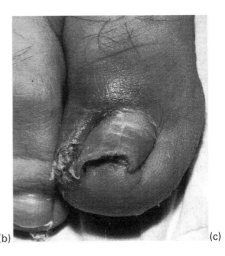

(a)   (b)   (c)

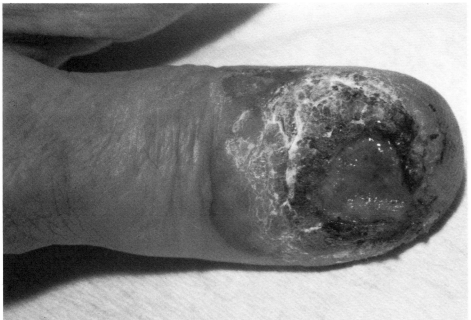

Fig. 17.4. (a) Mildly inflamed ingrowing toenail. (b) and (c) Grossly inflamed ingrowing toenail. Both of these toes can be easily treated by segmental phenolisation without waiting for the inflammation to settle. The resolution of the inflammation is rapid once the nail has been removed and the patient will be very much more comfortable after 24 h. Note that the nail in (c) has ingrown despite being cut straight across and being allowed to grow long.

Fig. 17.5. Squamous cell carcinoma present for 3 years in the dominant thumb. Treatment was with radiotherapy.

Fig. 17.6. (a–c) Removing a nail segment.

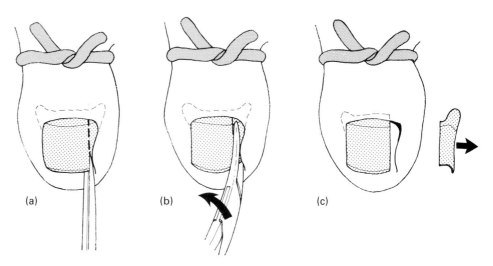

(a)   (b)   (c)

Removing a nail segment Simply removing a segment of nail will certainly allow rapid resolution of any inflammation but the patient should be made aware that the problem is very likely to recur after the nail grows back [1]. However, for an ingrowing toenail of only short duration or one following trauma with no previous history, this is an acceptable method of management. Any patient with longstanding or recurrent ingrowing toenail should be offered definitive treatment at the same time as removal of the nail segment.

After a digital nerve block, exsanguination and application of a tourniquet, a one fifth segment of nail is lifted from its bed using a mosquito artery clip. The nail is then split by cutting longitudinally down to and under the nail fold (Fig. 17.6a). Ordinary stitch scissors are quite adequate for most nails although special nail scissors or fine bone cutters may be necessary for the thickest nails. The segment of nail is then removed with an artery clip, using a twisting motion rather than a simple straight tug (Fig. 17.6b,c).

It is important to note that the proximal corners of the normal nail have rounded extensions that sit well into the lateral recesses of the nail germinal matrix. If the avulsed nail segment shows a sharp proximal edge then it is likely that the most proximal part of the nail has been left *in situ*. A retained fragment is likely when either the scissors have not cut back far enough to the proximal edge of the nail root or when the nail segment is pulled rather than twisted off.

Any retained fragment *must* be removed. It may be necessary to direct a pen light into the recess to visualise and confirm a retained fragment, and complete the proximal incision of the nail root with the scissors prior to attempted removal. The toe may be covered with a simple dry gauze dressing for a few days simply to soak up any exudate but may be washed at any time.

Definitive treatment for chronic or recurrent ingrowing toenails

A number of different methods of treating ingrowing toenails have been tried, including cryotherapy to granulations, insertion of cotton pledglets [2] under the nail edges to lift the nails, and insertion of plastic gutters [3] along the nail edge. However, segmental nail bed ablation with phenol (SNBAP) is simple and quick to perform and is the treatment of choice [4,5,6,7,8]. It has more than a 90 % success rate and can be easily repeated if necessary. It causes minimal pain when compared to surgical excision. Although wedge resection (Fig. 17.7) (or any of its modifications) is a common technique and involves excision of the nail, nail wall, and nail bed *en bloc* it should no longer be used as it is far more painful than SNBAP and there is no guarantee that the nail bed in the lateral recess will be completely excised. Lateral 'horns' may therefore result. (Note that the term *wedge excision* is often incorrectly applied to the simple removal of a segment of nail.)

Although the Zadik operation [9] (total nail bed excision) is still performed (and often under a general anaesthetic when it can be easily done using local anaesthesia), it is unnecessarily mutilating and painful and has no place in the routine management of ingrowing toenails (Fig. 17.8). Since ingrowing toenails are only caused by the edges of the nail digging into a bulky nail wall, there is no necessity to remove the central plate of the nail. Segmental nail bed excision under a local anaesthetic using Bonney's blue to paint and identify the germinal epithelium is the treatment of choice after failed phenol ablation. Total nail bed excision should be reserved for only very occasional use in troublesome onychogryphosis or very curved painful nails when phenol ablation has failed.

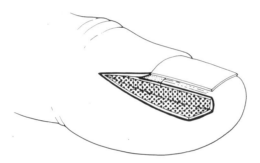

Fig. 17.7. Wedge excision of nail bed. This is an unnecessarily painful procedure and should be discarded in favour of the simpler and less traumatic SNBAP.

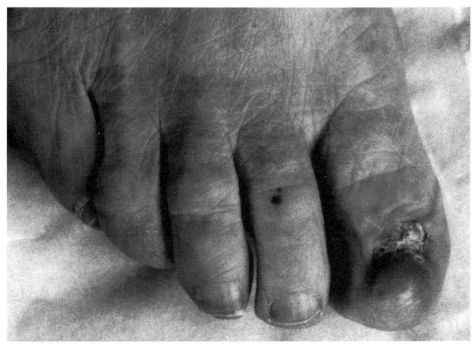

Fig. 17.8. Mutilating treatments have no place in the management of ingrowing toenails. This patient had a failed Zadik operation to her great toe. The horny outgrowths are clearly seen. In addition, the patient had an amputation of the distal phalanx of her ring toe for ingrowing toenail. Segmental nail bed phenolisation can be used on any toe and also on the fingers and thumb, if necessary.

Segmental nail bed ablation with phenol (SNBAP)

Phenol (80%) is a caustic liquid that can be applied to cauterise chemically the nail germinal matrix (Figs. 17.9, 17.10). Although phenol is customarily applied for 3 min, a 5 min application ensures against inadequate cautery and does not result in postoperative exudate any more than the shorter application. Methylated spirits neutralises phenol and is used to protect the surrounding skin.

SNBAP is *not a sterile procedure* and can be performed in the presence of heavy granulation tissue and contamination. In such cases, it is kinder and more effective to proceed directly to SNBAP rather than to use antibiotics.

The doctor should wear protective gloves and special care should be taken not to spill or splash the phenol. After a digital nerve block, exsanguination and application of a tourniquet, a one fifth segment of nail is removed. The toe is protected with a methylated spirit-soaked gauze swab and a cotton bud dipped in phenol is inserted into the lateral recess. The cauterised tissue soon appears grey-white. After 5 min the bud is removed and the toe swabbed with methylated spirits to remove any excess phenol. A dry gauze dressing is applied and mild analgesics such as Co-proxamol given for 24 h. Usually, the patient will report that

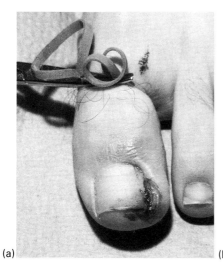 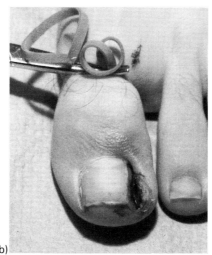 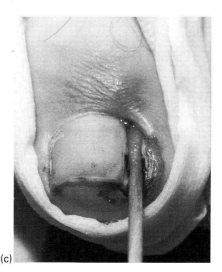

(a)   (b)   (c)

Fig. 17.9. Single edge segmental nail bed ablation using phenol: (a) tourniquet in place, (b) nail segment removed, (c) methylated-spirit-soaked swab around toe, (c) cotton bud dipped in phenol in lateral recess.

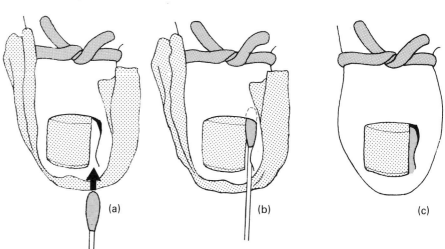

(a)   (b)   (c)

Fig. 17.10. Segmental nail bed ablation using phenol: (a) insertion of phenol bud, (b) phenol bud left in place for 5 min, (c) the phenolised nail bed.

by the next day the soreness from the operation is much less than the discomfort of the ingrowing nail prior to surgery. The dressing can be removed after a day or so and the foot washed normally. It will be necessary to use a light gauze dressing to absorb the exudate from the lateral recess but the toe should be dry after 1–2 weeks.

Sometimes the exudate may persist for a little longer. If, however, the exudate shows no sign of lessening or erythema and pain persists, it is likely that there is a retained fragment of nail or tissue debris in the lateral recess that must be removed before the toe will settle down.

The final result is not seen for about 3 months. Although slightly narrower than normal, the nail will be quite natural-looking (Figs. 17.11, 17.12).

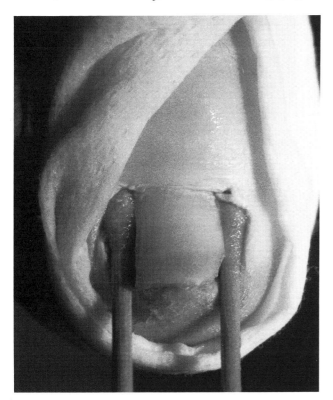

Fig. 17.11. Double-edge segmental nail bed ablation using phenol.

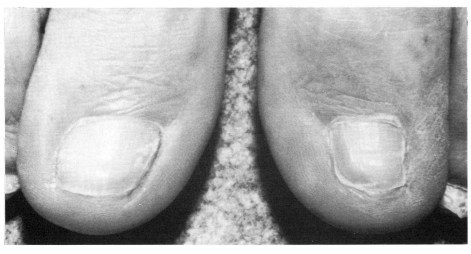

Fig. 17.12. Appearance 2 years after double-edge segmental nail bed ablation using phenol: the left great toenail is natural-looking but narrower than the untreated right great toenail.

Segmental nail bed excision

Segmental nail bed excision (Fig. 17.13) should be reserved for treatment of ingrowing toenails after failed SNBAP.

It is ordinarily quite difficult to distinguish germinal epithelium fragments from underlying tissues and hence incomplete excisions resulting in regrowths of

Fig. 17.13. (a–f) segmental nail bed excision. Retraction instruments not included to maintain clarity.

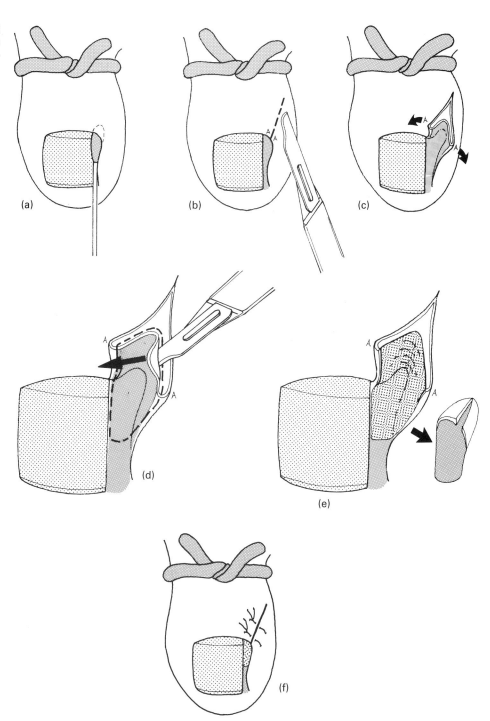

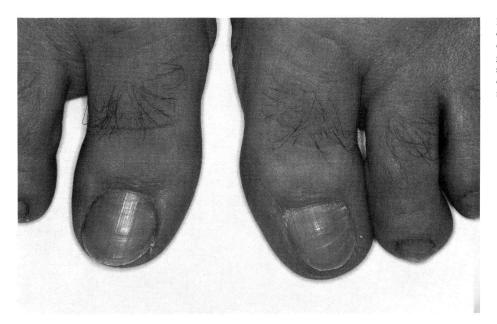

Fig. 17.14. Appearance 6 years after double-edge segmental nail bed excision for ingrowing toenail of left great toe. Note that only a thin segment of nail bed has been excised. This allows for a more natural-looking final result.

lateral 'horns' are not uncommon. However, accurate definition of the germinal epithelium can be achieved by first painting the lateral recesses with a cotton bud dipped in Bonney's blue.

After a digital nerve block, exsanguination and application of a tourniquet, a one fifth segment of nail is removed. A standard cotton bud is usually too bulky to insert adequately into the lateral recess and is likely to leave the depth of the recess unpainted. The bud should, therefore, be teased so that just a small amount of cotton is left on the wooden shaft.

The cotton bud is then dipped into Bonney's blue and inserted into the lateral recess. This paints the germinal epithelium and the sterile matrix. An oblique 10 mm incision is made at the nail fold angle, extending proximally but stopping short of the interphalangeal joint. The two skin flaps thus created are retracted and the blue germinal epithelium is seen and excised by sharp dissection. The median incision follows the line of the avulsed nail, extends to the proximal margin of the germinal epithelium and distally to just beyond the lunula. The dissection is carried out towards the nail wall and into the nail fold angle to ensure complete excision. It is usual to be able to excise the germinal epithelium in one block. However, if the epithelium is accidentally perforated, the blue paint easily identifies any residual germinal epithelium in the recess and this is excised. The skin flaps are replaced and sutured with 5/0 nylon. A paraffin gauze, gauze and crepe dressing is applied and the tourniquet removed.

Mild analgesics are given postoperatively and the patient's foot elevated for 24 h. The dressing is changed the next day and the sutures removed at 5–7 days.

As this procedure may be performed on both sides of the nail, leaving a good-sized central nail plate (Fig. 17.14), there is no justification for routine total nail bed excision for simple double-edge ingrowing toe nails.

Fig. 17.15. Onychogryphosis.

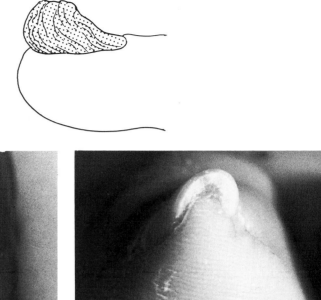

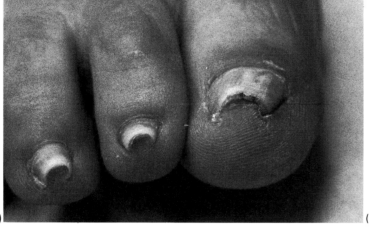

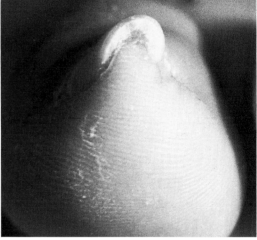

(a)   (b)

Fig. 17.16. Grossly curved nails. (a) If necessary, all of these nails can be treated by double-edge segmental nail bed ablation. (b) This great toenail was so curved and painful that the patient elected to have a total nail bed ablation. Leaving a thin central nail plate would look unsightly.

Onychogryphosis and grossly curved nails

Onychogryphosis is commonly found spontaneously in the elderly and occasionally in younger age groups after trauma (Fig. 17.15). It is still taught that these nails have to be treated by total nail bed excision or ablation. However, while it is often necessary surgically to treat these nails by reduction with small bone nibblers, combined with filing and regular chiropody to keep the nails under control, only when the trimmed nails are painful or are difficult or too time-consuming for the patient or chiropodist to attend to, need they be surgically treated. It is important to examine the leg circulation in the elderly, as toe surgery in the presence of arterial insufficiency may predispose to poor healing, chronic ulceration or gangrene.

Grossly curved nails are sometimes best treated by total nail bed ablation as leaving a very thin central nail plate would look unsightly (Figs. 17.16, 17.17).

Total nail bed phenolization

After a digital nerve block, exsanguination and application of a tourniquet, the whole nail is removed (Fig. 17.17a,b). The toe is protected with a methylated spirit-soaked gauze swab. A pledget of cotton wool dipped in phenol is placed on the top of the raw nail bed with the proximal portion of the pledget carefully tucked under the nail fold sulcus and the lateral ends inserted into the lateral recesses (Fig. 17.17c). After 5 min the pledget is removed and the toe swabbed

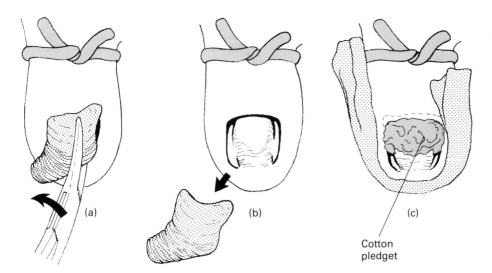

Fig. 17.17. (a–c) Total nail bed phenolisation.

Cotton pledget

with methylated spirit to remove any excess phenol. A dry gauze dressing is applied and mild analgesics such as Co-proxamol given for 24 h. The dressing can be removed after a day or so and the foot washed normally. It will be necessary to use a light gauze dressing to absorb the exudate from the lateral recesses, which will dry up after about 1–2 weeks.

Total nail bed excision

This may be performed if phenolisation fails. The technique is similar to segmental nail bed excision but flaps are raised on both sides of the nail and the whole of the germinal epithelium removed *en bloc* (Fig. 17.18a). Once the nail has been removed, the whole germinal epithelium is painted with Bonney's blue. The procedure is made easier if the dissection of the germinal epithelium is excised in two halves (Fig. 17.18b), starting in the midline, and proceeding laterally. Note

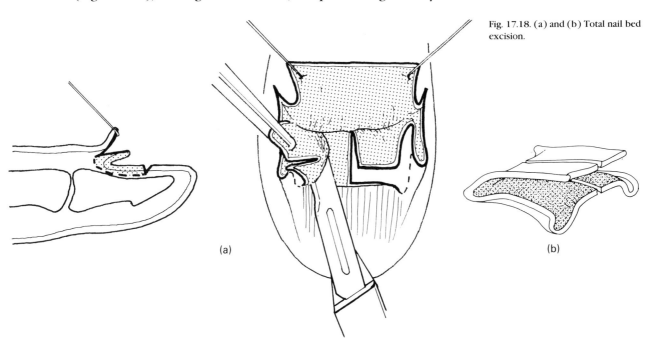

Fig. 17.18. (a) and (b) Total nail bed excision.

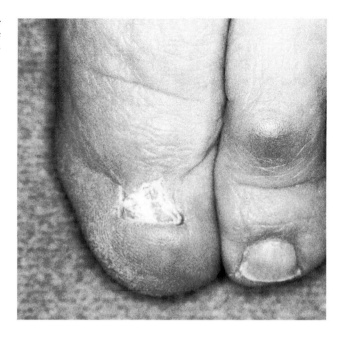

Fig. 17.19. Appearance 6 years after total nail bed excision for onychogryphosis. Note that there is no nail regrowth but the skin of the nail bed is thickened slightly.

that, although excision of the germinal epithelium prevents any nail regrowth, the skin of the nail bed will remain thickened to some degree but this does not normally cause any problem (Fig. 17.19).

References

1. Ingrowing toenails: the results of treatment. Palmer, B. V. & Jones, A. *British Journal of Surgery* (1979), **66**, 575–576.
2. Pledgets in ingrowing toenails. Connolly, B. & Fitzgerald, R. J. *Archives of Diseases in Childhood* (1988), **63**, 71–72.
3. Gutter treatment for ingrowing toenails. Wallace, W. A., Milne, D. D. & Andrew, T. *British Medical Journal* (1979), **ii**, 168–171.
4. The surgical management of ingrowing toenails. Murray, W. R. & Bedi, B. S. *British Journal of Surgery* (1975), **62**, 409–412.
5. Nail bed ablation – excise or cauterise? A controlled study. Andrew, T. & Wallace, W. A. *British Medical Journal* (1979), **ii**, 1539.
6. Surgical wedge excision vs phenol wedge cauterisation for ingrowing toenail. Varma, J. S., Kinnin-Month, A. W. G. & Hamer-Hodges, D. W. *Journal of the Royal College of Surgeons of Edinburgh* (1983), **28**, 331–332.
7. Surgical or phenol ablation of the nail bed for ingrowing toenails: a randomised control trial. Tait, G. R. & Tuck, J. S. *Journal of the Royal College of Surgeons of Edinburgh* (1987), **32**, 358–360.
8. Segmental phenolisation of ingrowing toenails: a randomised controlled study. Morkane, A. J., Robertson, R. W. & Inglis, G. S. *British Journal of Surgery* (1984), **71**, 526–527.
9. Obliterating the nail bed of the great toe without shortening the terminal phalanx. Zadik, F. R. *Journal of Bone and Joint Surgery* (1950), **32B**, 66–67.

18

Minor surgical procedures: Chronic skin ulcers

Corns

Corns are hardened areas of skin and usually develop secondarily to pressure either from inside (such as those under prominent metatarsal heads) or from outside (such as over the dorsum of the proximal interphalangeal joints of lesser toes that rub inside shoes (Fig. 18.1). When corns become chronic and painful and conservative measures fail, surgical treatment may be extremely effective. As with all problems due to pressure, removing the pressure is essential for resolution to take place and surgical excision should not be undertaken unless all tension and pressure from footwear can be avoided during the time of healing. Furthermore, except in selected cases, excision of corns underlying prominent metatarsal heads should be avoided as they are liable to recur because of the pressure effect.

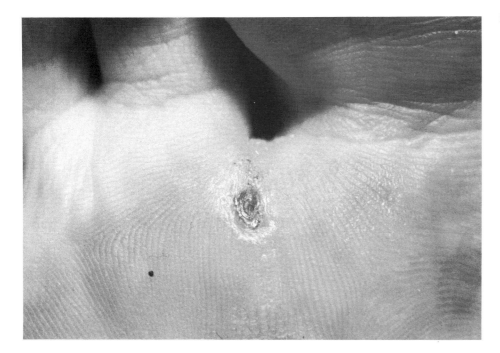

Fig. 18.1. Corn on sole of foot.

Fig. 18.2. (a–c) Taping corn on
dorsum of toe.

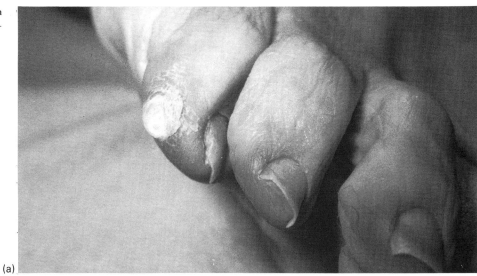

(a)

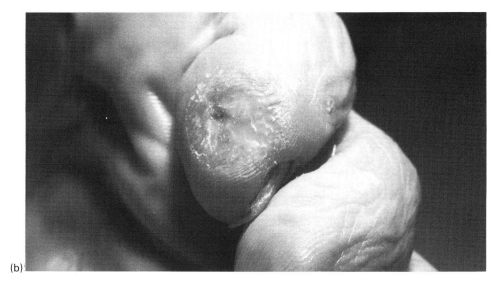

(b)

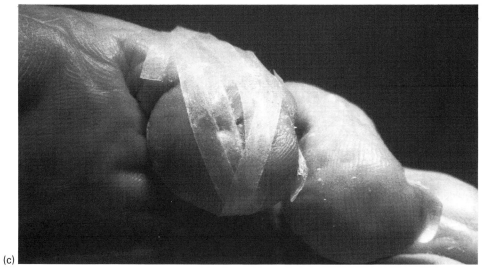

(c)

Sole of foot

A corn under a metatarsal head can be excised with a skin ellipse, as for any deep skin lesion. The incision should be longitudinal to allow easier closure and the dissection should remain within the subcutaneous fat and no deeper so as to avoid the underlying tendons and nerves.

Dorsum of toe

These commonly occur in association with clawing of the toes. The corn here is essentially a small pressure sore caused by friction with footwear. The first line of treatment should be aimed at avoiding any shoes that rub, and applying adhesive tapes across the corn to take up any skin tension. The tape is firmly placed on one side and gentle traction is applied so that the edges of the corn come together as much as possible (Fig. 18.2). It is not necessary to insist on complete approximation of the corn edges as, by avoiding pressure and tension, the corn will heal in a matter of 3–6 weeks. It may be necessary to change the adhesive tapes after every 1–2 weeks.

If the corn has a necrotic centre the edges can be excised in a very thin transverse ellipse and sutured with 5/0 nylon. It may be necessary to undermine the wound edges slightly to help closure without tension. Adhesive tapes are then applied to reduce further any tension (Fig. 18.3).

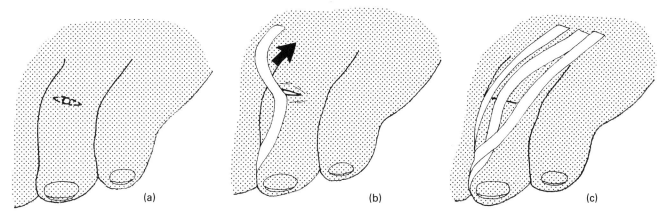

Fig. 18.3. Repair of corn on dorsum of toe (the digital tourniquet is omitted for clarity): (a) excision of corn as a thin ellipse with slight undermining of the wound edges, (b) the adhesive tape is placed on one side of the wound and pulled across to close the defect, (c) adhesive tapes in place.

Pinch grafts to a chronic ulcer

Venous leg ulceration is a common condition and repeated treatment with dressings and elevation can be very expensive in terms of time and labour. Pinch grafts are easy to produce and can be useful in helping to re-epithelialise large venous leg ulcers, provided that the ulcer is clean (Fig. 18.4).

Small full thickness grafts result in healing times that are equivalent to cultured skin equivalents [1] and are more readily obtained. Pinch grafts are very small pieces of full thickness skin and are taken by lifting the skin with the tip of a 21G

Fig. 18.4. A clean ulcer bed ready for
pinch grafting.

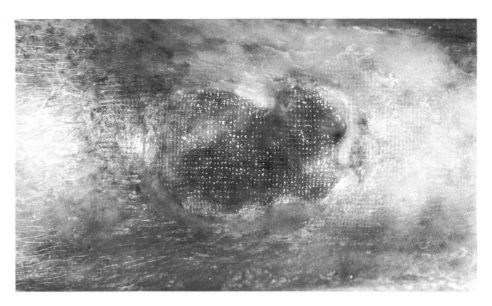

Fig. 18.5. Taking a pinch graft.

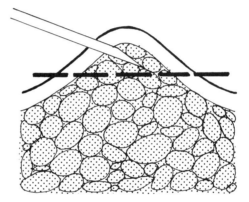

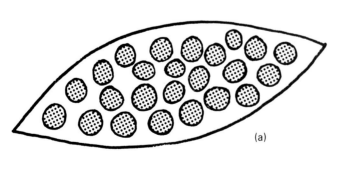

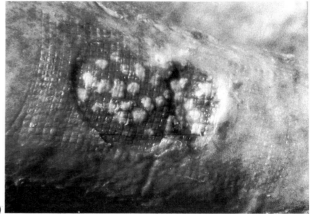

Fig. 18.6. (a) The donor area is
excised as an ellipse and sutured to
leave a linear scar. (b) Appearance
of pinch grafts on ulcer at 7 days.

needle and cutting horizontally just above the base of the cone with a no. 10
scalpel blade (Figs. 18.5, 18.6a).

If multiple pinch grafts are laid over a clean, granulating area, then, once taken,
the surrounding skin becomes epithelialised from around the graft islands. The
donor site can be left to heal by secondary intention but this will leave unsightly

scars. It is preferable to mark out an ellipse on the donor skin site, take the pinch grafts, excise the pock-marked ellipse of skin and close the defect, as when excising any skin lesion. This leaves a nice linear scar (Fig. 18.6a).

The pinch grafts can be placed in a gallipot of saline while the donor site is being repaired. They can then be taken out and placed onto the recipient granulations following which the grafts are covered with a paraffin gauze dressing. A support bandage is then applied to the recipient area and left for about 7 days (Fig. 18.6b) after which the dressings can be reapplied once or twice weekly as necessary. The patient should be encouraged to elevate the limb as much as possible to reduce any oedema, and treatment to the ulcer continued with support bandaging.

Pressure sore repair

Pressure sores are common in bedridden elderly or debilitated patients. Transporting these patients to the surgery can be very traumatic for them and difficult for the staff. However, surgery to small pressure sores can be performed in the patient's own bed. With careful technique, and attention to avoiding pressure during the healing period, it is possible to close a small long-standing pressure sore provided that all necrotic skin and tissue is removed and the skin edges can be brought together without undue tension. Debilitated and elderly patients are often thin and there is usually enough laxity in the skin to allow simple primary closure. This technique can avoid the necessity for turning a flap and general anaesthesia.

It may be necessary to debride the sore under wide infiltration anaesthesia as a first stage and then close the wound a week or so later (Fig. 18.7). It is surprising

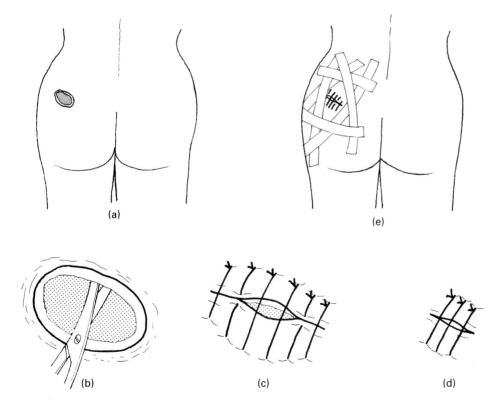

(a)

(e)

(b)

(c)

(d)

Fig. 18.7. (a) Pressure sore on buttock, (b) undermining edges, (c) suturing without excess tension, (d) and (e) resuture 10–14 days later to close further the defect.

Fig. 18.8. This left buttock pressure sore had been present for about 1 year in an elderly lady with multiple sclerosis. It was foul-smelling with a base of necrotic debris. The necrotic tissue was excised under wide infiltration anaesthesia and the wound closed progressively in three sessions over a 3 month period. The skin was still healthy and intact 18 months later.

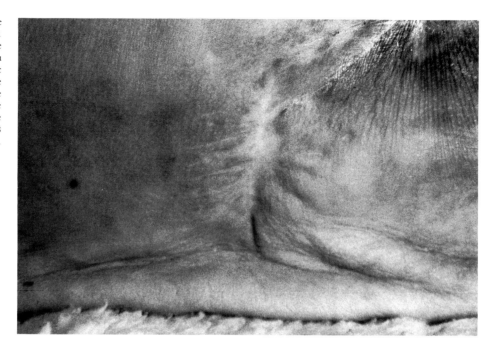

that, even with some degree of faecal soiling, a sore can be encouraged to heal with this technique (Fig. 18.8).

After wide infiltration of local anaesthetic a number of deep 2/0 or 0 braided nylon sutures should be inserted and clipped without tying (braided sutures are softer to lie on than monofilament; nylon causes less reaction than does silk). Once the last suture has been placed they can be tied while an assistant draws the wound edges together, thus removing the tension from the suture being tied. After suturing, tension should be further distributed by the application of wide adhesive tapes either side of, as well as across, the wound.

If some tension remains on the wound, it is not vital that the whole wound is closed completely. It is acceptable to reduce the size of the skin gap as much as possible and insert some further sutures a week or two later thus closing the gap progressively in two or three stages.

Reference

1. Grafting of venous leg ulcers: an intraindividual comparison between cultured skin equivalents and full-thickness skin punch grafts. Mol, M. A. E., Nanninga, P. B., Van Eendenburg, J. P., Westerhof, W. A., Mekkes, J. R. & Van Ginkel, C. J. W. *Journal of the American Academy of Dermatology* (1991), no. 1, 77–82.

19

Minor surgical procedures: Minor gynaecological surgery

Cervical polyp

These occur as distension cysts of the cervical glands or localised areas of hyperplasia of the stroma and epithelium in the cervical canal (Fig. 19.1). They may be brought to the attention by mucoid discharge or intermittent vaginal bleeding, often postcoitally. A small polyp with a thin stalk can be simply grasped with forceps and avulsed by twisting it repeatedly on its pedicle. If necessary, the base may be cauterised with a silver nitrate bud. The cervical canal may be gently dilated to exclude further unseen polyps. The polyp should be sent for histological examination and a cervical smear should also be taken. Patients with abnormal bleeding or larger polyps should be referred for excision and diagnostic curettage under a general anaesthetic.

Fig. 19.1. Cervical polyp.

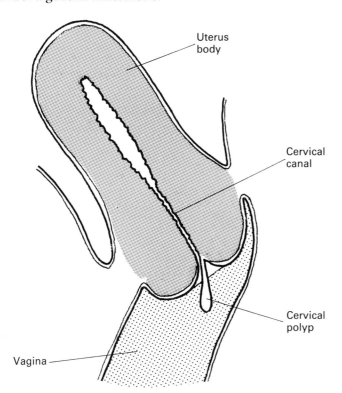

Uterus body

Cervical canal

Cervical polyp

Vagina

Fig. 19.2. The columnar epithelium
of the cervical canal abruptly
changes at the squamo-columnar
junction (arrowed) to squamous
epithelium of the cervix itself.

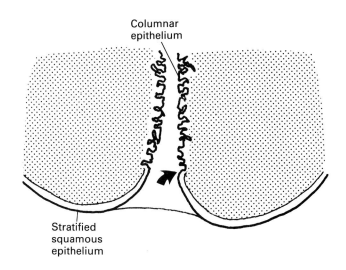

Cervical erosions

The columnar epithelium of the cervical canal abruptly gives way to squamous epithelium at the squamo-columnar junction (Fig. 19.2). The degree of eversion of the columnar epithelium is variable and the resultant 'erosion' does not normally need treatment unless the mucorrhoea from the exposed cervical cells is excessive or troublesome. A cervical smear should be taken prior to treatment and if necessary, minor degrees of erosion can be cauterised by the application of a silver nitrate stick or treated with a liquid nitrogen probe (see chapter 12), or by fulgaration using diathermy (see chapter 11). More marked erosions should be referred for specialist care as treatment may require a general anaesthetic and cervical dilatation to avoid cervical stenosis.

The patient should be warned to expect an increased amount of vaginal discharge for 1–2 weeks after treatment.

Urethral caruncle

This highly vascular pedunculated polyp usually arises from the mucosa of the posterior wall of the urethral meatus (Fig. 19.3). Being very tender it can cause

Fig. 19.3. Urethral caruncle.

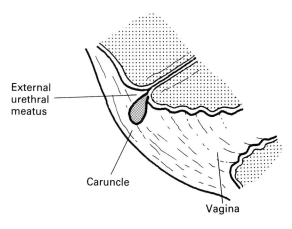

dysuria, bleeding or dysparunia. A small caruncle can be cauterised or excised using a local anaesthetic; larger lesions should be referred for treatment under a general anaesthetic.

Bartholin's cyst

Bartholin's glands lie on either side of the posterior part of the introitus and provide essential lubrication to the vagina and a cyst develops following blockage of the duct. If simple incision and drainage is used, there is a likelihood of recurrence and if the cyst is excised vaginal dryness may result. In order to prevent this happening, the cyst is deroofed from the introitus aspect and the cyst wall sutured to the surrounding vaginal skin with a 3/0 absorbable suture (marsupialisation) (Fig. 19.4). A small uninflamed cyst can be treated using wide local anaesthetic infiltration but larger infected cysts should be treated under general anaesthesia.

Prior to the procedure it is helpful to insert a small pack to distend the vagina and the sutures should be left long as they can be clipped and used for retraction. The sutures should be cut short at the end of the procedure. Marsupialisation maintains the function of the gland and widens the orifice, reducing the chance of further blockage.

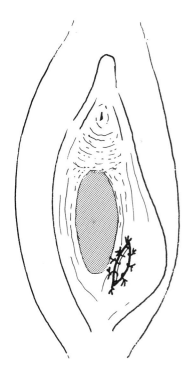

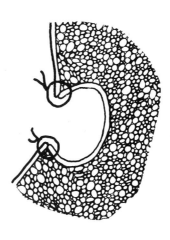

Fig. 19.4. Marsupialisation of Bartholin's cyst.

Insertion of depot hormone implant

Before starting hormonal replacement therapy (HRT) a woman must be fully informed of the benefits and associated potential risks. Hormone replacement has a number of benefits including improvement in skin health, vaginal lubrication and hot flushes, and also protection from osteoporosis and heart disease [1,2,3]. There may be a small increase in the risk of breast carcinoma, although the evidence is controversial. Women with an intact uterus require cyclical treatment with a progestagen (for 10–14 days per month) to avoid the risk of endometrial carcinoma but some women may find the resultant withdrawal bleeding unacceptable. For prevention of osteoporosis, HRT should be continued for 5–10 years after the menopause. The use of testosterone implants is not routinely recommended, although there is anecdotal evidence to suggest it is useful in patients with diminished libido.

There is a wide interpatient variation in response to any given hormone replacement preparation and it usually takes at least 3 months to assess a woman's response to treatment. Therefore, the first method of choice for hormone replacement in the menopause should be tablets or transdermal patches as the dose can be easily altered to suit the individual. Depot hormone preparations may allow better compliance in selected patients as the oestrogen is released slowly over a period of about 6 months.

Depot oestradiol pellets are available in 25, 50 and 100 mg strengths. Younger women generally require a higher dose. The pellets should be inserted either in the upper outer quadrant of the buttock or in the lower anterior abdominal wall.

Fig. 19.5. (a) and (b) Insertion of a depot hormone implant.

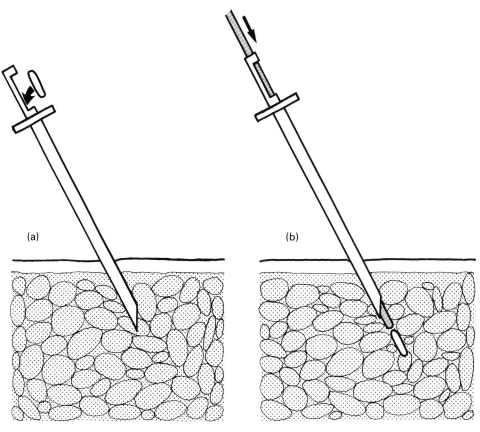

(a)   (b)

The site should be first infiltrated with a few millilitres of local anaesthetic and a small cut made in the skin with the tip of a scalpel blade. The trocar and cannula is then introduced through the incision and into the subcutaneous tissues. The trocar is removed, the hormone pellet is inserted into the cannula and the trocar or introducer is used to push the pellet into the subcutaneous tissue, after which the cannula is removed (Fig. 19.5). Note that the pellet should not be placed too deeply so that removal is still possible if required for any reason. Sutures are usually unnecessary, although adhesive tapes may be used to close the small wound. The wound should be covered with a small plaster or gauze for 24 h.

Intrauterine contraceptive device (IUCD)

It is essential to have adequate training before fitting an IUCD as complications are related to the inexperience of the fitter. In general, it is a good policy to become familiar with the feel and technique of inserting a particular IUCD and to use the same device as a routine. Prior to fitting an IUCD the patient should be counselled as to the different contraceptive options that are appropriate for her circumstances. Although in routine use current IUCDs may offer contraceptive efficiency at least equal to oral contraceptives [4], an IUCD is not 100 % effective and there is always a small chance of a pregnancy occurring. All women using IUCDs tend to have some pelvic discomfort and heavier periods and this tends to be more marked in nulliparous women. The use of levonorgestrel-containing IUCDs can reduce the menstrual loss and pregnancy rates. There is a small risk of uterine infection, although pelvic inflammatory disease is related more to risk factors such as multiple sexual partners and prevalence of causative organisms in the community than the use or non-use of an IUCD. Hence IUCDs are not advised in women who do not have a stable relationship. The use of an IUCD is associated with a small increased risk of ectopic pregnancy, and occasionally an IUCD is spontaneously expelled.

The cervix is most dilated at mid-cycle but an IUCD may be inserted at any time provided there is no suggestion of the patient being pregnant. If appropriate, it is recommended that an IUCD is inserted 6–8 weeks postpartum (the tissues are soft during this time and there is an increased risk of uterine perforation) although it can be inserted immediately after termination of pregnancy.

Copper-containing IUCDs may be left *in situ* for at least 5 years [5,6] and evidence shows that current copper devices are effective for up to 10 years (Fig. 19.6).

Fig. 19.6. (a) and (b) The Nova-T IUCD.

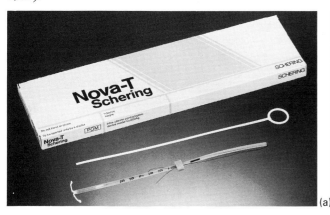

(a)

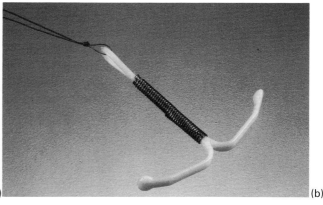

(b)

Contraindications and precautions IUCDs are contraindicated in women with undiagnosed genital bleeding, malignancy of the genital tract, vaginal or pelvic inflammatory disease, endometrial disease, Wilson's disease or allergy to copper. Relative contraindications include abnormalities of the uterine cavity, a history of ectopic pregnancy, immunosuppressive therapy, anaemia, menorrhagia, uterine fibroids, systemic corticosteroid therapy, recent cervical or vaginal infection and human immunodeficiency virus infection. Administration of prophylactic antibiotics prior to the procedure should be considered in women with rheumatic or congenital heart disease, or heart valve or other prostheses.

The nerve supply to the cervix is autonomic via the splanchnic nerves hence stretching of the cervix results in pain but cautery and biopsy is usually painless. The patient should be relaxed and reassured throughout the procedure and particular care should be taken not to apply too vigorous dilatation or traction on the cervix as this can trigger off a vasovagal attack. Resuscitation facilities should be readily available, including intravenous atropine for bradycardia and intravenous or rectal diazepam for seizures.

Fitting of an IUCD The patient should lie on her back with her knees bent and the buttocks near the end of the couch. A bimanual examination of the uterus should first be performed to assess the size, shape and direction of the uterus. A Cuscos speculum is inserted into the vagina, the cervix identified, and gentle traction is applied to the anterior lip of the cervix with a vulsellum forceps. This helps to align the long axis of the uterus with the vagina so making a more direct path for the IUCD (Fig. 19.7).

Fig. 19.7. IUCD correctly positioned.

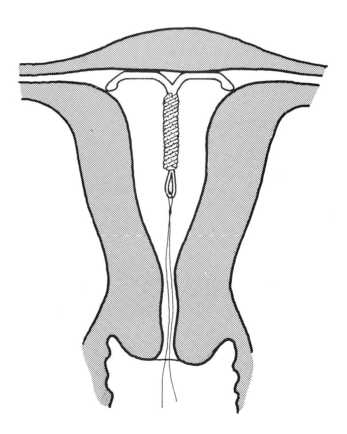

The utmost care should be used to insert the IUCD. Although vaginal and cervical asepsis is impossible and there is disagreement about the value of antiseptic preparation, nevertheless an aqueous antiseptic is advised. The depth and direction of the uterine cavity is then assessed with a uterine sound or the IUCD introducer itself. The directions given with the particular IUCD should be followed. Some IUCDs are pre-loaded, while others have to be loaded into the introducer. Making a slight bend in the introducer may make the insertion easier. The introducer is gently directed through the cervix until the fundus of the uterine cavity is felt. The IUCD is then released as the introducer is removed and the threads cut, leaving 2–3 cm protruding through the cervix. Since it is possible to place the device accidentally within the cervical *canal* itself, the cervical canal should be sounded after the procedure to ensure that the device has been correctly inserted. Since bleeding from a perforated uterus can be extensive, if there is any suggestion that the uterus has been perforated the patient should be referred urgently to a gynaecologist for laparoscopy.

The patient should be reviewed after 4–6 weeks and then annually, and should be asked to report at once if there is any suspicion of a pregnancy.

Removal of an IUCD Removal of an IUCD is usually straightforward if the threads are visible. If the threads are not seen they may be recovered by gentle probing with a thread retriever, blunt hook or cervical cytology brush. If the threads are not easily retrieved or there is doubt about whether the coil has been expelled, further probing should be avoided and the patient should be referred to a family planning clinic or gynaecologist for an ultrasound scan. In the meantime, the patient should be advised to use another form of contraception.

If a pregnancy occurs or is planned the patient should be referred to an obstetrician for assessment and removal of the IUCD. Although this procedure may itself entail a risk of causing an abortion, there is a greater risk of ectopic pregnancy occurring with an IUCD in place and retention of an IUCD in the uterus may increase the risk of sepsis and spontaneous abortion at a later stage. In addition, the long-term effects of intra uterine copper on the foetus are not fully known.

Episiotomy (Fig. 19.8)

Although it is less frequently performed than in the past, nevertheless an episiotomy should be considered when there is a risk of developing a perineal tear or foetal distress. However, episiotomy can have an adverse effect on the incidence of deep perineal lacerations [7]. In making the episiotomy the 'medio-lateral' incision is commonly preferred but neither the medio-lateral or mid-line episiotomy invariably protects against anal sphincter trauma [8].

The perineal repair should be made in three layers: vaginal epithelium, perineal muscles, and skin. The method described uses an absorbable subcuticular suture for the perineal skin as this results in less pain compared to interrupted skin sutures. Recently, the use of tissue adhesive to the skin has been shown to give good results [9]. The mother should lie on her back in the lithotomy position or in her bed with the knees bent and the hips flexed and abducted. The skin should be prepared with aqueous antiseptic and towels arranged to expose the perineum.

Fig. 19.8. Episiotomy, surgical
anatomy.

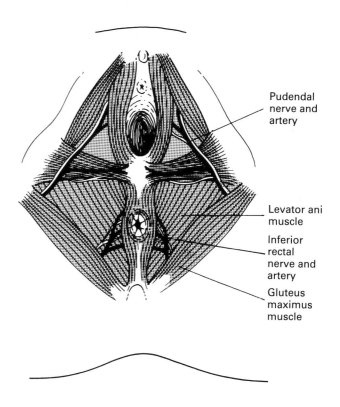

Pudendal
nerve and
artery

Levator ani
muscle

Inferior
rectal
nerve and
artery

Gluteus
maximus
muscle

Episiotomy incision Local anaesthetic should be infiltrated into the tissues and the perineal skin is put under tension by inserting the index and middle fingers of the left hand into the vagina. The fingers are spread out pointing posteriorly, the incision is made starting in the mid-line at the fourchette, and directed posterolaterally, avoiding the anal sphincter (Fig. 19.9a). Either a scalpel or scissors may be used but care should be taken to make a 'clean' cut and to avoid multiple snips that might result in a ragged incision.

Episiotomy repair Before proceeding to the repair, it is essential to examine the area thoroughly to define the extent of any damage. If necessary, a finger should be inserted into the rectum to assess the state of the anal sphincter and mucosa, after which the gloves are changed. A torn anal sphincter should be repaired only by an experienced surgeon.

The tissues will be oedematous and friable and are likely to swell further later. It is important to handle the tissues gently and close any dead space to minimise postoperative pain, and the risk of haematoma or infection. However, great care should be taken to ensure that any repair does not result in a tight introitus. A three-layered closure is essential as failure to repair the perineal muscles will result in a weak pelvic floor. All bleeding points should be picked up with artery clips and tied with a 3/0 absorbable suture. The key to easy access and repair is to place a large gauze pack (with a tail and a clip on its end) high up in the vaginal vault so the vagina is distended, and uterine blood is prevented from oozing into the operative field. Starting at the apex of the vaginal part of the incision, a continuous 0 absorbable suture is placed and tied at the fourchette. Large bites should not be taken in order to avoid narrowing the vagina. The knot is not buried as this may result in a painful scar at this point. It is essential to close the apex of the

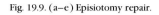

Fig. 19.9. (a–e) Episiotomy repair.

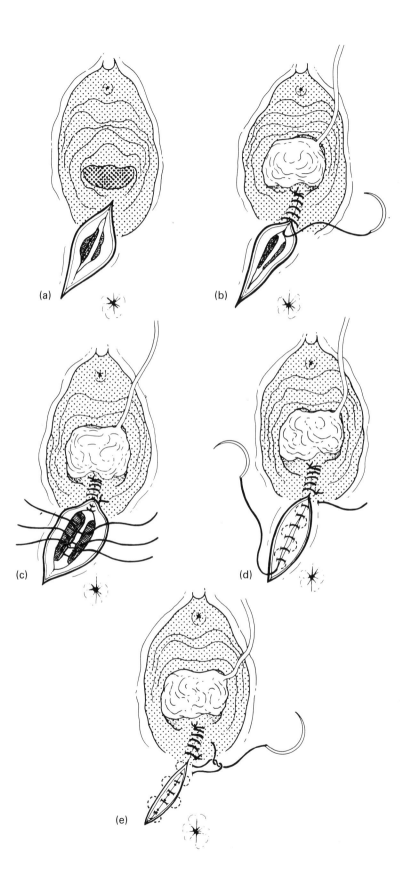

(a)

(b)

(c)

(d)

(e)

vaginal wound. If the apex cannot be seen, a suture should be placed as high as possible and traction on the suture should allow the apex to be seen and closed (Fig. 19.9b).

The edges of the perineal muscles and anal sphincter are identified and interrupted size 1 absorbable sutures on a strong needle are placed in the perineal muscles. The sutures should be inserted and clipped without tying so as to allow each suture to be placed under direct vision. The sutures are then individually tied and cut (Fig. 19.9c). The skin is then closed with a continuous subcutaneous and subcuticular 2/0 absorbable suture on a cutting needle. The needle is inserted in the skin to one side of the fourchette, taken to the apex of the perineal wound in the subcutaneous layer (Fig. 19.9d) and then taken back to the fourchette as a subcuticular suture. The ends are then tied above the skin (Fig. 19.9e).

Finally, a finger is inserted into the rectum to ensure that it has not been caught up in any of the deep sutures and the vaginal vault pack is removed. No special aftercare is required and a shower may be permitted as soon as required. Pelvic floor exercises should be encouraged as soon as the mother is able to do so.

References

1. Type III collagen content in the skin of postmenopausal women receiving oestradiol and testosterone implants. Savvas, M., Bishop, J., Laurent, G. *et al. British Journal of Obstetrics and Gynaecology* (1993), **100**, 154–156.

2. Individualising HRT. Gangar, K. & Key, E. *Practitioner* (1993), **237**, 358–360.

3. Hormone replacement therapy (part 1). *Merec Bulletin* (1993), **4**, 5–7.

4. Intrauterine contraceptive devices – a reappraisal. Bronham, D. R. *British Medical Bulletin* (1993), **49**, 100–123.

5. Five years experience of intrauterine contraception with the Nova-T. Fugere, P. *Contraception* (1990), **41**, 1–7.

6. Five years' experience of intrauterine contraception with the Nova-T and Copper-T-200. Luukkainen, T., Allonen, H., Nielsen, N-C., Nyren, K. G. & Pyörälä, T. *American Journal of Obstetrics and Gynaecology* (1983), **147**, 885–892.

7. Advantage or disadvantage of episiotomy compared with spontaneous perineal laceration. Larsson, P. G., Platz-Christensen, J. J., Bergman, B. & Wallstersson, G. *Gynecologic and Obstetric Investigations* (1991), **31**, 213–216.

8. Association of epsiotomy and delivery position with deep perineal laceration during spontaneous delivery in nulliparous women. Borgatta, L., Piening, S. L. & Cohen, W. R. *American Journal of Obstetrics and Gynaecology* (1989), **60**, 294–297.

9. The use of Histoacryl for episiotomy repair. Adoni, A. & Anteby, E. *British Journal of Obstetrics and Gynaecology* (1991), **98**, 476-478.

20

Minor surgical procedures: In the male

Circumcision

The vast majority of boys will have fully retractile foreskins by the age of 3–4 years. Circumcision may be advisable if the foreskin cannot be retracted enough for the glans to be kept clean, or if there are recurrent attacks of balanitis, or paraphimosis. However, there is probably an unnecessary number of circumcisions performed and, in selected cases, a safe alternative is 'preputial plasty' for patients with tight but unscarred foreskins [1]. This is essentially a small dorsal slit (see below) and involves a longitudinal dorsal incision of the constricting band followed by transverse suture and results in a fully mobile foreskin.

Circumcision is normally performed under general anaesthetic but can be performed under a local anaesthetic in adults. However, circumcision under local anaesthetic should not be undertaken by an inexperienced doctor. The sensation to the distal two thirds of the penis is supplied by the dorsal nerve of the penis, which is a branch of the pudendal nerve (Fig. 20.1). The proximal part of the penis is supplied by branches from the ilioinguinal nerve. These nerves are blocked using a ring of local anaesthetic (*without* adrenaline) infiltrated around the midshaft or base of the penis, taking special care around the ventral mid-line to

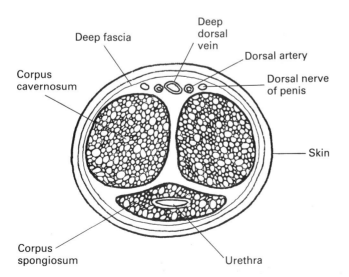

Corpus cavernosum

Deep fascia

Deep dorsal vein

Dorsal artery

Dorsal nerve of penis

Skin

Corpus spongiosum

Urethra

Fig. 20.1. Nerve supply of the penis.

Fig. 20.2. Circumcision: guillotine
method.

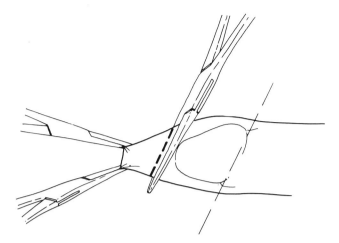

avoid the urethra, which is very superficial. Although the guillotine method is classically described for infants (Fig. 20.2), the formal dissection method is advised in all age groups as this reduces the possibility of leaving redundant preputial skin or of injury to the glans.

The penis should be cleansed with aqueous antiseptic and exposed through a paper towel. The tip of the prepuce is grasped with two artery clips and gently stretched. Dorsal and ventral mid-line cuts are made with scissors extending proximally to 5 mm of the coronal sulcus, taking care to avoid entering the urethra with the tip of the scissors (Fig. 20.3a). Any remaining smegma is then cleared.

Enough skin should be left to cover the erect penis and this is assessed by pulling the penis straight before the prepuce is excised. The prepuce is trimmed parallel to the coronal sulcus with scissors (Fig. 20.3b). Note that once the prepuce has been excised bleeding can be steady from a number of points so a number of artery clips should be available to clip and tie these points. All points that are bleeding are ligated with 3/0 absorbable sutures (Fig. 20.3c). The skin edges are then sutured with 3/0 absorbable sutures, starting by matching up the dorsal and ventral mid-lines (Fig. 20.3d). These two sutures are left long and held with artery clips to stabilise the penis while the rest of the sutures are inserted (Fig. 20.3e). It is advisable to probe the urethra gently with a lubricated bougie or artery clip to confirm that it has not been accidentally caught by one of the ventral sutures. The suture line may be sprayed with a plastic spray followed by a gauze swab when dry. All dressings are notoriously difficult to hold in place. The patient may shower after 24 h and mild analgesics should be given for the first few days.

It is quite normal for the operative site to be quite swollen during the first week. However, the judicious application of ice packs can be extremely helpful in reducing the swelling. Complete healing usually takes 2–3 weeks.

Dorsal slit

It is sometimes necessary to perform a dorsal slit (Fig. 20.4) on an elderly debilitated man with incontinence and marked phimosis prior to catheterisation. It is possible to do the procedure in a nursing home in the patient's own bed.

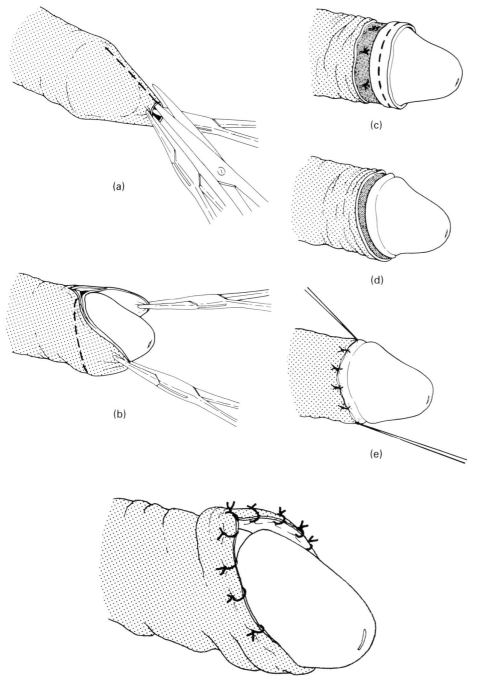

Fig. 20.3. Circumcision: (a) dorsal slit, (b) prepuce trimmed parallel with the coronal sulcus, (c) all bleeding points are ligated and the deep skin layer is trimmed, (d) the appearance prior to suture, (e) skin closure.

(a)

(c)

(d)

(b)

(e)

Fig. 20.4. Dorsal slit.

The penis should be cleansed with aqueous antiseptic and exposed through a paper towel and local anaesthetic (*without* adrenaline) infiltrated around the midshaft or base. Two artery clips are then loosely applied to the prepuce so as not to crush the skin. One blade of a pair of scissors is introduced under the dorsal prepuce, and care taken not to enter the external urethral meatus itself. A dorsal slit is then made, stopping a few millimetres from the corona. Any points that are bleeding are picked up with artery clips and tied off with absorbable sutures.

Interrupted sutures are then used to close the deep and outer edges of the cut prepuce. There often remains a problem due to soiled underwear around catheters. Therefore, rather than using absorbable sutures (which can take 2–3 weeks to dissolve) it may be wise to use nylon sutures and remove them after 7 days. A catheter may be inserted immediately the dorsal slit has been completed. As with circumcision it is quite normal for the operative site to be quite swollen during the first week, and the judicious application of ice packs can be extremely helpful in reducing the swelling.

Vasectomy

Although vasectomy is generally a simple procedure, on occasion it can be surprisingly difficult for even the experienced surgeon to locate the vas. The operation should not be performed without adequate surgical experience.

The procedure is easily performed under simple local anaesthesia and sedation is only necessary for the more anxious patient. The patient must be examined at the initial consultation as very anxious patients, and those in whom the vas is

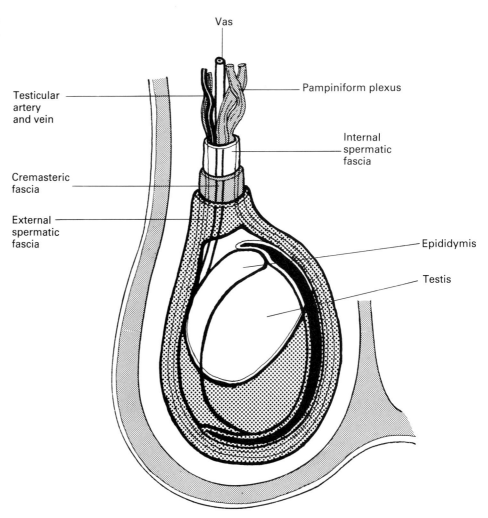

Fig. 20.5. Surgical anatomy: the scrotal contents.

Vas

Pampiniform plexus

Testicular artery and vein

Internal spermatic fascia

Cremasteric fascia

External spermatic fascia

Epididymis

Testis

difficult to identify, are best dealt with under general anaesthesia. The patient should be fully informed that the operation is permanent but there is a very small chance of natural reversal. In addition, although vasectomy may be technically reversed there is no guarantee that a reversal will be effective. Failure of reversal can be due to the formation of sperm antibodies in the seminal plasma. It may be advisable for some patients to consider cryopreservation and banking of semen prior to vasectomy [2].

Patients often enquire about the risk of cancer after vasectomy. Cancer of the testes is a rare condition and current evidence does not support the idea that vasectomy increases the incidence of testicular carcinoma [3,4]. Recently there has been reported a link between vasectomy and prostatic carcinoma [5,6], but the risk is regarded as small and should not deter patients from vasectomy, which is essentially a very safe form of contraception. It is helpful to supply the patient with an information leaflet (see p. 291).

Although not legally necessary it may be wise to obtain written consent from both partners.

With experience, the doctor will be able to perform the operation through a very small incision. Commonly, two separate incisions are used, but it is possible to perform the operation through a single central incision.

Preparing the patient The patient should be asked to shave the scrotal skin from the level of the penis downwards. If this is done 2 days prior to the surgery the antiseptic paint will not sting as any small abrasions of the skin will have had time to heal. Vasectomy is one of the few local anaesthetic operations for which the patient should not take anything by mouth except a light drink for 4 h prior to the procedure. It is vitally important to reassure the patient as soon as he arrives in the operating room. Even the most hardy man is likely to be feeling very uneasy inside.

The patient should be examined prior to any injection in order to locate the position of the vas on each side. It is vitally important to ensure that the patient is warm and relaxed and that the room is well ventilated. If the patient is cold or anxious the scrotum will become bunched up, making the operation more difficult. If the room is stuffy, the patient may unexpectedly feel faint during the procedure. It is pleasant for both the patient and surgeon to be able to listen to a radio tuned into a music station, and the surgeon or nurse should make a positive effort to chat with the patient and reassure him throughout the operation.

It is worth emphasising again that it is *vitally important* for the patient to be at ease during a vasectomy as anxiety coupled with any abdominal ache caused by traction on the spermatic cord can lead to a vaso-vagal attack and cardiac arrest.

Local anaesthetic The nerve supply to the anterior one third of the scrotal skin is from the ilioinguinal nerve and the genital branch of the genitofemoral nerve. The posterior two thirds are supplied by branches of the perineal nerves and branches of the posterior femoral cutaneous nerve. The nerve supply of the spermatic cord and testes is via the T10 and T11 segments through fibres from the renal and aortic plexuses accompanying the testicular artery. Thus, the scrotal skin and cord structures have to be separately anaesthetised.

There are a number of techniques available. One method involves injecting the local anaesthetic into the skin of the scrotum, locating the vas, making a further injection around the vas and using any additional injection as the operation proceeds. This is an acceptable method but it has the risk of handling and clamping unanaesthetised tissue, with its inherent pain and complications. It is preferable and kinder to inject the cord structures at the scrotal neck (below and medial to the pubic tubercle) and allow the local anaesthetic time to work before proceeding. This is the method that is described below.

The local anaesthetic is injected prior to the formal skin preparation and it is essential to allow 5–10 min before proceeding with the operation. The spermatic cord is felt at the scrotal neck and 5 ml of 1% *plain* lignocaine injected in and around it. This anaesthetises the scrotal contents. Then 2.5 ml of 1% lignocaine (with or without adrenaline) is injected into the anterior scrotal skin at the sites of the proposed skin incisions (Fig. 20.6).

Fig. 20.6. Injection of local anaesthetic: Ⓐ around the cord structures at the scrotal neck, and Ⓑ into the anterior scrotal skin.

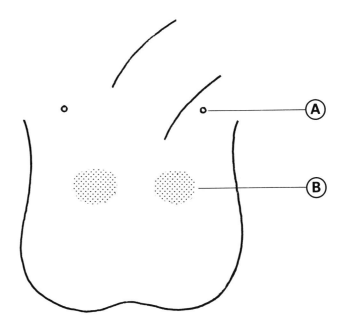

Skin preparation A paper towel is placed under the buttocks as the skin preparation is liable to seep downwards. The skin is prepared with povidone iodine or chlorhexidine and the scrotal skin isolated through the centre of a paper drape.

The operation Starting with the right side, a 1 cm incision is made in the anaesthetised anterior scrotal skin. The skin here is very lax hence it has to be steadied with the fingers of the left hand or with forceps. Although the aim is to avoid any large veins, this is not always possible but any bleeding can be easily controlled with artery clips. With the index and middle fingers behind the scrotum and the thumb in front, the vas is then identified, isolated and steadied. The vas is then grasped with vasectomy forceps or Allis forceps introduced through the scrotal incision (Figs. 20.7, 20.8).

Extreme care should be taken at this point to ensure that the cord structures are fully anaesthetised. Before the vas is firmly gripped, the Allis forceps should be gently closed onto the vas and if sensation is still present, a few millilitres of plain

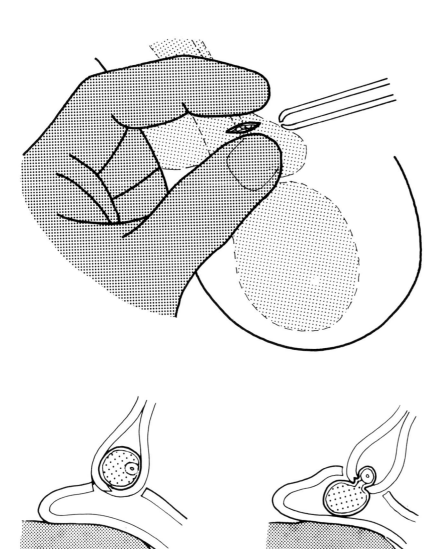

Fig. 20.7. The vas is isolated between the fingers and thumb and grasped through the scrotal incision with Allis forceps.

Fig. 20.8. Hooking out either the spermatic cord or only the vas.

lignocaine are injected into the cord and time allowed for anaesthesia to take effect. The vas is then delivered through the skin incision (Fig. 20.9a,b).

At this point the vas will still be covered by the spermatic cord fascia (external, cremasteric and internal spermatic fascia). By means of a scalpel, a longitudinal incision is made through the fascial coverings to expose the vas (Fig. 20.9c,d). An artery clip is then placed onto the vas, which is gently teased out of the fascia by blunt dissection with non-toothed forceps (Fig. 20.9e,f). Care should be taken not to tear the nearby veins. If a vessel is torn, it should be clipped and tied with catgut. Haemostasis is vital as any oozing can result in a painful scrotal haematoma and at all stages of the operation it is wise always to have an artery clip attached to the cord fascia to avoid the risk of the vas falling back and being lost inside the scrotum.

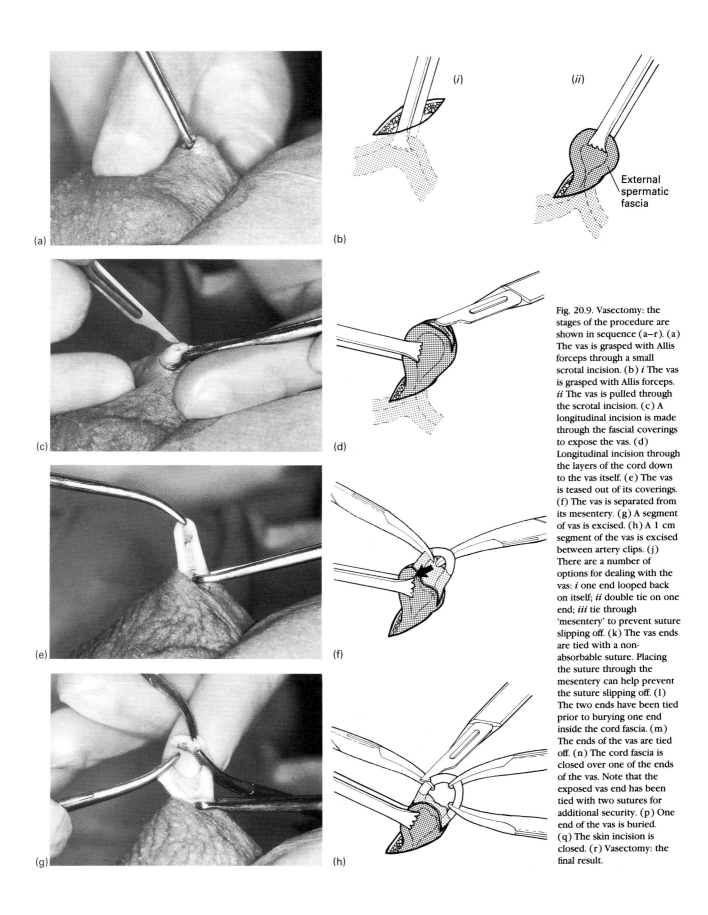

Fig. 20.9. Vasectomy: the stages of the procedure are shown in sequence (a–r). (a) The vas is grasped with Allis forceps through a small scrotal incision. (b) *i* The vas is grasped with Allis forceps. *ii* The vas is pulled through the scrotal incision. (c) A longitudinal incision is made through the fascial coverings to expose the vas. (d) Longitudinal incision through the layers of the cord down to the vas itself. (e) The vas is teased out of its coverings. (f) The vas is separated from its mesentery. (g) A segment of vas is excised. (h) A 1 cm segment of the vas is excised between artery clips. (j) There are a number of options for dealing with the vas: *i* one end looped back on itself; *ii* double tie on one end; *iii* tie through 'mesentery' to prevent suture slipping off. (k) The vas ends are tied with a non-absorbable suture. Placing the suture through the mesentery can help prevent the suture slipping off. (l) The two ends have been tied prior to burying one end inside the cord fascia. (m) The ends of the vas are tied off. (n) The cord fascia is closed over one of the ends of the vas. Note that the exposed vas end has been tied with two sutures for additional security. (p) One end of the vas is buried. (q) The skin incision is closed. (r) Vasectomy: the final result.

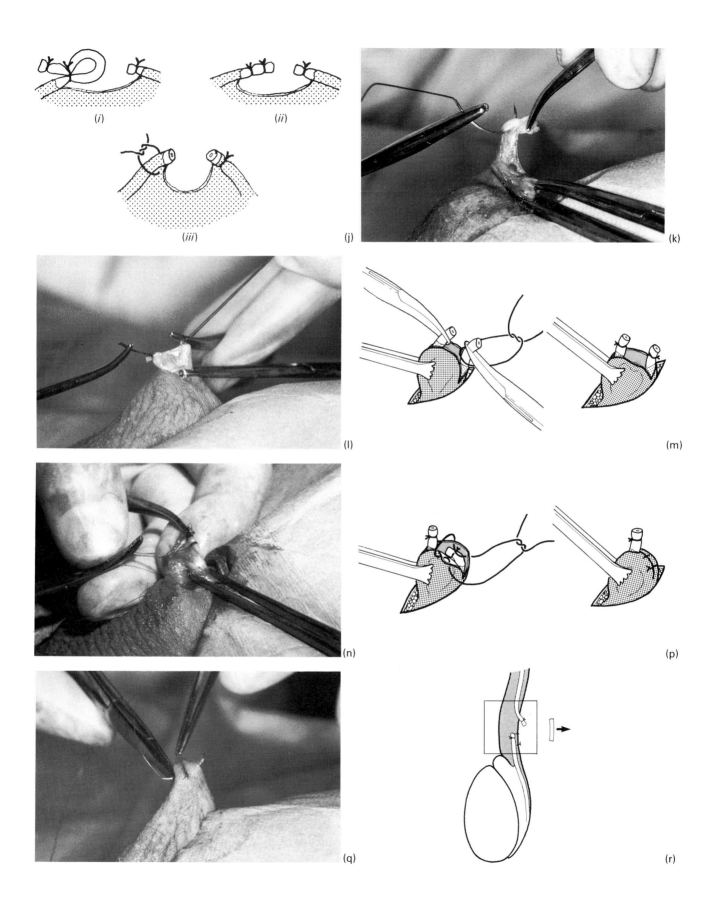

(i)

(ii)

(iii)

(j)

(k)

(l)

(m)

(n)

(p)

(q)

(r)

When 2 cm of vas had been delivered an artery clip is placed at each end and a 1 cm segment excised with scissors or scalpel (Fig. 20.9g,h). The segment is sent for histological examination.

A number of methods are available for dealing with the cut ends of the vas. Some doctors prefer simple diathermy of the lumen without ligation, using a needle point introduced into the centre of the vas. Others prefer to ligate the vas with an absorbable suture. These two methods rely on scarring to seal the vas. Generally, however, it is advisable to ligate the vas with a non-absorbable suture, with further security being gained by closing the cord fascia over one end of the vas. This last method is now described (Fig. 20.9j,i,ii,iii).

The vas is *gently* crushed with an artery clip and then tied with a 2/0 braided nylon suture (Fig. 20.9k,l,m). Care should be taken as it is easy to cut through the vas completely if the crushing or tying is too vigorous. To ensure against the tie slipping off, a suture may be inserted through the 'mesentery' next to the vas itself, and then tied. An artery clip should be placed on the suture of one end of the vas and an absorbable 3/0 suture used to close the cord fascia over the other end of the vas, thus burying one end (Fig. 20.9n,p). In this way any possibility of spontaneous union is minimised as the two ends of the vas are tied and also separated by a tissue plane.

A final check is made to ensure that all bleeding has been arrested and the vas and cord are then allowed to fall back into the scrotum. A check is made to ensure that a suture has not accidentally tied the inner scrotal wall to the vas and cord structures (it should be possible to pick up the scrotal skin without any pulling on the testes).

Two or three 5/0 nylon skin sutures are inserted into the skin (catgut tends to cause pricking and takes a few weeks to dissolve). These should take up the whole thickness of the scrotal wall to ensure against any deep oozing (Fig. 20.9q,r).

The scrotum is cleaned of any excess skin preparation. A few gauze swabs are placed over the wound and held in place by the underwear.

Postoperative care The patient may shower after 24 h, by which time the wounds will have become sealed.

After the operation the patient should be advised to rest for 24–48 h and avoid playing with children and dogs. Mild analgesics such as Co-proxamol should be prescribed for use if necessary. Often no analgesia is required at all. It is normal for the scrotum to be bruised and swollen afterwards because of the laxity of the skin and this may give rise to a dragging or heavy sensation.

The skin sutures should be removed after 7 days, at which time the scrotum can be examined and specimen containers given for subsequent semen samples.

Semen tests Opinions differ about when the sperm test should be done, how many tests should be done and how they should be interpreted.

Although it is commonly stated that azoospermia (as distinct from the absence of motile sperms) may take 30–40 ejaculations, azoospermia can result in most men after as few as 10 post-vasectomy ejaculations [7].

However, a man with non-motile sperms is sterile because non-motile sperms cannot penetrate cervical mucus [8] and the sperm tail must beat vigorously for the sperm to penetrate and fertilize an ovum [9]. The disappearance of motile sperms is unrelated to the number of ejaculations and usually occurs by the 15th day after vasectomy [10].

Some clinics insist on a period of 3–4 months before the first test, arguing that earlier tests may fail to detect some cases of recanalisation. However, there is little information in the literature on this subject. Late spontaneous recanalisation can occur [11,12] and the overall failure rate is influenced by the experience of the surgeon. Evidence from a large series spanning a 17 year period shows that tests based on the absence of motile sperms can be done 4 weeks after vasectomy, regardless of the number of post-vasectomy ejaculations [13]. The author's practice is to arrange semen tests between approximately 6 and 8 weeks after the operation.

Patient information leaflet
Vasectomy

Before proceeding
You must be sure about the operation because, although vasectomy can be reversed, for a number of technical reasons there can be no guarantee that fertility will be regained. In addition, there is always a very small chance of the tubes joining up again despite adequate surgery. Vasectomy has no effect on sexual function and there is no evidence to suggest that vasectomy is associated with an increase in risk of disease. In particular, there is no known association with testicular cancer.

Preparation
You should shave the skin of the scrotum from the side of the penis downwards (it is not necessary to shave the pubic hair). This should be done 2 days before the operation so as to allow time for any abrasions to heal.

Operation
Vasectomy is a simple procedure and is usually performed under a local anaesthetic. The operation involves removing a short section of the vas (the tube that carries the sperms from the testes) and tying of the loose ends. This is normally done through two very small cuts in the front of the scrotum. You will be awake throughout the whole procedure and should feel no pain at all. Occasionally however, a little dragging sensation may be felt in the stomach when the vas is handled.

Afterwards
After the operation you should rest for 24–48 hours and avoid playing with children and dogs. You will be given some mild pain killers to take if necessary. It is normal for the scrotum to be bruised and swollen afterwards but this is only because the skin is so soft in that area. You may take a shower after 24 hours, by which time the wounds will have essentially sealed. If your stitches are to be removed this will be done after 7 days and you will then be given specimen containers for your subsequent semen samples.

Semen tests
Semen tests will be arranged approximately 6 and 8 weeks after resumption of sexual relations. These samples should be sent directly to the hospital pathology department as soon after production as possible.

Normal contraceptive methods *must* be continued until your doctor has informed you that two consecutive semen samples are clear.

The patient should be advised that normal contraceptive methods *must* be continued until he has been informed that two consecutive semen samples show no motile sperms. Although the chance of recanalisation occurring between two samples taken 2 weeks apart must be extremely small, two samples are routinely taken for medico-legal purposes.

Sperm samples should be examined as soon after production as possible, but in any case, within 12 hours of collection (on the basis that at room temperature it takes about 12 hours for the percentage of motile sperms to be halved, with little change in their motility [*14*]. Motile sperms should be sought by examining a number of high power fields. Centrifugation is not necessary as only motile sperms are of importance and occasional non-motile sperms can be found in centrifuged samples in 10% of men 12 months after vasectomy [*15*].

References

1. Saving the normal foreskin. Cuckow, P. & Mouriquand, P. *British Medical Journal* (1993), **306**, 459–460.

2. Reversing vasectomy. Cahills, D. J., Wardle, P. G., Coulson, C., Harris, S., Ford, W. C. L. & Hull, M. G. R. *British Medical Journal* (1992), **305**, 52.

3. Incidence of disease after vasectomy: a record linkage retrospective cohort study. Nienhuis, H., Goldacre, M., Seagroatt, V., Gill, L. & Vessey, M. *British Medical Journal* (1992), **304**, 743–746.

4. Vasectomy and testicular cancer. West, R. R. *British Medical Journal* (1992), **304**, 729.

5. A prospective cohort study of vasectomy and prostatic carcinoma in US men. Giovannuci, E., Ascheria, A., Rimon, E. B., Colditz, G. A., Stampfer, M. J. & Willett, W. C. *Journal of the American Medical Association* (1993), **269** 873–877.

6. A retrospective cohort study of vasectomy and prostatic carcinoma in US men. Giovannuci, E., Ascheria, A., Rimon, E. B., Colditz, G. A., Stampfer, M. J. & Willett, W. C. *Journal of the American Medical Association* (1993), **269**, 878–882.

7. Disappearance rate of spermatozoa from the ejaculate following vasectomy. Freund, M. & Davis, J. E. *Fertility and Sterility* (1969), **20**, 163–170.

8. Swimming rate of bull spermatozoa in various media and the effect of dilution. Tampion, D. & Gibbons, R. A. *Journal of Reproduction and Fertility* (1963), **5**, 259.

9. Sperm molitilty. Amelar, R. D., Dubin, L. & Schoenfeld, X. X. *Fertility and Sterility* (1980), **34**, 197–215.

10. Evolution of the properties of semen immediately following vasectomy. Jouannet, P. & David, G. *Fertility and Sterility* (1978), **29**, 435–441.

11. Late failure of vasectomy after two documented analyses showing azoospermic semen. Philip, T., Guillebaud, J. & Budd, D. *British Medical Journal* (1984), **289**, 77–79.

12. Late failure after vasectomy. Sherlock, D. J. & Holl-Allen, R. T. J. *British Medical Journal* (1984), **289**, 318–319.

13. Earlier testing after vasectomy, based on the absence of motile sperm. Edwards, I. S. *Fertility and Sterility* (1993), **59**, 431–436.

14. Factors affecting sperm motility. In vitro change in motility with time after ejaculation. Makler, A., Zaidise, I., Paldi, E. & Brandes, J. M. *Fertility and Sterility* (1979), **31**, 147–154.

15. Non-motile sperms persisting after vasectomy: do they matter? Edwards, I. S. & Farlow, J. L. *British Medical Journal* (1979), i, 87–88.

21

Minor surgical procedures: Minor cosmetic procedures

The greatest care needs to be taken when a doctor is performing any procedure for cosmetic purposes. In particular, surgery on the face and eyelids should only be undertaken by an experienced doctor and only the simplest and smallest lesions should be tackled in general practice. Nevertheless, many unsightly lesions may be significantly improved by the application of some simple methods.

Since all surgery results in scarring to some degree, it is essential that the patient should be given a full understanding as to the timescale and likely appearance of the final result.

Hypertrophic and keloid scars

Hypertrophic and keloid scars should not be treated by simple excision alone as recurrence is inevitable. Hypertrophic and keloid scars (Fig. 21.1) on the head and neck and anything other than small scars on the body should be referred to a specialist. However, small hypertrophic and keloid scars in areas on the body not subject to tension can be treated by injection of steroids (see chapter 7), cryotherapy (see chapter 12), or excision in association with injection of a depot corticosteroid (e.g. 20–40 mg of methyl prednisolone) into the wound edges prior to suture [1]. Before the operation, the patient should be fully informed that

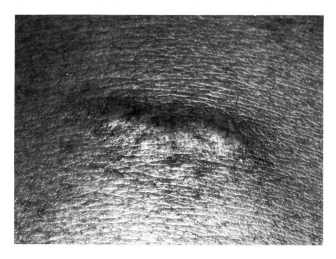

Fig. 21.1. Keloid scar on the shoulder which may be softened and flattened by intralesional injection of a depot steroid. Excision in this case should be avoided because of the likelihood of skin tension.

even with careful technique a keloid or hypertrophic scar may recur and may occasionally be worse than before excision. The injection of depot steroid at the time of the excision is the most important injection but the steroid injection may be repeated a number of times postoperatively at monthly intervals. This technique does not interfere with healing of the wound itself.

Xanthelasma

These lesions are commonly seen on the eyelids and the fatty deposits lie very superficially in the skin. They can be treated by a number of methods.

Small lesions may be excised as with any skin lesion but special care should be taken as the eyelid skin is very lax and the excision of larger amounts of skin may pull the lid margin to cause ectropion. As an alternative the xanthelasma can be simply evaporated by superficial diathermy or electrocautery through the thin overlying skin (Figs. 21.2, 21.3).

The application of 50% trichloroacetic acid or pure phenol directly onto the xanthelasma patch results is a slough that peels off after a number of days. This method should not be used by the inexperienced doctor as the utmost care must be exercised when using caustic liquids near the eyes (which should be closed and protected by a swab), and the surrounding normal skin should be protected by a layer of collodion. More than one application may have to be used.

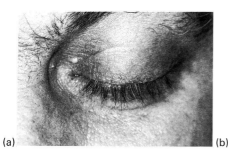
(a)

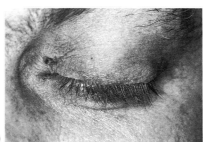
(b)

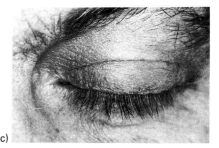
(c)

Fig. 21.2. (a–c) A small area of xanthelasma easily treated by diathermy.

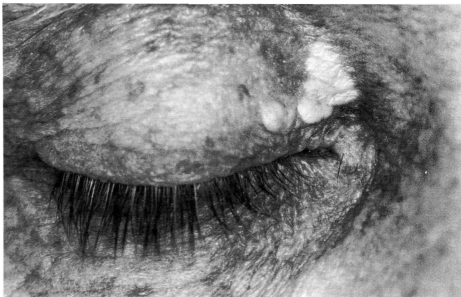

Fig. 21.3. An extensive area of xanthelasma unsuitable for treatment by the inexperienced doctor.

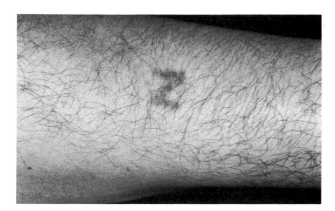

Fig. 21.4. This simple tattoo can be easily excised by following its pattern to leave an irregular scar.

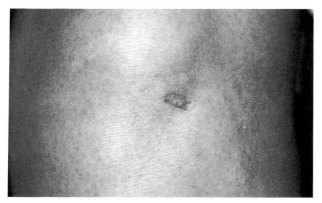

Fig. 21.5. This tattoo (which followed an abrasion on the knee) can be easily excised.

Tattoos

Minor small tattoos (either cosmetic or those following abrasions) can be excised as in an excision biopsy with a minimal ellipse of normal skin. A simple small irregular tattoo may be excised by following its pattern to leave an irregular scar (Figs. 21.4, 21.5). Special care needs to be taken to avoid stretching of the excision scar by using long-lasting subcutaneous sutures in areas that are subject to tension (such as the knee). In addition, care should be taken when suturing the tips of small triangular flaps of skin, where a modified Donatti suture is useful.

Anything other than small and easily excised tattoos should be referred to a specialist for removal by laser, dermabrasion or skin grafting. In particular, beware tattoos such as the typical swallow over the web space between the thumb and index finger. These should not be excised as there is little spare skin available.

Accessory auricle

Accessory auricles are commonly found just anterior to the tragus. Since these congenital lesions may be associated with abnormalities of the middle and inner ear the hearing should always be tested by audiometry. However, simple accessory auricles are, for practical purposes, merely small pedunculated papillomata and can be tied off. Larger lesions are likely to contain a core of cartilage and should be excised with a very small ellipse of skin.

Accessory nipple

Accessory nipples are commonly found along the mid-clavicular line and may be found in the axilla. If unsightly or troublesome, they are usually small enough to be easily removed with an ellipse of skin and they should be sent for histological examination (Fig. 21.6).

Fig. 21.6. Accessory nipple.

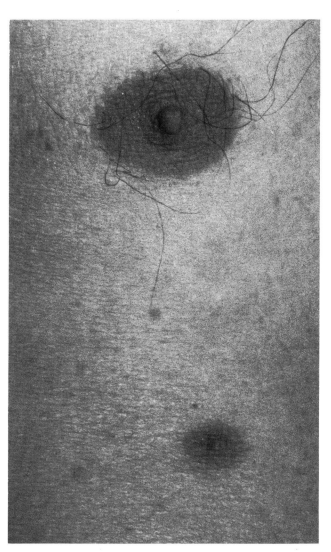

Varicose veins

Varicose veins and thread veins may be treated provided there is no saphenofemoral or saphenopopliteal incompetence. However, the treatment of veins requires meticulous assessment and is therefore very time consuming. Before the operation, it is vitally important that the patient is given an understanding of the likely result of treatment and, in particular, that recurrences are possible. Although not essential, it is helpful to take photographs in order to compare the appearances before and after treatment.

Multiple ties

Segments of varicose veins may be dissected out and excised through multiple small incisions, provided that there is no saphenofemoral or saphenopopliteal incompetence (Figs. 21.7, 21.8a). The veins should be first carefully marked out while the patient is standing. Local anaesthetic is then infiltrated around the proposed incision sites and the skin prepared and paper towels arranged to expose the leg. A small incision is made in the skin in the line of the skin creases and the underlying vein isolated by blunt dissection with an artery clip (Fig. 21.8b). The artery clip is then placed onto the vein and gentle traction combined with further blunt dissection will allow a loop of vein to be pulled out of the wound (Fig. 21.8c). Care should be taken not to pull too hard or to try to extract too long a segment as varicose veins are weak and thin walled, and liable to tear easily. Artery clips are then applied as far apart on the ends of the vein as possible and the vein gently crushed. The artery clips are then taken off and replaced a few

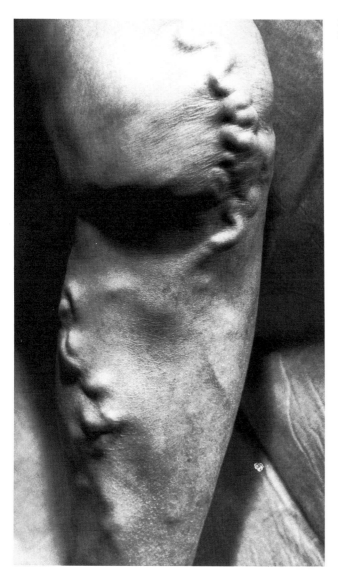

Fig. 21.7. These varicosities of the long saphenous system are not suitable for simple multiple ties as the cause is saphenofemoral incompetence.

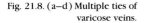

Fig. 21.8. (a–d) Multiple ties of
varicose veins.

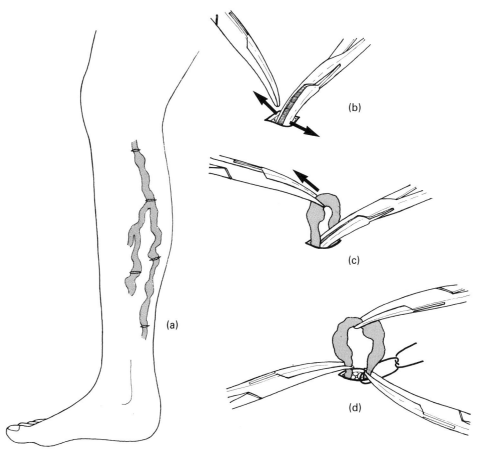

millimetres along the vein, and an absorbable 3/0 suture used to tie the vein at the crushed points, below the artery clips (Fig. 21.8d). The segment of vein is then excised with scissors or a scalpel. A final check is made to ensure that the ties are secure and the artery clips are removed. If the vein does tear or retracts into the wound and continues to bleed then the corner of a gauze swab should be inserted into the wound and pressure applied to either side of the wound for a few minutes. The swab should then be slowly removed so as not to disturb any clot and the end of the vein grasped with an artery clip. The vein can be tied or, if that is not possible, it should be twisted a few turns with the artery clip, and left for another few minutes after which haemostasis is usually achieved and the artery clip can be removed. If necessary, and if the subcutaneous tissue will hold a suture, the area may be undersewn with an absorbable suture.

An alternative technique of excision of varicose veins is to twist the vein segment a few turns around an artery clip and avulse a segment of vein. However, this method is liable to result in brisk bleeding and is not recommended unless the practitioner is familiar with the technique.

The skin is closed with either a 5/0 nylon suture, absorbable subcutaneous suture or adhesive tapes. A light dressing and bandage is applied for a few days, after which the wounds can be exposed if required and a shower taken. If nylon sutures are used they should be removed at 4–5 days to minimise suture markings and the wounds supported with adhesive tapes for a few more days.

Injection of varicose veins

Sclerosant injections can be used to treat varicose veins below the knee and also for persistent lower leg veins after saphenofemoral or saphenopopliteal ligation (Fig. 21.9). Sclerosant injections should not be used in the presence of saphenofemoral or saphenopopliteal incompetence as the persistent back-pressure will make recurrence inevitable. Commonly used sclerosants are sodium tetradecyl (STD) and ethanolamine oleate. For large veins 3% STD solution is used and the 0.5% solution is used for injecting venules and spider veins (Fig. 21.10). STD is available in 1 ml ampoules and 30 ml vials. Ethanolamine oleate 5% is available in 2 and 5 ml ampoules. Reactions are rare but resuscitation equipment should be available at hand in case of anaphylaxis.

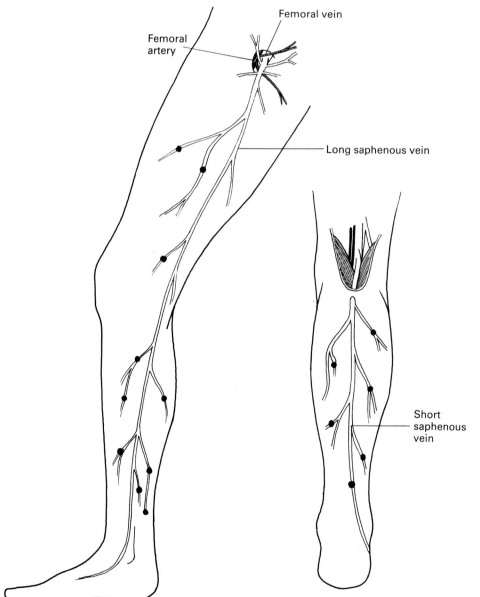

Fig. 21.9. Varicose veins: anatomy showing common perforator sites.

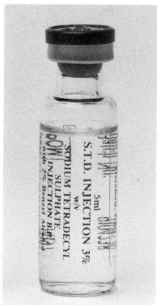

Fig. 21.10. Sodium tetradecyl for injection into varicose veins.

Although the technique is both simple and safe, care should be taken, as extravasation can cause necrosis of tissues and the patient should be warned that occasionally some persistent brownish staining of the overlying skin may result despite a correctly sited injection. The injection causes damage to the intima and the resultant fibrosis, in association with compression bandaging, results in permanent occlusion of the vessel. The procedure is contra-indicated in patients in whom there is aching and oedema that does not go down after rest and elevation and therefore where there is doubt about deep vein patency. Such cases should be referred to a specialist for investigation and assessment prior to any treatment.

Sclerotherapy should not be used in the following conditions

1. Saphenofemoral or saphenopopliteal incompetence.
2. Persistent leg oedema.
3. Recurrent phlebothrombosis.
4. Difficulty in palpating perforators.
5. Where ulceration is present.

These patients should be referred for full assessment.

Patients using oral contraceptives should stop their use for 4–6 weeks prior to treatment. Allergy is rare, but it is necessary to have adrenaline, chlorpheniramine and hydrocortisone available in case of anaphylaxis.

Although incompetent perforators may be identified by serial tourniquets at different levels, the palpation method is sufficient for this procedure. With the patient in a standing posture, finger-tip pressure over the sites of bulbous veins allows the openings in the deep fascia to be felt, and the perforator sites ('blow outs') are marked out.

A number of 1 or 2 ml syringes with 25G needles are prepared with 0.5–1 ml of STD and some lengths of adhesive tape are stuck onto rolls of gauze or cotton wool balls and placed conveniently at hand.

With the patient standing on a footstool and next to the couch, a perforator site is punctured and a little blood is withdrawn to confirm that the needle tip is in the vein. No injection is made at this point but the syringe is then taped to the skin and the procedure is repeated with the other perforators. Four to five sites can be injected at one time. The patient is then asked to lie on the couch and the leg elevated to empty the veins. A portion of a crêpe bandage (or a self-adhesive bandage such as the Secure forte) is then applied around the foot and ankle and left. Some 2 cm of the lowermost vein segment is then isolated at either side of the needle with the fingers and 0.5–1 ml of STD injected slowly (Figs. 21.11, 21.12).

The needle is withdrawn and a gauze roll or cotton wool ball is taped in place and the crêpe bandage applied over the site. The procedure is repeated for the other veins, working upwards, and the bandage wound around after each injection. An elasticated stocking is then applied over the bandage. The patient is encouraged to walk a good distance daily. It is customary to retain the bandages for 6 weeks but they often work loose and are then ineffectual. There is good

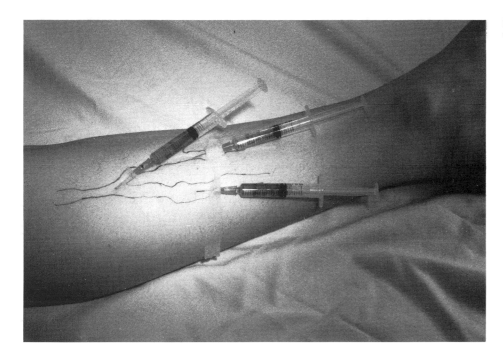

Fig. 21.11. Injection into varicose veins.

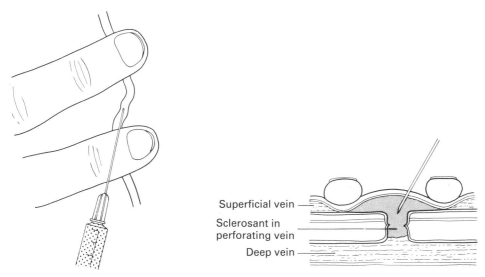

Superficial vein
Sclerosant in perforating vein
Deep vein

Fig. 21.12. Injection into varicose veins.

evidence to show that bandaging for only 3 days is equally effective and greatly reduces the inconvenience to the patient [2].

Thread veins

Thread veins are often extensive and are far more time consuming to treat than injection or excision of larger veins. However, treatment of unsightly flares can make a marked difference to the appearance. Thread veins may be treated either by meticulous small monopolar diathermy burns using a very fine 32G solid needle or by injection using a number of sclerosant preparations such as hypertonic saline, glycerine, aethoxlerol and STD through a fine 28 or 32G needle [3].

Whichever method is used, it is important for patients to understand that unless the treated area is very small not all the vessels will disappear and that there are likely to be some recurrences.

Diathermy treatment If the area involved is limited, some patients will tolerate the treatment without a local anaesthetic. However, thread veins often appear fanwise over large areas of skin and the area has to be anaesthetised first using either wide infiltration or a topical preparation such as EMLA cream, but the latter is unpredictable in the depth of its effect. The diathermy current should be adjusted to a low position at first and then slowly increased to the desired level. The thread veins are extremely superficial and the needle tip should be placed just through the skin and onto the vein. A very short duration current is passed and the vein will be seen to blanch and partially evaporate. A series of 'spot welds' are made along the lengths of the veins (Figs. 21.13, 21.14).

At least two or three sessions are usually required and some 3–6 weeks are necessary between treatments to allow any crusts to separate and the full result of a particular treatment to be seen.

Immediately after treatment the vein may disappear completely. After some minutes erythema and a wheal will appear. By the end of the treatment session the whole treated area will show superficial swelling and erythema and this will gradually subside over the ensuing days. Multiple small crusts will appear at the treatment sites and these will take 3–4 weeks to disappear completely. The procedure is time consuming and a number of sessions are necessary to deal with all the tributaries. The patient should be reviewed after 2–4 weeks, at which time any remaining veins can be treated. The patient should be warned that there will occasionally be very tiny multiple scars left at the site of the diathermy burns, but these are usually hardly noticeable and are trivial compared to the original fan of ugly veins.

Fig. 21.13. (BELOW LEFT) Thread veins.

Fig. 21.14. (BELOW RIGHT) Diathermy to thread veins showing the immediate wheal.

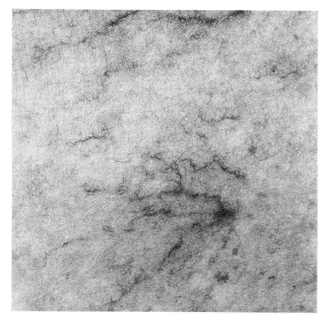

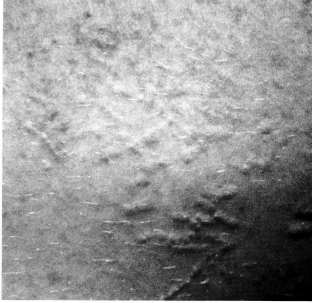

Sclerosant injection A magnifying loupe is essential. The patient will usually easily tolerate the multiple very slight pin pricks. As the thread veins are extremely superficial, the needle should be placed onto the skin surface above a vein and the skin is then gently punctured. In doing so the needle tip will immediately enter the vein lumen. Only the bevel tip of the needle should enter the vein – any more and the needle will almost certainly exit the lumen on the other side of the vein. Each small injection will flow into two or three tributaries and as the injections proceed, any excess sclerosant lying on the skin is mopped up with a gauze swab. Care should be taken not to inject the sclerosant into the skin itself. The procedure is time consuming and a number of sessions are often necessary to deal with all the tributaries. Immediately after the injection the veins will be seen to blanch as the sclerosant flows through. After some minutes erythema and a wheal will appear. By the end of the treatment session the whole treated area will show superficial swelling and erythema and this will gradually subside over the coming days. No compression is necessary. The patient should be reviewed after 2–4 weeks at which time if any veins remain they should be injected.

References

1. Management of keloids by surgical excision and local injections of steroid. Singleton, M. A. & Gross, C. W. *Southern Medical Journal* (1971), **64**, 1377–1381.
2. Prolonged bandaging is not required following sclerotherapy of varicose veins. Fraser, A., Perry, E. P., Hatton, M. & Watkin, D. F. L. *British Journal of Surgery* (1985), **72**, 488–490.
3. Small vessel sclerotherapy: an overview. Duffy, D. M. *Advances in Dermatology* (1988), **3**, 221–242.

SECTION V

22

Minor casualties: Simple wounds and burns

Simple wounds

Assessment

Simple lacerations can be easily dealt with in the surgery (Fig. 22.1). More complicated wounds should be referred to the local accident and emergency department. Elective surgical wounds are clean but, for practical purposes, all traumatic wounds are potentially infected. All grossly contaminated, crushed or neglected wounds should be considered as infected.

The examination of all wounds should include the depth, degree of contamination, presence or absence of any foreign body, damage to underlying nerves, tendons or vessels, bones and joints. Often, a full assessment cannot be made until the area is anaesthetised, but nerve and tendon function should be assessed prior to infiltration of any local anaesthetic. To minimise the pain of injection, the local

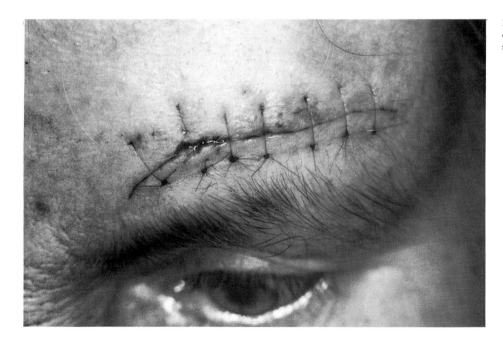

Fig. 22.1. A simple laceration, easily dealt with in the general practice setting.

anaesthetic should be infiltrated from within the wound itself. In children it is preferable to drip local anaesthetic into the wound itself and this may avoid the necessity for injection altogether (see chapter 6).

Sometimes, however, if seen soon after the accident, small uncomplicated wounds (particularly on the scalp after blunt injuries) can be sutured without any local anaesthetic infiltration. Beware lacerations over the hand and digits as these are likely to give rise to tendon injuries (Fig. 22.2).

Fig. 22.2. All wounds need careful examination. This small cut in the wrist could easily have transected the median nerve.

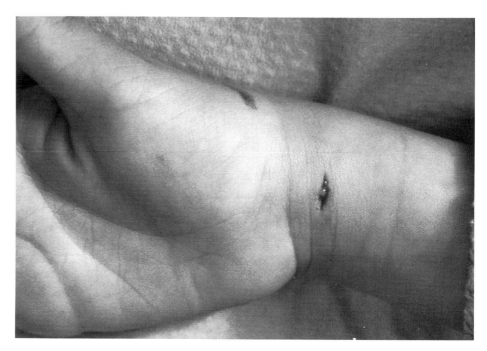

Debridement

The wound should be irrigated using a gauze swab soaked with 0.5% aqueous chlorhexidine or 1% aqueous povidone iodine. Cotton wool balls should be avoided as the fibres tend to be left in the wound. Foreign material, grit, and debris should be removed with forceps or a wet gauze swab. Any devitalised skin and tissue should be excised and in addition, antibiotics and tetanus prophylaxis should be considered (see opposite).

Repair and closure

The wound edges should be correctly aligned by suturing angles and landmarks first. Particular care should be taken to avoid undue tension in the wound edges as any subsequent swelling is likely to be greater than after a clean surgical incision. Occasionally, after a wound has been closed, some of the sutures may be seen to be too tight or poorly positioned. These should be removed and replaced. Bleeding can often be a problem during the suturing but this can be minimised by inserting part of a gauze swab into one end of the wound while the other end is

---

Tetanus prophylaxis [1]

Adsorbed tetanus vaccine (0.5 ml) should be given by intramuscular or deep subcutaneous injection. Because of the risk of developing hypersensitivity reactions, a tetanus vaccine reinforcing dose (booster) should not be given less than 10 years after the last dose. The following should be given in addition to wound toilet:

Less than 10 years since last tetanus booster
Simple clean open wounds
  No further action required.
Simple potentially contaminated or contaminated wounds
  Benzylpenicillin or other appropriate antibiotic.
Serious potentially contaminated or contaminated wounds
  1. Tetanus immunoglobulin.
  2. Benzylpenicillin or other appropriate antibiotic.

More than 10 years since last tetanus booster
Simple clean open wounds
  Tetanus vaccine booster dose.
Simple potentially contaminated or contaminated wounds
  1. Benzylpenicillin or other appropriate antibiotic.
  2. Tetanus vaccine booster dose.
Serious potentially contaminated or contaminated wounds
  1. Tetanus immunoglobulin.
  2. Benzylpenicillin or other appropriate antibiotic.
  3. Tetanus vaccine booster dose.

No previous tetanus immunisation
Simple clean open wounds
  1. Tetanus vaccine booster dose.
  2. Arrange course of tetanus vaccine.
Simple potentially contaminated or contaminated wounds
  1. Benzylpenicillin or other appropriate antibiotic.
  2. Tetanus vaccine booster dose.
  3. Arrange course of tetanus vaccine.
Serious potentially contaminated or contaminated wounds
  1. Tetanus immunoglobulin.
  2. Benzylpenicillin or other appropriate antibiotic.
  3. Tetanus vaccine booster dose.
  4. Arrange course of tetanus vaccine.

Tetanus immunoglobulin should also be considered for patients with wounds more than 6 hours old before treatment, and those with contaminated puncture wounds.

---

being sutured. It is often better to start suturing at the upper end of the wound and work downwards. If suturing is commenced from the lower end of the wound, blood from bleeding at the upper end will tend to flow down and obscure the field of view.

Special considerations

Crushed lacerations Since crushed wounds generally heal poorly and tend to swell considerably, it is sometimes better to avoid sutures and undue tension. Instead, the wound may be covered by a paraffin tulle dressing and elevated, and consideration given to delayed closure after a few days.

Tooth bites Lacerations from human and animal bites are always heavily contaminated and should not normally be closed primarily unless they are obviously clean (Fig. 22.3). If these wounds are closed one end may be left unsutured to allow drainage. In addition, broad spectrum antibiotics and metronidazole (for anaerobes) should be considered. Special care should be taken with bites over the finger and hand joints. In such cases an infection should be referred early as this may herald septic arthritis [2].

Fig. 22.3. Hamster bite to thumb.

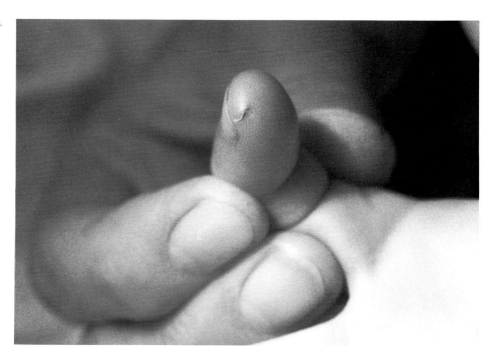

Scalp Scalp wounds tend to bleed profusely. If necessary, bleeding may be controlled to some degree by applying artery clips to larger cut vessels. Common lacerations only need skin sutures but longer wounds should be closed in two layers, with an absorbable suture to the epicranial aponeurosis (Figs. 22.4, 22.5, 22.6).

Tissue adhesive can be used for small wounds, particularly in children. Alternatively, in selected cases small scalp wounds may be closed by twisting a number of hair strands and knotting them together across the wound. The knots may be secured by either using a plastic spray or tissue adhesive.

Forehead Particular attention should be paid to ensuring that any frown lines are matched up accurately. Often in the elderly, when the skin is lax, the wound can be easily closed with adhesive tapes.

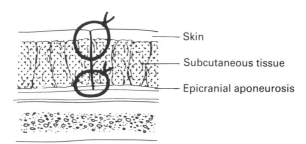

- Skin
- Subcutaneous tissue
- Epicranial aponeurosis

Fig. 22.4. Suture of scalp in two layers.

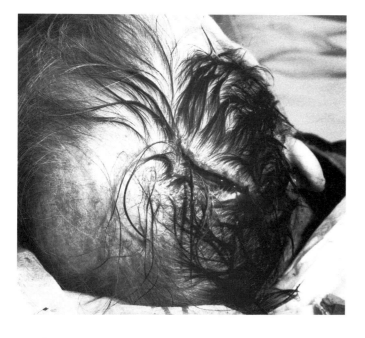

Fig. 22.5. (FAR LEFT) Scalp laceration.

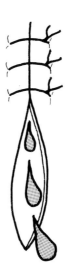

Fig. 22.6. Start suturing at the upper end of a wound to avoid obscuring the field with blood.

Eyebrows It is essential to ensure that there is accurate approximation of the eyebrow hair line to avoid any ugly step deformities.

Face Fine (5/0) sutures should be used to minimise suture marks. Lacerations of the eyelids, and near the lachrymal ducts should be referred to the accident and emergency department.

Chin Sutures are usually unnecessary as these wounds can often be easily closed with adhesive tapes (Fig. 22.7). Tissue adhesive is an alternative, if available, provided there is no undue tension. The mandible and temperomandibular joints should be examined for signs of bone injury after any blunt injury to the chin.

Tongue Small lacerations caused by the teeth can be left alone to heal spontaneously. Larger wounds should be referred to the accident and emergency department.

Lip Wounds caused by penetration of incisor teeth should be cleaned, examined to exclude foreign particles or tooth fragments and can almost always be left to heal spontaneously without sutures (Fig. 22.8). Large lacerations of the lip should be closed in three layers, mucosa, muscle and skin (Figs. 22.9, 22.10).

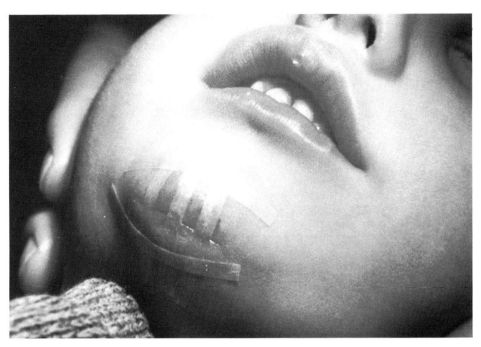

Fig. 22.7. Chin laceration closed with adhesive tapes.

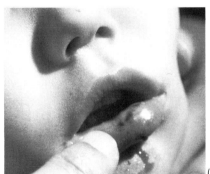 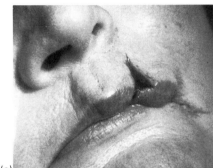 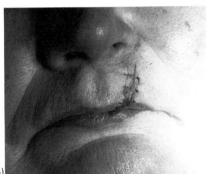

(a)   (b)

Fig. 22.8. (ABOVE) Lower lip laceration caused by upper incisor teeth.

Fig. 22.9. (a) and (b). (ABOVE, CENTRE AND RIGHT) Lip laceration involving skin only, caused by dog bite. Always start the skin closure with alignment of the vermillion border.

Fig. 22.10. (RIGHT) Suture of lip laceration.

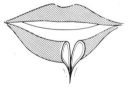 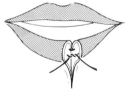 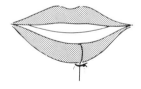

Fingers and hand Careful examination must be made prior to the use of any local anaesthetic to exclude nerve or tendon injury (Fig. 22.11). Nerve and tendon injuries should be referred. When lacerations in fingers are to be sutured, it is often useful to exsanguinate the finger and apply a rubber band tourniquet after a digital nerve block. The wound can then be accurately sutured without any bleeding. It is important to be aware that, if a laceration of a tendon is sustained while the digit is either flexed or extended, the laceration of the tendon may not lie directly below the skin wound (Fig. 22.12). Any wound over a tendon should therefore be examined while the digit is flexed and extended.

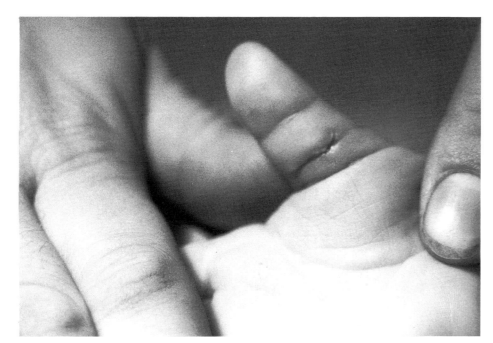

Fig. 22.11. Wounds can be deceptive. This laceration of thumb resulted in transection of the tendon of flexor policis longus.

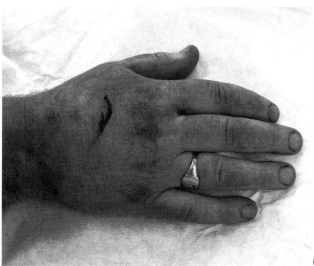 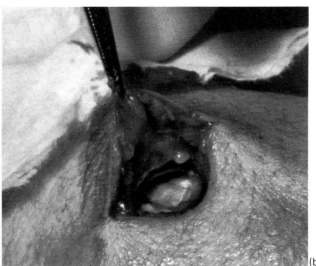

(a) (b)

Simple flap lacerations involving the terminal pulp can usually be held in place with the use of adhesive tapes, although larger flaps may require sutures.

Amputations involving loss of small areas of the terminal pulp can usually be allowed to heal by secondary intention. Larger areas of skin loss and amputations through the terminal phalanx should be referred to an accident and emergency department for either grafting or revision of the tip.

Feet Puncture wounds with nails are a common problem. Fortunately, most of these puncture wounds will heal with antibiotic cover. A magnesium sulphate dressing may be helpful and incision and drainage or exploration is usually unnecessary. Exploration of puncture wounds is seldom necessary unless there is any suggestion of a retained foreign body or infection. Such cases may require

Fig. 22.12. (a) and (b). Laceration on the back of the hand. Note that tendon lacerations can be found in the presence of some active finger extension because of the action of the interossei and the tendinous bands between the extensor tendons. The extensor tendons are easily seen on opening the wound after infiltration with local anaesthetic but in this case, the tendon lacerations are hidden from view, being proximal to the wound.

Fig. 22.13. (a) and (b). This infant
was limping for few days after
treading on a needle. Gentle probing
of the puncture site allowed the
needle to be removed without a
local anaesthetic.

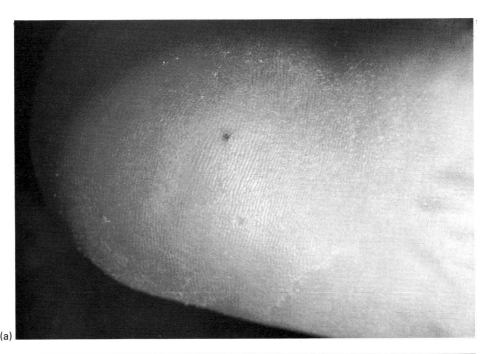

(a)

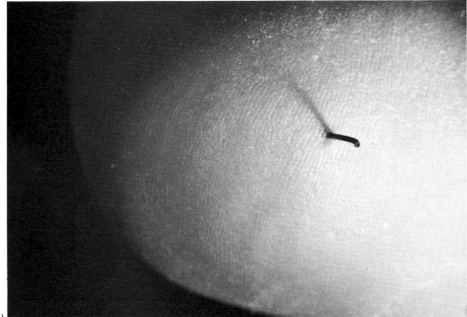

(b)

X-rays and should be referred to an accident and emergency department. Sometimes, however, a foreign body can be easily removed without local anaesthetic
(Fig. 22.13).

Pretibial lacerations Relatively thin flap lacerations are common on the shins,
especially in the elderly. Most of these flaps can be laid back in place and
supported with adhesive tapes, taking care to unfurl any edges.
    A paraffin tulle dressing should be placed over the tapes, followed by a

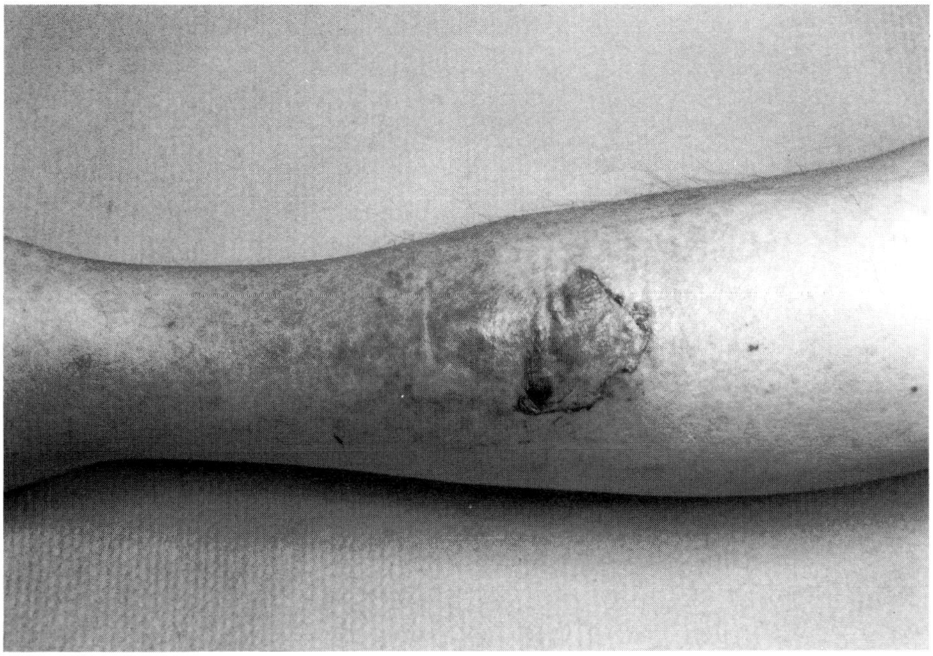

Fig. 22.14. This thin distally based flap is associated with swelling and bruising immediately below it. This flap is liable to necrose and leave a raw granulating area.

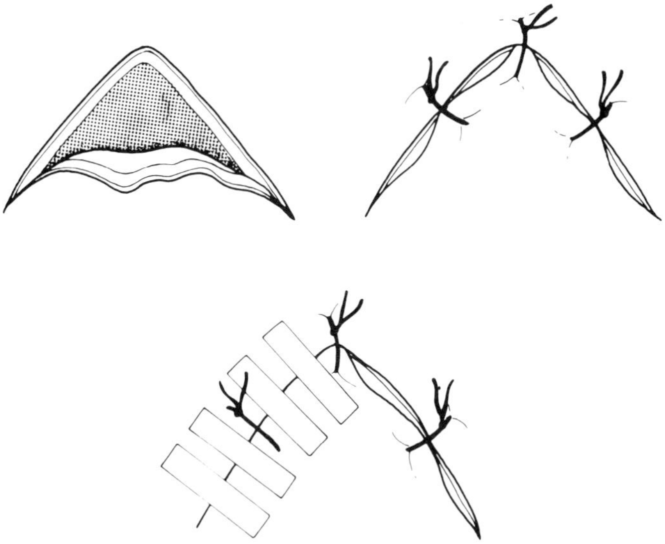

Fig. 22.15. Pretibial laceration with temporary sutures.

protective wad of gauze, the dressing should be taped in place and the ankle and lower leg should be supported with a crêpe or tube bandage. The leg should be elevated as much as possible to reduce swelling and to encourage healing.

In general, sutures should be avoided as they tend to cut through, especially at the vulnerable apex of the flap (Fig. 22.14). However, sometimes a few temporary sutures may be inserted to help to approximate the skin edges. These can be removed once the adhesive tapes have been applied (Fig. 22.15). If the flap shows marked venous congestion, it can be excised at its base, defatted and laid back as a full thickness graft. Thick flaps can be loosely sutured and given additional support with adhesive tapes (Fig. 22.16).

Fig. 22.16. (a–c) Thick flap with sutures and adhesive tapes.

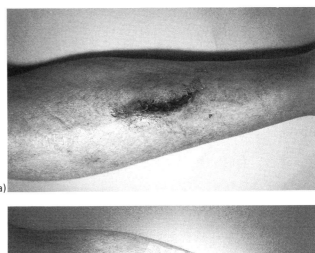

(a)

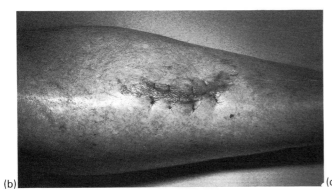

(b)

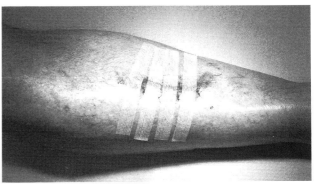

(c)

Fig. 22.17. The skin of this flap has necrosed leaving a dry crust. The crust can be left alone but any persistent pain it is likely to indicate that there is some underlying pus or haematoma.

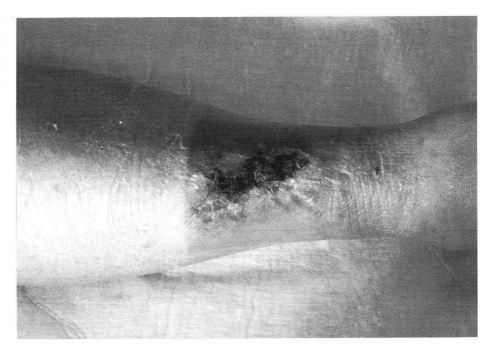

Bleeding from a tooth socket Occasionally, blood will continue to ooze out of a socket some hours after tooth extraction. Although it is often recommended that a suture should be inserted across the cavity, in practice it is usually effective to instil 1 or 2% lignocaine with 1:200000 adrenaline into a small wad of gauze, place it in the cavity, and ask the patient to bite on it for 5–10 min.

If a suture has to be inserted, it may be placed quickly and tied over a small wad of gauze without the need for any further local anaesthetic. Prior to the insertion of the suture, a wad of gauze should be placed in the buccal side of the gum to allow room for the needle to pass through (Fig. 22.18). The suture can be removed after 3–4 days.

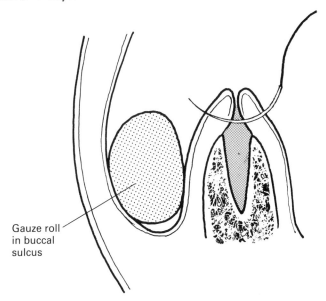

Fig. 22.18. Suture for bleeding from a tooth socket.

Gauze roll in buccal sulcus

Simple burns

All scalds and burns should be immediately cooled with clean water. If the skin is red and sensitive, the damage is likely to be superficial (Fig. 22.19). However, if the skin is grey or charred and insensitive the damage is deep. Deep dermal, full thickness and more extensive burns should be referred to an accident and emergency department. Likewise, electrical burns are usually deep dermal or full thickness and, unless small, they too should be referred (Fig. 22.20).

Simple scalds and burns resulting in superficial erythema do not need to be covered but may be made more comfortable with the use of an antiseptic cream such as Flamazine (silver sulphadiazine). With minor burns on the hand it is almost always more convenient to avoid bulky dressings or occlusion in plastic bags or gloves. Such methods should be reserved for more serious or extensive burns. Superficial blisters can be left intact, exposed and allowed to dry spontaneously. However, the blisters can be drained and excised if large or intrusive. The resulting raw surface can be covered with a paraffin tulle dressing or with Flamazine cream covered with ordinary gauze. The dressing should be left in place for 5–7 days and not changed unless obviously stained or foul-smelling. If the dressing is changed too frequently this merely disturbs the growing epithelium and can result in unnecessary bleeding and delayed healing. The skin can be left exposed once the skin has epithelialised and is dry.

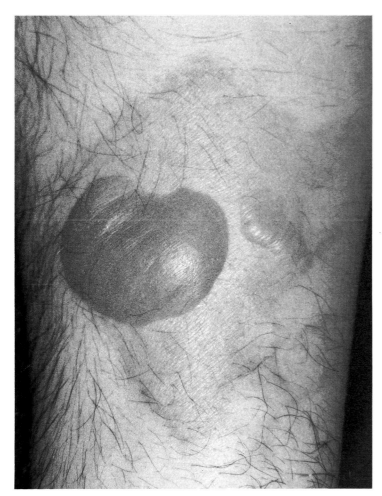

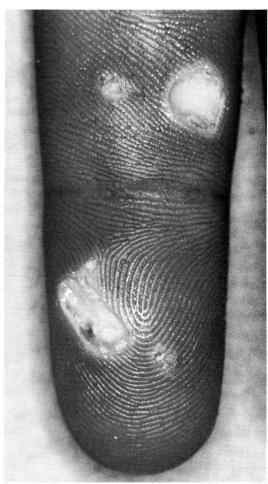

Fig. 22.19. (ABOVE) Superficial blistering on the arm caused by steam. This can be treated by Flamazine or paraffin tulle dressings, allowing the blisters to burst or shrivel spontaneously.

Fig. 22.20. (ABOVE, RIGHT) Full thickness electrical burns on the fingers. These burns should be referred for specialist care.

Non-accidental injury

Any doctor who has to deal with injuries from time to time should be alert to the possibility of non-accidental injuries. A number of suggestive signs are listed below. In addition, a child who has been unloved and repeatedly battered may show little trust and have an attitude of 'frozen watchfulness'. Any battered child is at serious risk and, even if the presenting lesion is minor, the doctor should arrange for the child to be admitted to hospital without delay.

Features suggestive of non-accidental injury

1. Nature of the injury does not correlate with history.
2. Bruises at various stages of healing.
3. Unexplained delay in bringing child to the doctor.
4. No explanation for a particular injury.
5. Homogeneously burned surface.
6. Burns with straight edges.
7. Child has attitude of 'frozen watchfulness'.

References

1. Tetanus vaccine and immunoglobulin. *British National Formulary 1993*, pp. 464, 467. British Medical Association and Royal Pharmaceutical Society of Great Britain: London.
2. Septic arthritis of the hand. de Vries, H. & Van der Werken, C. *Injury* (1993), **24**, 32–34.

23

Minor casualties: Infections and haematomata

Abscesses

In the early stages (before the appearance of pus) acute suppurative inflammation may be aborted by the use of antibiotics. At this time there is nothing to be gained by incision into the inflamed tissues. However, once there is pus, it should be drained as soon as possible in order to limit the extent of any tissue damage. Although superficial abscesses will demonstrate fluctuation, where the abscess is bound by dense fibrous tissue (e.g. breast) or is deep (e.g. ischiorectal) fluctuation may be absent.

Infections and abscesses in the middle third of the face should be treated actively and urgently with antibiotics and/or drainage because of the risk of cavernous sinus thrombosis. Examination should be made to exclude signs of ascending lymphangitis (Fig. 23.1), which usually indicates a *Streptococcus pyogenes* infection, which should be treated with penicillin.

Fig. 23.1. Ascending lymphangitis.

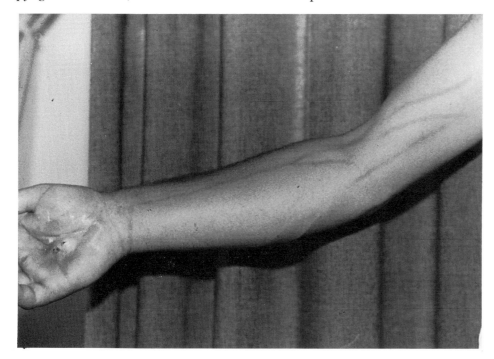

Treatment of infections and abscesses in the limbs should always be accompanied by elevation if possible (to reduce swelling and pain).

It is traditionally recommended that patients with skin sepsis should be screened for diabetes. However, unselected screening of all such patients yields only a slightly higher number of cases of abnormal glucose tolerance than in controls and it may be more prudent to screen selectively all patients over 40 years of age who present with skin sepsis [1].

Anaesthesia

Deep abscesses will usually require referral for a general anaesthetic. Superficial abscesses may be drained using 'dome infiltration' (Figs. 23.2a,23.2b), wide infiltration, or with entonox, if available. The use of ethyl chloride spray to numb the skin by cooling should be avoided, as it is both crude and unsatisfactory. Occasionally, when the abscess is pointing and the overlying skin is very thin and necrotic, the dome can be incised quickly without any anaesthesia.

When the overlying skin is thin and not necrotic, dome infiltration of a small quantity of local anaesthetic can be used. Only perhaps 0.25–0.5 ml is necessary and this only causes a transient sharp pain as the skin is seen to blanch. Almost immediately the dome can be punctured with a no. 11 blade, releasing the pus.

Wide infiltration is necessary when the dome of the abscess is thick or indurated (Fig. 23.3). The infiltration should be wide of the inflammation, because injecting into red, inflammed skin is extremely painful. Adequate time should be allowed for the anaesthetic to work and this usually takes a few minutes longer than in normal skin. In addition, since inflamed skin is more vascular, any anaesthetic effect will be relatively short-lasting.

Fig. 23.2. (a) Dome infiltration anaesthesia. (b) This axillary abscess was easily drained using dome infiltration.

There are two basic methods of closure after drainage of abscesses. The tried and tested method is one of incision and drainage followed, if necessary, by the insertion of a paraffin tulle wick for 24–48 h. An alternative is treatment with intramuscular antibiotics 1 h before incision, drainage and curettage, followed by

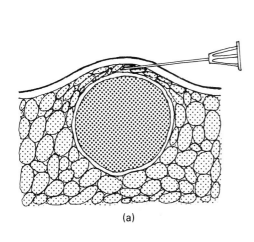

(a)

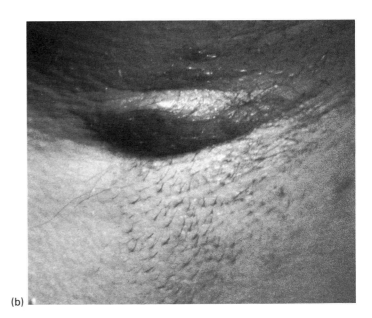

(b)

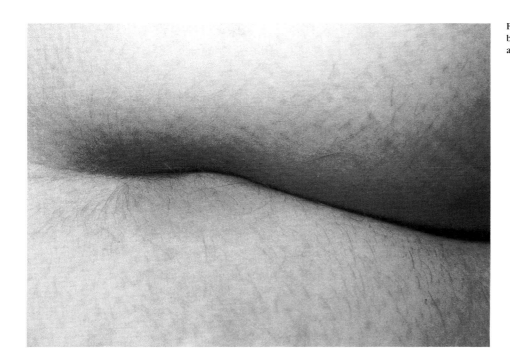

Fig. 23.3. This natal cleft abscess can be drained using wide infiltration anaesthesia.

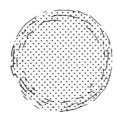

Fig. 23.4. Deroofing of abscess or simple incision.

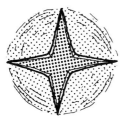

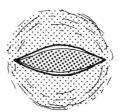

primary suture to obliterate the cavity. The latter method, although effective, is time consuming and requires meticulous technique to clear the cavity of all pus and debris.

If the cavity is large or the skin necrotic a cruciate incision is performed and the corners removed. Alternatively, skin excision may be avoided by making the incision long enough to gape open and prevent premature closure (Fig. 23.4). This method is preferred in areas where there is little spare skin, such as the sole of the foot and fingers.

Boil

Boils can usually be simply drained with a stab incision following dome infiltration. Deroofing is not usually necessary (Fig. 23.5).

Carbuncle

A carbuncle is a specific form of staphylococcal skin infection that results in multiple loculations of pus, often pointing at a number of places. These multiple sites can often be incised without local anaesthetic. If used, however, the local anaesthetic should be injected wide of the inflamed area and the separate loculi deroofed. Sinus forceps should be used to remove as much debris and pus as possible. It is common to find that the pus in a carbuncle is not liquid but often forms a plug that can be lifted out as thick globules (Fig. 23.6). Although antibiotics are not generally required once an abscess is drained, a carbuncle is a particularly persistent infection and an anti-staphylococcal antibiotic such as flucloxacillin should be given to hasten resolution. A paraffin tulle wick may be necessary for 24–48 h.

Fig. 23.5. This abscess developed at the site of a chicken pox lesion and was easily drained by dome infiltration and drainage.

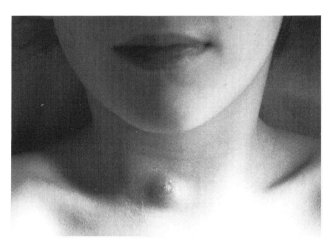

Fig. 23.6. (a) and (b) Antibiotics are often of secondary importance to debridement. This carbuncle had a central plug which could be lifted out with forceps. Following this resolution was rapid.

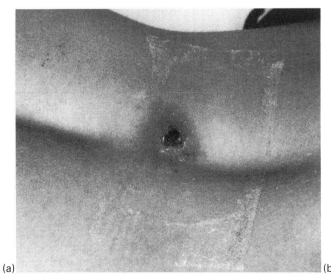

(a)

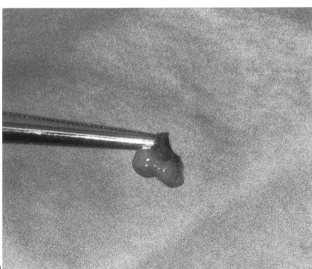

(b)

Infected sebaceous cyst

An infected cyst can usually be drained by using dome infiltration. Unless as sometimes happens, the cyst wall fragments lie loose in the cavity and are easily extracted, it is often kinder not to scrape the inside of the cavity in an attempt to remove cyst wall remnants. Instead, the contents can be allowed to drain and the wound allowed to close spontaneously. Any residual cyst can be more easily and less painfully removed after 4–6 weeks when the acute inflammation has resolved (see chapter 16).

Acute paronychia

Acute paronychia is usually caused by a staphylococcus and if seen early, it may be aborted with the use of an antibiotic such as flucloxacillin or erythromycin. Usually, when the skin is thin, devitalised and insensitive an acute paronychia can be drained without a local anaesthetic. Sometimes, however, simple drainage with or without resection of a sliver of nail has to be performed under a digital nerve block. Antibiotics are not usually necessary and resolution is rapid once the pus has been drained (Figs. 23.7, 23.8, 23.9, 23.10a,b).

Figs 23.7 (BELOW, LEFT) and 23.8. (BELOW, CENTRE AND RIGHT) Early acute paronychia: careful examination and gentle probing with a no. 11 blade can often yield a small bead of pus.

Fig. 23.9. (BOTTOM, LEFT) Extensive acute paronychia: sometimes a sliver of nail has to be removed to allow for adequate drainage.

Fig. 23.10. (BOTTOM, CENTRE AND RIGHT) Extensive acute paronychia in (a) adult and (b) infant.

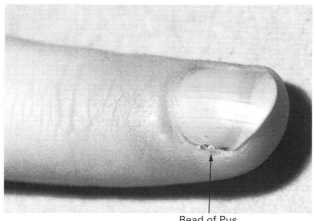
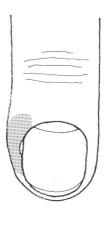
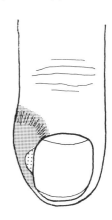

Bead of Pus

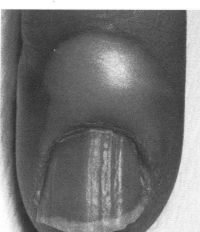
(a)

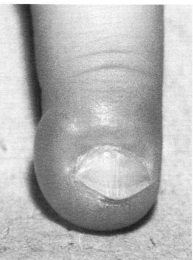

(b)

Pulp space abscess

The skin over the pulp spaces is tethered to the underlying bone by fibrous bands. Because of this, pus may be trapped deep in the tissues and point to the surface as a 'collar-stud' abscess. This is usually caused by *Streptococcus pyogenes* and penicillin cover should be considered. The deep pocket of pus should be drained with a probe or sinus forceps under a digital nerve block (Fig. 23.11).

Fig. 23.11. Pulp space abscess.

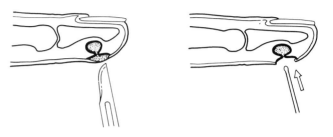

Stye

This is the result of suppuration within a lash follicle (Fig. 23.12). In the early stage it may be aborted with the use of flucloxacillin. Sometimes, drainage of pus may be effected by simply pulling out the affected eyelash. Incision and drainage may be necessary for larger styes using local anaesthetic infiltration into the eyelid. Antibiotic eye ointment (e.g. Chloramphenicol 1%) should be used for a few days to prevent any conjunctivitis.

Fig. 23.12. Stye.

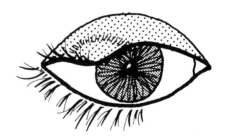

Tooth abscess

This should be treated with penicillin along with metronidazole to deal with anaerobes. If there is no resolution the patient should be advised to see a dentist for drainage or extraction.

Breast abscess

Unless small and superficial, in which it can be treated like any other superficial abscess, a breast abscess (Fig. 23.13) should be referred to an accident and emergency department for incision and drainage under a general anaesthetic.

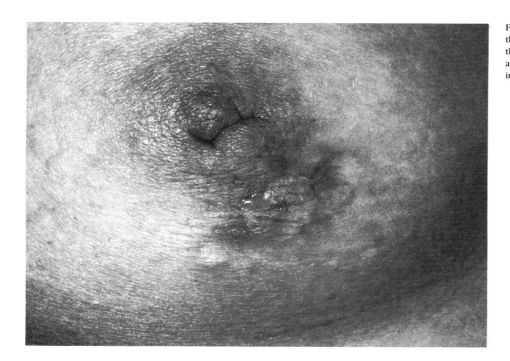

Fig. 23.13. This breast abscess below the nipple was discharging through the nipple itself. It was opened up and allowed to heal by secondary intention.

Pilonidal abscess

An acute pilonidal abscess can be drained in the same way as other abscesses but unless all the hair nests are removed and all the sinus tracks excised, the condition is likely to persist as a chronic sinus. Unless very small, a pilonidal sinus is best excised under general anaesthesia with injection of methylene blue to stain all the sinus tracks.

Perianal abscess

Small superficial perianal abscesses can be drained following dome infiltration. Note that the urethra is vulnerable when an anterior perianal abscess is incised in the male. Larger or deeper abscesses should be referred to an accident and emergency department.

Granulomata

Pyogenic granuloma

This persistent overgranulation tissue usually follows a small wound caused by a splinter or involving foreign particles. Occasionally, a pyogenic granuloma may appear without apparent cause. Small lesions can be cauterised with a silver nitrate stick but this can be quite uncomfortable and is often ineffective. The lesion should preferably be curetted and cauterised under a local anaesthetic.

Fig. 23.14. This bleeding lesion had been present for only a few weeks on the chest of a 7 year old boy. It was excised with a small ellipse of normal skin. Histological examination confirmed it to be a pyogenic granuloma.

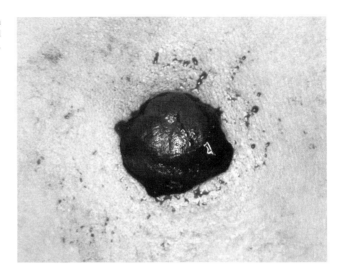

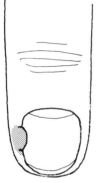

Fig. 23.15. Paronychial overgranulation.

Occasionally a very large pyogenic granuloma may look more sinister (Fig. 23.14). These lesions should be excised with an ellipse of normal skin and sent for histological examination.

Paronychial overgranulation (Fig. 23.15)

This condition follows nail trimming that leaves a lateral spicule, or appears after the penetration of a small splinter. Simple cautery with a silver nitrate stick is usually ineffective and it is often preferable to remove a small sliver of the nail under a digital nerve block and cauterise the lesion. Failure to remove a sliver of nail is likely to perpetuate the condition as the edge of the nail acts like a foreign body against the inflamed and swollen tissue.

Haematomata

Subungual haematoma

A subungual haematoma is usually caused by a crushing injury. A minor fracture of the terminal tuft is of no practical importance. However, if the injury has been more severe, the patient should be referred to an accident and emergency department for an X-ray.

The pressure of the subungual blood causes extreme pain and throbbing but this can be easily and quickly relieved by gently drilling two holes with a 21G needle (Figs. 23.16, 23.17). There is no need to use the relatively frightening methods of the heated paper clip or electrocautery. The patient can be reassured that the needle will simply drill through the nail and not through into the finger tip below. Drilling can stop once the nail is adequately perforated but often the blood ceases to come out if the needle is removed. Therefore, the needle should be left

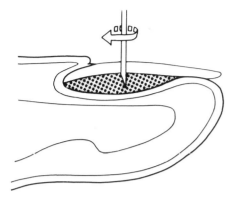

Fig. 23.16. Subungual haematoma.

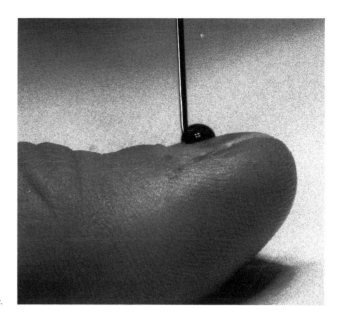

Fig. 23.17. Drilling a subungual haematoma with a 21G needle.

in situ and, if necessary, gently turned one way or other to allow the blood to seep out. If the blood merely forms a small bead around the needle and does not flow out, it is often helpful to wipe it away with a wet swab, which encourages more blood to exit.

Usually there is great relief of the pain as soon as blood is released. The hand should be rested in a high sling for 24–48 h until the throbbing has settled and simple analgesics given e.g. Co-proxamol.

If the subungual haematoma is large it is likely that the nail will eventually separate and a new one will grow in 6–8 weeks. When seen after a few days the nail may be lifting off its bed and it can often be removed completely without a digital nerve block by incising the devitalised skin around the whole nail perimeter with a scalpel blade.

Thrombosed external haemorrhoid

This can be extremely painful and the patient often declines to take a seat in the waiting room. The patient should be examined in the left lateral position and it may be helpful for an assistant to retract the upper buttock to allow adequate access. Entonox, if available, can be a useful adjunct to local anaesthetic. A small quantity of local anaesthetic is injected into the skin of the dome of the haemorrhoid. This only causes a transient sharp pain. Almost immediately the dome can be incised with a no. 11 or no. 15 blade. Often the blood has clotted and a gentle squeeze is necessary to evacuate it. The haematoma is often loculated and the separate loculations have to be individually incised (Figs. 23.18, 23.19). The raw area should be covered with a paraffin tulle dressing and the patient is allowed to bathe normally. The dressing should be changed daily and there should be gradual steady resolution over the following 4–5 days.

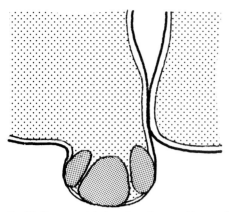

Fig. 23.18. (ABOVE) A thrombosed external haemorrhoid is often loculated and the compartments have to be separatedly incised.

Fig. 23.19. (RIGHT) Thrombosed external haemorrhoid.

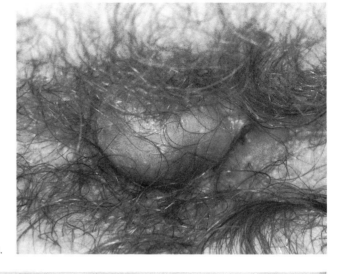

Fig. 23.20. This pretibial haematoma was evacuated after dome infiltration.

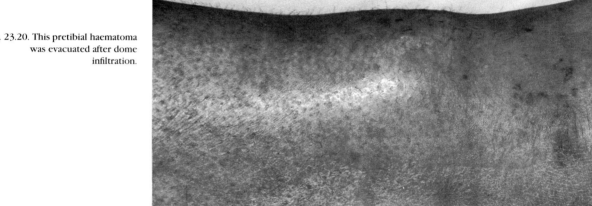

Subcutaneous haematoma

A blunt injury to the shin or forehead can often result in a subcutaneous haematoma. Small haematomata should be treated initially with ice following which they can be left to resolve spontaneously. If the haematoma is sizable or painful it can be evacuated through a small incision after injecting 1–2 ml of local anaesthetic into the skin over the dome of the swelling (Fig. 23.20). It is usually necessary to insert a pair of sinus forceps into the wound to evacuate the blood, which may be very thick or clotted. Provided the forceps do not scrape the floor of the haematoma cavity, they can be tolerated very well. Once the blood has been removed the cavity should be kept open with a paraffin tulle wick, which can be removed after 24 h. A wad of gauze can be taped to the haematoma site to help to provide pressure to occlude the cavity together with a bandage or elasticated stocking. If the haematoma is on the leg, the limb should be elevated to help to minimise swelling.

Reference

1. The value of screening for diabetes in patients with skin sepsis. Baynes, C., Caplan, S., Hames, P., Swift, R., Poole, S., Wadsworth, J., Touquet, R. & Elkeles, R. S. *Journal of the Royal Society of Medicine* (1993), **86**, 14–15.

24

Minor casualties: Foreign bodies

Eye

The eye should always be examined carefully under a good light, preferably one with a magnifying lens. A foreign body may lodge under the upper eyelid, in the cornea, or occasionally in the scleral conjunctiva. A simple speck or a simple abrasion can be easily treated in the surgery. A deeper or central foreign body or corneal abrasion should be referred for ophthalmic care.

Subtarsal speck (Figs. 24.1, 24.2)

Even the tiniest speck hidden under the upper eyelid can cause intense pain. Examination of the eye for a foreign body cannot be considered to be complete without eversion of the upper lid. The eye should be everted by asking the patient to look downwards and gently pulling the upper lashes while applying pressure against the upper lid with a finger tip or cotton bud. Topical anaesthesia is not usually required but may be necessary if there is intense blepharospasm. The speck can be simply lifted off with a cotton bud. The eye may then be stained with

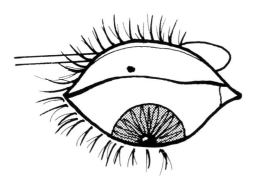

Fig. 24.1. Subtarsal speck.

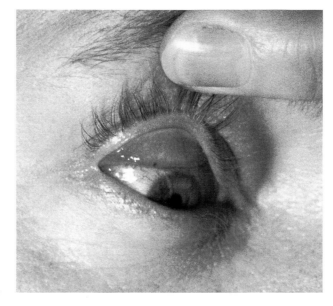

Fig. 24.2. Subtarsal speck.

a fluoroscein paper and examined in a blue light to exclude any corneal abrasions. A simple speck that has been present for a short while with no corneal abrasion needs no treatment but merely its removal. A speck that has been present for more than a few hours or has caused a corneal abrasion should be treated with an antibiotic ointment for a few days. Occasionally, a patient may present with symptoms and signs suggesting subtarsal dust but any particles may be too small to be easily seen. In such cases immediate relief may be obtained by gently wiping the underside of the eyelid with a moist cotton bud.

Corneal speck (Fig. 24.3)

A recent corneal speck or one that has floated into the eye is likely to be easy to remove in the surgery. A speck that has been present for some hours or has hit the eye with speed, as from machinery, is likely to be more difficult to remove. Such a case should be referred for ophthalmic care.

The cornea is first anaesthetised with topical 0.5% amethocaine. The patient should be warned that this can be extremely painful for a few seconds, after which the pain will pass and the cornea will usually be completely numb after 3–5 min. The patient should be asked to fix his or her gaze on some convenient object in order to keep the eye still and a cotton bud used gently to lift the speck off. Sometimes the speck may be slightly adherent, in which case it can be removed with the tip of a 21G needle. Metal foreign bodies may leave a 'rust ring' that may be difficult to remove initially but the ring is often easier to remove after 48–72 h. Until the local anaesthetic has worn off, the eye should be covered with a patch, which may be retained if the eye is more comfortable with the lid closed. Antibiotic ointment should be given for 5–7 days. A corneal speck always leaves some degree of an abrasion but this usually heals very quickly over a few days. However, a corneal laceration caused by abrasion with a finger nail, although usually quick to heal, can sometimes result in serious permanent damage to the cornea, particularly when over the central part of the cornea. These abrasions should be referred for ophthalmic care (Fig. 24.4). Although corneal abrasions are customarily treated with antibiotic eye ointment and an eye pad, there is evidence that corneal oxygenation is lower when an eye pad is used and that the cornea will heal more quickly if the eye is treated without a pad [1].

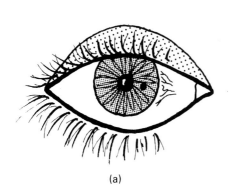

(a)

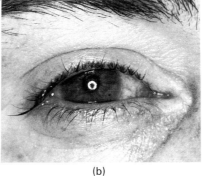

(b)

Fig. 24.3. (a) and (b) Corneal speck.

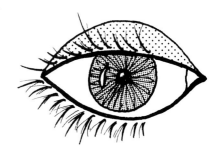

Fig. 24.4. Corneal laceration.

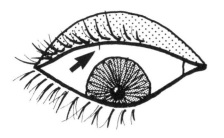
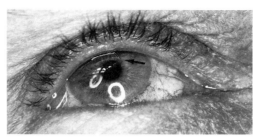

Fig. 24.5. Ingrowing eyelash.

Fig. 24.6. Ingrowing eyelash.

Ingrowing eyelash (Figs. 24.5, 24.6)

An ingrowing eyelash can be extremely painful for the patient and extremely difficult to identify and remove without a good light, magnification and a good pair of eyelash forceps that are able to grip right at their very tips. The offending hair is usually only a few millimetres long and so fine that it cannot be grasped with a fine artery clip. Recurrent ingrowing eyelashes should be referred to the ophthalmic department for fine needle diathermy to the offending follicles.

Ear

Unless easy to see and grasp, foreign bodies in the ear should be referred to the ear, nose and throat (ENT) department. The foreign body is usually a bead or a wad of cotton wool that has been pushed too far inwards. After first looking in the ear with an auroscope to see the exact orientation, the foreign body is usually easy to remove with fine forceps. In order to get a more direct access it is often necessary to draw the tragus forwards or the pinna backwards as appropriate. A small or deeper foreign body may be removed by syringing the canal. Once the foreign body is removed it is essential to examine the ear for any retained fragments or damage.

Embedded ear stud (Figs. 24.7, 24.8)

Commonly, inexpensive ear studs cause inflammation and the resultant swelling can envelope and bury the ear stud. Sometimes, with a little patience, the stud can

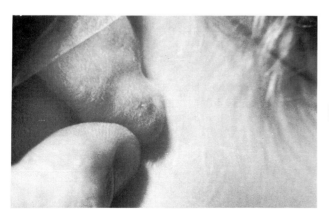
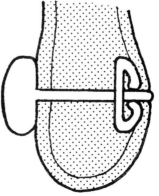

Fig. 24.7. Embedded ear stud. Only the reflection from a tiny portion of the stud is visible.

Fig. 24.8. Embedded ear stud.

be removed with a fine artery clip without a local anaesthetic. At other times the ear lobe has to be first anaesthetised by injection in the soft skin around the base of the ear.

Nose

Like foreign bodies in the ear, unless easy to see and grasp, foreign bodies in the nose should be referred to the ENT department. Small children often push things into the nose (Fig. 24.9). Beads and crayons and toy fragments can usually be removed with an artery clip, fine non-toothed forceps or a blunt hook. It is most important to spend a little time to quieten the child and it is essential to have the head held firmly and still. Any child presenting with a foul nasal discharge is likely to have a retained foreign body and should be referred to a specialist for examination.

Fig. 24.9. Bead in nostril.

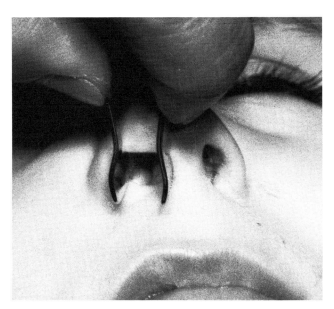

Subungual splinter (Fig. 24.10)

If a portion of the splinter is still protruding it may be withdrawn with splinter forceps, an artery clip or a hook made by bending the tip of a 21G needle. Withdrawal should be made as quickly as possible to minimise pain. Often, however, the splinter breaks off leaving very little to grasp. Sometimes trimming away the overhanging nail will allow enough purchase to pull the splinter out. Deeper splinters will need to be removed after administration of a digital nerve block.

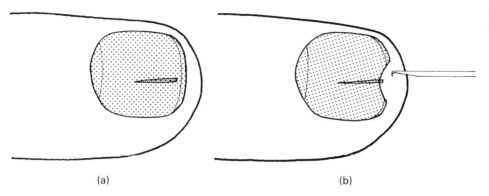

Fig. 24.10. (a) and (b) Subungual splinter.

(a)   (b)

Bamboo/wood splinters

Care should be taken with these foreign bodies as they often splinter during removal and it is not uncommon for a fragment to be retained after removal of what seems to be the whole piece. The wound should be examined and cleaned after local anaesthetic infiltration and left open (in order to allow drainage) rather than sutured.

Fish hooks

A fish hook has a barbed tip so that it cannot be simply withdrawn through its entry site. However, after a local anaesthetic, it can be easily pushed through the skin and removed after first cutting the eye end (Fig. 24.11). Fish hooks are always dirty and antibiotic treatment for a few days should be considered.

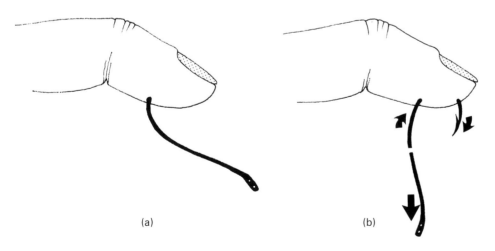

Fig. 24.11. (a) and (b) Removal of fish hook in finger.

(a)   (b)

Fig. 24.12. Granulating wound in thumb 2 months after accidental high pressure injection of paint into the terminal pulp.

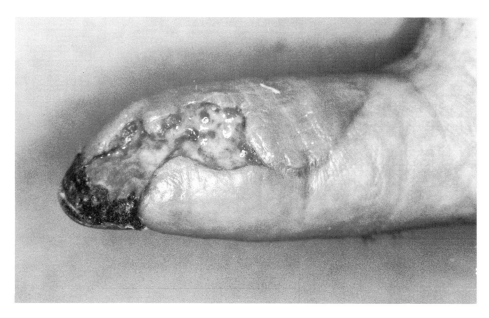

Paint or oil from pressure guns

Paint or oil can be accidentally injected under high pressure and may leave only a deceptively small entry wound. These injuries can result in serious damage and should be referred urgently for formal surgical exploration and debridement (Fig. 24.12).

Reference

1. No eye pad for corneal abrasions. Kirkpatrick, J. N. P., Hoh, H. B. & Cook, S. D. *Eye* (1993), **7**, 469–471.

25

Minor casualties: Epistaxis

Management

Epistaxis commonly occurs spontaneously and in the majority of patients the site of the bleeding can be easily identified in the lower anterior part of the septum (Little's area) (Fig. 25.1). In older patients the site of the bleeding may be higher up or posterior and inaccessible. If the bleeding is not readily controlled by cautery or a pack, the case should be referred to an ear, nose and throat specialist. A bismuth iodoform paste pack (BIPP) is both antiseptic and comforting. The pack should be first inserted along the floor of the nose and then layered successively until the whole nasal cavity is filled (Figs. 25.2, 25.3).

When Little's area is being cauterised the patient should lie supine with the head slightly propped up. A cotton wool pledget, or ribbon gauze soaked in 2% lignocaine with 1 : 200 000 adrenaline should be inserted into the anterior part of the nose and a paper tissue should be placed below the nostrils to prevent the ribbon gauze from dangling over the mouth. The nostrils should then be pinched gently for at least 5 min because adequate time must be allowed for the surface anaesthesia to work and for haemostasis. During this time, the cessation of any blood dripping down the back of the throat will confirm that the site of the bleeding is indeed anterior. Bleeding from a high or posterior site will not be controlled by such a simple anterior pack. Since it is not uncommon for the

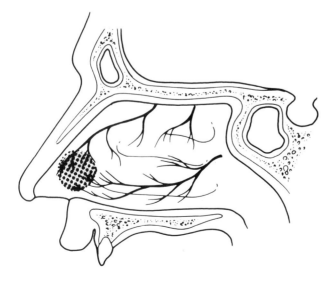

Fig. 25.1. Little's area.

Fig. 25.2. The nasal pack should be first inserted along the floor of the nose and then layered successively until the whole nasal cavity is filled.

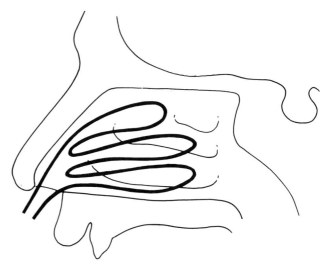

Fig. 25.3. Nasal pack held in place with tape to allow a clear airway to the unaffected side.

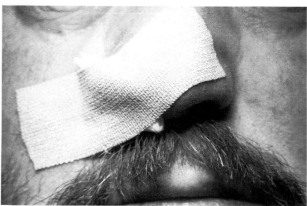

patient to retch and vomit large clots of blood from earlier bleeding, it is a sensible precaution for the doctor to wear a plastic apron to protect against any spray of blood. While the anaesthetic is working, additional ribbon gauze and cotton buds should be made ready at hand.

After a while, the pack is gently removed and the patient's head is extended and turned to one side. A nasal speculum is inserted and the nose inspected with a good light. Either the site of the bleeding will be seen in Little's area or it will be obvious that the bleeding is coming from an inaccessible site. If the site of bleeding is accessible it should be cauterised. However, cautery will be extremely difficult or impossible in the presence of any persistent bleeding. If anterior bleeding persists it may be worth re-packing and waiting longer, or it may be best to leave a pack *in situ* for 24–36 h.

Cautery may be carried out using either electrocautery, a silver nitrate stick or diathermy. However, the silver nitrate stick is the gentlest method and should be used if there is minimal bleeding. Electrocautery or diathermy is likely to cause some pain, despite the topical anaesthesia, but they are more effective methods if the bleeding continues and the patient is cooperative and able to withstand the discomfort.

Unless it is obvious that the bleeding is permanently arrested, the nose should be packed with a BIPP for 24 h.

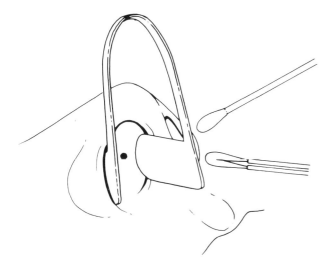

Fig. 25.4. Treatment of epistaxis using electrocautery.

Electrocautery (Fig. 25.4)

Before switching on the current, it may be necessary first to bend the cautery tip
to a favourable angle. If there is still a slight amount of bleeding, a cotton bud may
be applied to the site to mop up any blood and then quickly removed before the
cautery is applied. Care should be taken to avoid burns to the skin of the nostril by
positioning the cautery tip inside the nose before switching on the current. If the
bleeding is not controlled easily, the cautery may be applied around the edges of
the site of the bleeding rather than the doctor continuing to apply the current to
the same spot. Excessive use of cautery must be avoided because of the risk of
septal perforation.

Silver nitrate (Fig. 25.5)

Chemical cautery can only be used if there is little or no active bleeding. Care
should be taken to prevent the silver nitrate from trickling down into the depths

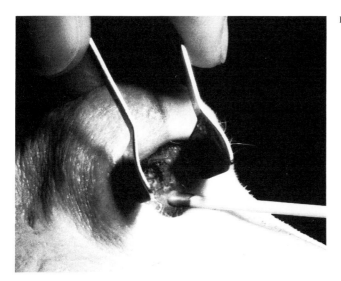

Fig. 25.5. Treatment of epistaxis using silver nitrate.

of the nose and so it may be helpful to adjust the patient's head position such that the septum is horizontal. In addition, it may be possible to insert a small pack beyond the site of the bleeding to prevent the silver nitrate from flowing away deeper into the nose. The stick is applied directly onto the site of the bleeding and the area will be seen to turn white almost immediately. An application of 5–10 s is usually sufficient, but sometimes a broader area needs to be cauterised using a number of applications.

Fig. 25.6. Treatment of epistaxis using bipolar diathermy.

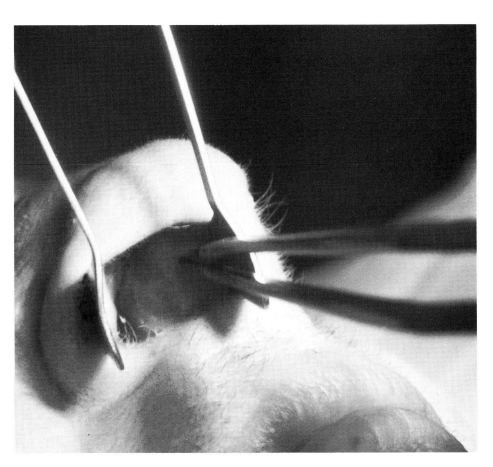

Diathermy (Fig. 25.6)

Provided the bleeding is not rapid, diathermy allows the greatest control in the treatment of epistaxis and either the bipolar or the unipolar mode may be used.

26

Minor casualties:
Emergency laryngotomy

Emergency laryngotomy (Cricothyroidotomy)
(Figs. 26.1, 26.2, 26.3)

Acute upper airway obstruction often occurs when there are no proper resuscitation facilities or equipment at hand. Laryngotomy is a quick and safe method of securing the airway in acute upper airway obstruction by introducing two large 12G intravenous cannulae through the cricothyroid membrane (Fig. 26.2). There is no risk to the vocal cords at this level and neurovascular injury can be avoided by keeping in the mid-line. Minor bleeding may occur due to injury to the small cricothyroid artery that lies on the superior part of the cricothyroid membrane.

   Prior local anaesthetic infiltration should be used if available and if time permits.

   The patient will be either supine or propped up against a convenient support. The cricothyroid membrane is identified by sliding a finger down from the

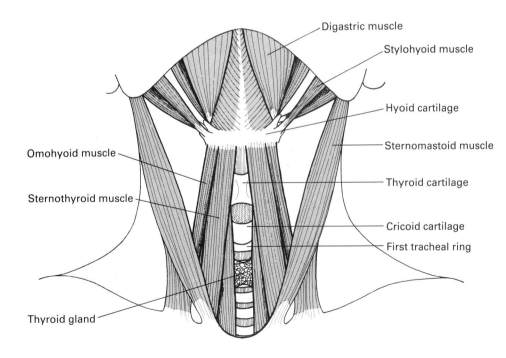

Digastric muscle

Stylohyoid muscle

Hyoid cartilage

Sternomastoid muscle

Omohyoid muscle

Thyroid cartilage

Sternothyroid muscle

Cricoid cartilage

First tracheal ring

Thyroid gland

Fig. 26.1 Laryngotomy (cricothyroidotomy): surgical anatomy.

Fig. 26.2. Laryngotomy (cricothyroidotomy) using intravenous cannulae.

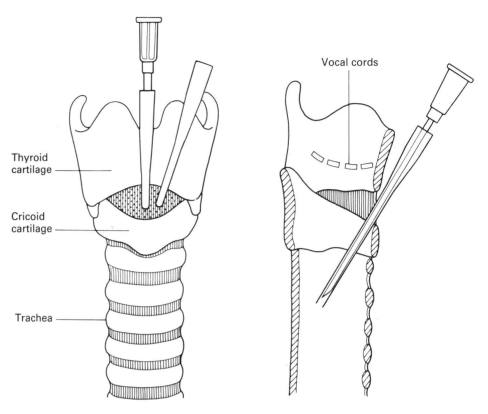

Thyroid cartilage

Cricoid cartilage

Trachea

Vocal cords

Fig. 26.3 Laryngotomy (cricothyroidotomy) cannula.

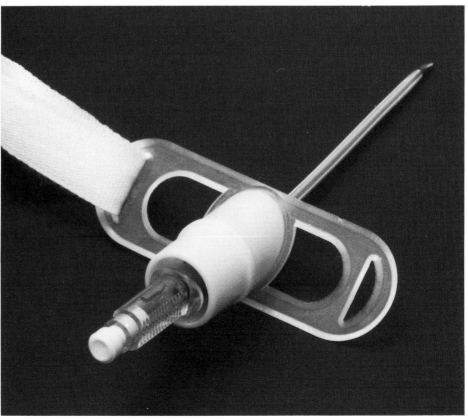

prominence of the thyroid cartilage into the gap between the thyroid and cricoid cartilages. The skin is incised with a no. 11 blade to ease the insertion of the cannulae, which should be aimed downwards and caudally. Once the crico-thyroid membrane is pierced, the trocar is withdrawn and the cannula passed down into the trachea. Once the airway is secure, oxygen can be given and arrangements can be made to transfer the patient to hospital.

Purpose-made laryngotomy sets (also called cricothyroidotomy sets or mini-tracheostomy sets) are available that allow a small bore tube to be inserted through the cricothyroid membrane using a flexible introducer (Fig. 26.3). If no cannulae are available, then the skin and cricothyroid membrane must be perforated with any sharp instrument, and any convenient tube used to maintain the airway.

Appendix 1

Instrument and equipment suppliers

United Kingdom

Operating room fittings

The Plinth Co: Wetheringsett Manor, Wetheringsett, Stowmarket, Suffolk IP14 5PP.
Daray Lighting Ltd: 7 Commerce Way, Stanbridge Road, Leighton Buzzard, Bedfordshire LU7 8RW.

Resuscitation equipment

Vitalograph Ltd: Maids Moreton House, Buckingham MK18 1SW.

Disposable electrocautery

Warecrest Ltd: Unit D4 Cowdray Centre, Cowdray Avenue, Colchester, Essex CO1 1BW.
A–Z TEC Medical Supplies: 360 Cheriton Road, Folkestone, Kent CT19 4DU. (Also cricothyroidotomy catheter.)

Diathermy

Schuco International London Ltd: Lyndhurst Avenue, London N12 0NE.

Surgical instruments

Rocket of London: Imperial Way, Watford, Hertfordshire WD2 4XX.
Chas Thackray Ltd: PO Box HP 171, I Shire Oak Street, Leeds LS6 2DP.
John Bell & Croyden: Chatham Street, Reading, Berkshire RG1 7HT.

Equipment, instruments and disposables

Porter Nash Medical: Freepost 18, London W1E 1YZ.
Also at 116 Wigmore Street, London W1H 9FD.
Pulse Doctor's shop: Morgan Grampian House, 30 Calderwood Street, London
SE18 6QH.
Doctor Bylines: Room 1617, Quadrant House, Sutton, Surrey SM2 5AS.
GP Equipment: 30 Lancaster Gate, London W2 3LP.
PracticePLUS: De Puy Healthcare, 45 Great George Street, Leeds LS1 3BB.
Timesco Surgical & Medical: Timesco House, 176 Pentonville Road, London N1
9JP.

Autoclaves

Prestige Ltd: 23–26 High Street, Egham, Surrey TW20 9DU.
Eschmann Bros & Walsh: Peter Road, Lancing, West Sussex. (Little Sister, SES 2000
autoclaves.)
Goldsworth Engineering: 1/7 Cherry Street, Woking, Surrey GU21 1EE. (Instaclave
autoclave.)

Histoacryl tissue adhesive

Davis & Geck Ltd: Fareham Road, Gospot, Hampshire PO13 0AS.

Cryotherapy equipment

Practice Management Systems: 145b Hughenden Road, High Wycombe, Bucks
HP13 5PN. (Cry-Ac.)
Downs Surgical plc: Church Path, Mitcham, Surrey CR4 3UE. (Frigitronics equip-
ment.)

United States

Disposable electrocautery

Aaron Medical Industries: PO Box 261196, Tampa, Florida 33685, USA.

Diathermy

Birtcher Corporation: 4051 N. Arden Drive, El Monte, CA 91734, USA.

Cryosurgical instruments

Brymill Corporation: PO Box 2392, Vernon, Connecticut 06066 USA.

Appendix 2

Minor surgery list: United Kingdom National Health Service

Para 42 Schedule 1 (minor surgical procedures for which payment may be made).

Injections

Intra-articular
Periarticular
Varicose veins
Haemorrhoids

Aspirations

Joints
Cysts
Bursae
Hydrocoeles

Incisions

Abscesses
Cysts
Thrombosed piles

Excisions

Sebaceous cysts
Lipomas
Skin lesions for
   histological
   examination
Intradermal naevi,
   papilloma,
   dermatofibroma, and
   similar conditions
Warts
Removal of toenails
   (partial and complete)

Curette, cautery and cryotherapy

Warts and verrucae
Other skin lesions,
   e.g. molluscum
     contagiosum

Other

Removal of foreign
   bodies
Nasal cautery

Index